Orthopaedic Biomechanics: Mechanics and Design in Musculoskeletal Systems

Donald L. Bartel

Dwight T. Davy

Tony M. Keaveny

PEARSON
Prentice Hall

Upper Saddle River, New Jersey 07458

Library of Congress Cataloging-in-Publication Data

Bartel, Donald L.
  Orthopaedic biomechanics : mechanics and design in musculoskeletal systems / Donald
L. Bartel, Dwight T. Davy, Tony M. Keaveny.
    p. ; cm.
  Includes bibliographical references and index.
  ISBN 0-13-008909-5
  1. Musculoskeletal system—Mechanical properties. 2. Orthopedic surgery. 3. Total
knee replacement. 4. Biomechanics. 5. Human mechanics. I. Davy, Dwight T. II.
Keaveny, Tony M. III. Title.
  [DNLM: 1. Musculoskeletal Physiology. 2. Arthroplasty, Replacement, Hip. 3.
Arthroplasty, Replacement, Knee. 4. Biomechanics. 5. Orthopedic Fixation Devices.
WE 102 B283o 2006]
  RD732.B37 2006
  617.4'7—dc22

                                                             2005058676

Vice President and Editorial Director, ECS: *Marcia J. Horton*
Senior Editor: *Holly Stark*
Executive Managing Editor: *Vince O'Brien*
Managing Editor: *David A. George*
Production Editor: *Daniel Sandin*
Director of Creative Services: *Paul Belfanti*
Creative Director: *Jayne Conte*
Cover Designed: *Bruce Kenselaar*
Art Editor: *Greg Dulles*
Manufacturing Manager: *Alexis Heydt-Long*
Manufacturing Buyer: *Lisa McDowell*

© 2006 by Pearson Education, Inc.
Pearson Prentice Hall
Pearson Education, Inc.
Upper Saddle River, New Jersey 07458

The author and publisher of this book have used their best efforts in preparing this book. These efforts include the development, research, and testing of the theories and programs to determine their effectiveness. The author and publisher make no warranty of any kind, expressed or implied, with regard to these programs or the documentation contained in this book. The author and publisher shall not be liable in any event for incidental or consequential damages in connection with, or arising out of, the furnishing, performance, or use of these programs.

Pearson Prentice Hall™ is a trademark of Pearson Education, Inc.

Printed in the United States of America

2 3 4 5 6 7 8 9   10 09 08 07

ISBN 0130089095

Pearson Education Ltd., *London*
Pearson Education Australia Pty. Ltd. *Sydney*
Pearson Education Singapore, Pte. Ltd.
Pearson Education North Asia Ltd., *Hong Kong*
Pearson Education Canada, Inc., *Toronto*
Pearson Educación de Mexico, S.A. de C.V.
Pearson Education—Japan, *Tokyo*
Pearson Education Malaysia, Pte. Ltd.
Pearson Education, Inc., *Upper Saddle River, New Jersey*

To

Joanne
Kathlene
Shui

Contents

9 Total Hip Replacements 290

10 Total Knee Replacements 314

11 Articulating Surfaces 335

Preface

This book has grown out of class notes and text material developed for the courses we teach in orthopaedic biomechanics at Cornell University, Case Western Reserve University, and the University of California–Berkeley. It is aimed primarily at engineering students who would like to learn more about the mechanical and structural aspects of the skeletal system along with the analysis and design of orthopaedic implants that are used to repair the system when it is damaged. We think the book will also be of interest to orthopaedic surgeons who wish to learn more about mechanics and design in the musculoskeletal system than is usually provided in the typical biomechanics short course.

Most of the students in our classes have taken prerequisite undergraduate, introductory courses in dynamics and strength of materials. Typically, these are senior-level engineering or first-year graduate students. However, we have also had a number of students over the years who have successfully negotiated the course without this background, but with the commitment and determination to learn the necessary fundamentals of mechanics as they go. A background in physiology, biology, or anatomy is not assumed. We have provided the essentials needed as part of the text, which we have found to be sufficient for our own students.

We hope this book achieves three goals. The first is to present applications of mechanical engineering in orthopaedic biomechanics. During the past 30 years, orthopaedic practice has been strongly influenced by contributions from mechanical analysis and design. It is hoped that students will find these applications interesting and that some will be inspired to make orthopaedic biomechanics a career.

The second goal is to encourage students to think qualitatively about complex biomechanical systems by quantitatively studying relatively simple, idealized models of these systems. Quantitative modeling is a continuing theme throughout the book. In the courses we teach, this has been reinforced by posing open-ended questions and mini-projects. Such assignments are, of course, more difficult to create and execute, and they are time consuming to evaluate. However, the benefits outweigh the cost because they require the student to create simple models of complex systems and to think rigorously about them in terms of basic engineering principles. The exercises at the end of each chapter help prepare students to address more open-ended questions.

And a third goal is to enhance the student's general expertise in the area of mechanics. The study of the skeletal system provides an interesting context in which to review and restate topics such as basic rigid body dynamics and beam theory. We also introduce mechanics topics that are new to the typical undergraduate such as composite beam and beam on elastic foundation theories, both very useful for the analysis and design of bone-implant systems.

The book has two parts. In the first, Chapters 1–6, we cover fundamental background material: an introduction to the musculoskeletal system (Chapter 1), determining loads and motions (Chapter 2), the structure and properties of bone and soft tissue (Chapters 3 and 4), and stress analysis of biomechanical systems

(Chapters 5 and 6). The material on loads and motion (Chapter 2) and on structural analysis (Chapters 5 and 6) are designed to provide an opportunity for students to develop confidence and competence in applying fundamental concepts of mechanics to biomechanical systems. Furthermore, they also provide a common approach and notation for students who come from a variety of introductory courses. The remaining chapters introduce applications of the fundamentals addressed in the first part of the book. Chapter 7 provides a basic introduction to bone-implant systems, which is followed by chapters on fracture fixation devices, hip replacements, knee replacements, and articulating surfaces.

The material can be organized in a number of ways for courses with particular emphases. For example, although the chapters provide a logical progression, the topics in Chapters 5 and 6 can also be addressed in parallel with the applications presented in the later chapters. The book is generally broader than any of the courses we have offered, which at one time or another have stressed dynamics, bone mechanics, or bone-implant systems. But while the text is quite broad, there are parts of this fascinating field that we have only touched upon lightly or not even covered. What we present represents our interests and areas of expertise and doesn't attempt to cover the entire field of musculoskeletal biomechanics and orthopaedic design and engineering. A number of other works are referenced in the text to help direct the student to other sources. It should be noted also that we have stayed away from subjects that are still controversial. Our philosophy was to focus on fundamental topics that have stood and will stand the test of time. As such, this is not a survey of current research, but indeed much more of a traditional textbook.

Many people have contributed directly and indirectly to the development of this text and the courses from which it grew. We would like to thank the students who have taken our courses, asked good questions, and ferreted out errors as we developed the manuscript. The graduate students who have served as teaching assistants to us in teaching our courses over the years also deserve special mention. Indeed, all three of us have been influenced by colleagues and graduate students far too numerous to list. We thank them all for what they have taught us as we worked and learned together. We would, however, like to thank several individuals specifically. First, we thank our colleagues Clare Rimnac and Ken Mann for their important contributions to the section on implant materials. We also thank post-doctoral trainee Chris Hernandez, and graduate students Jenni Buckley and Eric Nauman for their contributions to the tissue mechanics sections. Special thanks to Ginny Giles and Judy Thoroughman for their valuable assistance and their patience in dealing with word processors and professors as the book took form. Finally, we would like to thank our families for their support during the course of this project. Perhaps this book will give them additional insights into what has occupied our time and energy as we have pursued various aspects of the fascinating world of biomechanics.

DONALD L. BARTEL
Cornell University

DWIGHT T. DAVY
Case Western Reserve University

TONY M. KEAVENY
University of California at Berkeley

The Musculoskeletal System

This book is for people who are interested in applying the principles of engineering mechanics to analyze the mechanical and structural functions of the musculoskeletal system, including the design of orthopaedic devices that are used to treat skeletal diseases or repair damage to the skeleton. We can do this because the skeletal system is a machine. That is, it is a combination of rigid or resistant bodies having definite motions and capable of performing useful work. The links of this machine are the bones along with the soft tissue structures that are associated with them. These links are connected to each other at joints that enable the body to move quickly in a relatively agile manner and transmit large forces from link to link.

In general, the relative motion between bones is not as precisely defined as the motions between the links of most engineered machines. The hip joint is an exception. It is a ball and socket joint, and the motion between the femur and the pelvis at the hip is well defined. The knee joint, however, allows at least five degrees of freedom, and six if separation of the femur and the tibia is included. The motion at the knee is constrained by soft tissue structures: the ligaments that connect bone to bone, the joint capsule that encloses the joint space, the menisci between the femur and the tibia, and the tendons that connect the muscles to the bone and transmit the muscle forces across the joint. It is possible to describe the general characteristics of the motion of the knee joint under the loads associated with normal daily activities to a precision sufficient for purposes of analysis and design. Under other loading conditions, however, the precise relative motions of the joint and the contact forces across the joint depend upon the functional loads applied to the skeleton.

In most machines, it is possible to consider the kinematics of the mechanism without regard for the external loads acting on it and the internal forces transmitted from link to link. Such is not the case with biological joints. Because kinematic constraint at the joint is provided in part by elastic structures, which are much less stiff than the bony links, the loads across the joint and the motion of the joint are coupled. Changes in force will produce changes in joint motion, and changes in the relative motion between the bones will result in changes in joint forces.

One may be tempted to say, as a colleague once did, that when analyzing the skeletal machine instead of an engineered machine, only the nouns are different; the verbs are the same. This is not quite the case. Most engineering analyses of machines are done for devices we design; and we design them so the analysis tools we have available are applicable. When analyzing the skeletal system, we are confronted with a machine we did not design and one that is, in many ways, more complex than the machines we produce. Consequently, we are often confronted with the need to first understand the basic functioning of the skeletal system by using fundamental principles of mechanics.

Skeletal loads and motions vary from individual to individual and from time to time in a particular person. The structural characteristics of the skeleton also change with time. There are changes with disease and aging that we might wish to avoid or inhibit, but there is also the remarkable ability of the skeleton to heal damage. Even more remarkably, the skeleton has the ability to adapt to changing demands—the geometry and mechanical properties of bones and soft tissues change when the loading changes.

It would be nice, at least in some cases, to precisely estimate the motion, stresses, and deformations in a particular individual for specific circumstances. Of course, this is not practical, and our modeling of disease and damage must be done while realizing the uncertainties of intersubject and intrasubject behavior. Often, precise measures of stresses or motions in particular situations are unnecessary. What is needed, instead, are models that describe the fundamental behavior of the system. To this end we can use basic concepts from dynamics and strength of materials to understand many of the effects of damage and disease and to evaluate the methods and techniques used to restore function. The choice of model is critical in this endeavor and is one of the underlying themes of subsequent chapters. First, we need to look in more detail at several aspects of this wonderful machine.

1.1 | Anatomical Overview

Engineering analysis of the skeletal system is a relatively recent activity and involves collaboration with physicians and life scientists who understand in depth the anatomical and physiological details of the body. To be effective collaborators, we each need to learn something of the language of the other. But the anatomy of the musculoskeletal system is not a part of most engineering or biomedical engineering curricula, although, increasingly, an introduction to biology is either expected or required. Consequently, in this section we provide an overview of the anatomy of the musculoskeletal system, along with the associated terminology, to give sufficient background for the topics introduced in subsequent chapters. The scope is necessarily very general and emphasizes the systems and subsystems we have chosen to address in the rest of the book. There are any number of good reference books on anatomy and physiology available for those who would like to see these topics and others in greater depth.

Bones of the Skeleton.   There are 206 bones in the human skeleton (210 if we count the two sesamoid bones that lie under the head of the first metatarsal in each foot in most people) (Figure 1.1). The axial skeleton, the skull, the vertebral column, and the thorax consist of 80 bones. The spine (Figure 1.2) consists of 33 vertebrae in three sections: 7 in the cervical spine (the neck), 12 in the thoracic spine (surrounding the chest and rib cage), 5 in the lumbar spine (the lower back), 5 in the sacral spine (which are fused), and 4 in the coccygeal region. The appendicular skeleton has 126 bones. There are 4 bones in the pectoral girdle, 60 bones in the upper limbs, 2 bones in the pelvic girdle, and 60 bones in the lower limbs.

Bones come in a wide variety of shapes and sizes, but most fall into three groups. Long bones, such as the femur, the tibia, and the humerus, are long in one direction and have cross sections in the central shaft that are tubular. Short bones, such as the bones of the wrist and the ankle, are bones or portions of bones that have about the same dimensions in all directions; the other bones of the hand and foot fall somewhere between long and short bones (Figures 1.3 and 1.4). Flat bones (sometimes called tabular bones), which make up portions of the skull, the scapula, the pelvis, and the transverse and spinous processes of vertebrae, are much smaller in one dimension than in the others. Irregular bones are those that do not fit neatly

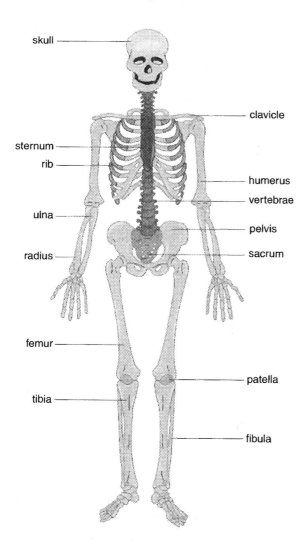

FIGURE 1.1 A frontal view of the adult skeleton.

FIGURE 1.2 A side and frontal view of the spinal column. C: cervical region, T: thoracic region, L: lumbar region.

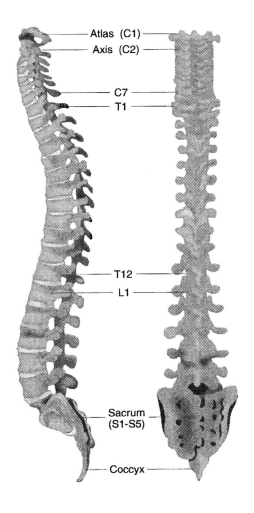

FIGURE 1.3 The bones of the foot and ankle joint.

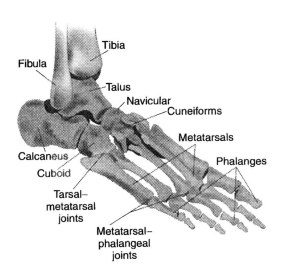

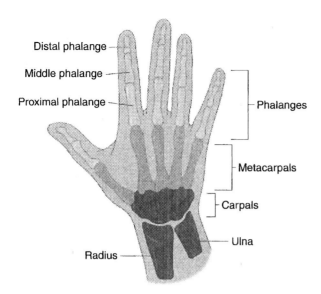

FIGURE 1.4 The bones of the hand and wrist joint.

into the first three categories and include the vertebral bodies and the posterior vertebral elements (Figure 1.5).

Anatomical Terms. When we discuss the bones of the human skeleton, it is often useful to distinguish between different regions of the bone. The following terms are commonly used when discussing the subjects considered in this book:

- **Proximal aspect:** Nearest to the top of the body. Usually only used in conjunction with the bones of the appendicular skeleton. Thus, we talk of the proximal femur, which is at the hip joint.
- **Distal aspect:** The opposite of proximal—nearest the bottom of the body. Again, this term is normally used in conjunction with the bones of the appendicular skeleton. The distal femur, for example, is at the knee joint.
- **Inferior:** Beneath or lower. Used to denote the bottom or underside of a tissue or structure. Especially important when discussing bones of the axial skeleton.
- **Superior:** Opposite of inferior; same rules of usage.

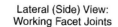

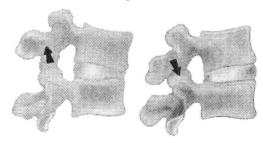

FIGURE 1.5 Spinal motion segment. A motion segment consists of two vertebral bodies with posterior elements and the intervening disc. With forward flexion (left), the facet joints tend to seperate, and with extension (right) they tend to compress.

- **Lateral:** The part closest to the outside of the body or farthest from the body's midline. So the lateral aspect of the femur is on the outside of your (left or right) thigh.
- **Medial:** Opposite of lateral—the part closest to the inside or midline of the body. Note that lateral and medial are referenced to the midline of the body, not to either the left or right sides.
- **Anterior:** Before or in front.
- **Posterior:** Behind or in back.
- **Dorsal:** Near or on the back.
- **Ventral:** Near or on the anterior or lower surface of an animal opposite the back.

To describe motions of the skeleton, we must first define the anatomic position and the three anatomic planes. In the **anatomic position**, the individual is standing with head and palms facing forward (Figure 1.1). **The frontal (coronal) plane** divides the body front–back, the **sagittal plane** divides the body left–right, and the **transverse plane** divides the body top–bottom. For example, a biceps curl is a motion in the sagittal plane; twisting one's head to the side is a motion in the transverse plane. In order to describe motions in these planes, we use the following terms:

- **Flexion:** A folding movement in which the anterior angle between two bones is decreased (except in the knee and toes, in which case the angle is measured posteriorly). It generally means that you are moving a bone closer to the body with respect to its anatomical position.
- **Extension:** The opposite of flexion—an increase in the anterior angle between two bones (except in the knee and toes, in which case the angle is measured posteriorly).
- **Abduction:** Movement away from the midline of the body, usually in the frontal plane.
- **Adduction:** Movement toward the midline of the body, usually in the frontal plane.
- **Hyperextension:** Continuation of motion beyond the anatomic position.
- **Lateral flexion:** Movement of the spine to the right or left, in the frontal plane.
- **Supination:** A movement of the forearm to rotate the hand into the anatomic position. For example, this would be a clockwise rotation of the right forearm (looking down the arm).
- **Pronation:** Opposite of supination—a movement of the forearm to rotate the hand so that the palm faces backwards.
- **Dorsiflexion:** Rotation of the ankle about a transverse axis so that the toes move upwards (away from the ground) in the sagittal plane. Used only for the ankle.
- **Plantar flexion:** Opposite of dorsiflexion—rotation of the ankle so that the toes move toward the ground. Used only for the ankle.
- **Inversion:** Rotation of the foot inward and upward (in the frontal plane).
- **Eversion:** Rotation of the foot outward and upward (in the frontal plane).

In addition to these terms, there are a number of other specialized terms for specific motions of specific bones; books on functional anatomy can be consulted for a more comprehensive list.

1.2 | The Functions of the Musculoskeletal System

The musculoskeletal system has four main functions; the first two are physiological in nature, the second two, mechanical:

- hematopoiesis
- mineral storage
- protection of the vital organs
- support and motion

Hematopoiesis

Trabecular bone, the spongy, highly porous bone found at the ends (epiphyses) of the long bones, the vertebrae, and several other locations (skull, pelvis, sternum) provides sites for the formation of red blood cells, a process known as hematopoiesis. This occurs only in the red bone marrow. Yellow bone marrow, which is found in the middle (or diaphysis) of most long bones, serves primarily as a storage area for fat cells.

Mineral Storage

The skeletal system also has an important physiological function in that it acts as a mineral bank, especially for calcium and phosphorous. Bone is made up primarily of a mixture of collagen (a compliant and ductile protein polymer) and hydroxyapatite (a brittle calcium phosphate ceramic). Approximately 99 percent of the calcium in the human body is stored in the skeleton. One of the ways that the body regulates the level of these minerals in the bloodstream is by a continuous process of remodeling (the resorption and formation of bone tissue). If the body falls short of its daily calcium intake via the gut, it will turn to the bones to get what it needs. Thus, individuals with calcium-deficient diets are at risk of losing bone mass, which in turn would lead to weakening of their bones. Since calcium absorption decreases with aging, elderly people are advised to increase their daily intake of calcium to help reduce the risk of osteoporotic bone fractures.

Protection of the Vital Organs

In order to protect the vital organs such as the brain, heart, spinal cord, and lungs, the skeleton has developed various structures that allow it to absorb large amounts of energy, yet remain lightweight. For example, the cranial bones of the skull have a sandwich construction consisting of a stiff cortical shell surrounding a relatively compliant trabecular bone core, called the diploe (Figure 1.6). The outer cortical shell distributes external forces evenly to the underlying trabecular bone, which absorbs most of the energy on compression. The ribs and sternum protect the lungs and heart in a similar manner as do the spine and pelvis their respective soft tissue organs.

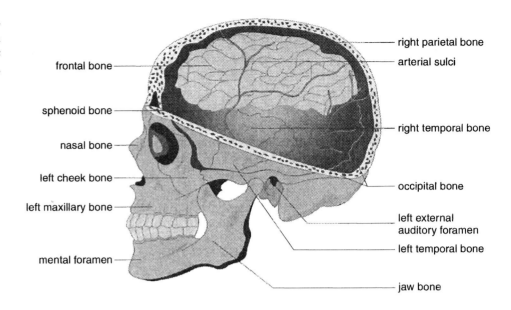

FIGURE 1.6 Sagittal cross-sectional view of the human skull. (*Atlas of the Human Body.* Harper Perennial, New York, 1989.)

frontal bone

sphenoid bone

nasal bone

left cheek bone

left maxillary bone

mental foramen

right parietal bone

arterial sulci

right temporal bone

occipital bone

left external auditory foramen

left temporal bone

jaw bone

Support and Motion

As suggested previously, the primary function of the skeletal system addressed in this book is its ability to provide force and motion for mobility and to take care of the functions of daily living. The functions of daily living vary, of course, from individual to individual. For some, it is a matter of simple survival; for others, it may include strenuous activities such as high-performance athletics. The bones and joints operate together as levers, with the muscles providing the active torque about the joint. When the muscles contract, they produce forces that cause a bone or an entire limb to rotate about a joint, thereby generating movement. For example, when the biceps contract, the forearm rotates about the elbow joint, an action known as flexion (Figure 1.7). Since muscles are usually attached (or inserted) quite close to the joint, there is a mechanical disadvantage at most joints—the muscle must pull with a force that is much larger than the external load. Therefore, the joint loads (internal forces) are much larger than the functional loads (the external forces on the skeletal system).

This is easily visualized by imagining holding a weight in the hand (the functional load) with the upper arm vertical and the forearm horizontal. The moment arm for the biceps muscle is a small fraction of the moment arm for the weight in the hand.

Even in activities such as normal gait, the loads across joints are surprisingly large. For example, hip joint loads have been measured to be two to three times body weight for level walking at constant speed. The largest loads on the foot in this case are only about 1.2 times body weight. The loads on joints of athletes may be much greater. For example, when a professional basketball player jumps to dunk the ball, the load on the foot has been measured to be as high as 13 times body weight. It is no wonder that these individuals often end up with damaged joints.

The advantage of having the tendons close to the joint is that small excursions of the muscle (changes in length) can produce large angular motions at the joint; the skeleton is designed both to provide fast motion and to withstand large loads. We

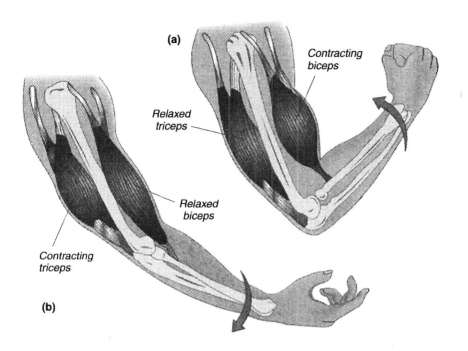

FIGURE 1.7 Flexion (a) and extension (b) of the elbow joint. In each case, the agonist muscles contract and the antagonist muscles relax, all in a highly coordinated fashion.

will see that muscles can only produce large loads when they are moving slowly. Speed is only possible when the loads are light. All in all, the skeletal muscles are amazingly efficient actuators that one would be hard pressed to duplicate with any engineered device of similar size and weight.

1.3 | Bones

It is important to distinguish between bones, the structures, and bone tissue, the material from which bones are made. There are two basic types of bone tissue. Cortical, or compact bone, is the most dense bone in the skeleton. The diaphysis, or central shaft, of a long bone such as the femur or tibia is made of cortical bone. Cancellous bone (or trabecular or spongy bone) is much less dense than cortical bone and is found in the epiphyseal regions at the ends of long bones, within the very thin cortices of vertebral bodies, and between the more dense outer layers of bones such as the skull and pelvis.

Since we will be dealing primarily with long bones throughout this book, they warrant a closer look (Figure 1.8). The shaft, or diaphysis, of a long bone grows from its ends at growth plates. The growth plates eventually close when the individual has matured. The epiphyses, or large ends of the bone, grow from separate ossification centers. The metaphysis is the region between the diaphysis and the epiphysis.

The medullary, or marrow cavity, of a long bone is filled with yellow marrow that consists of fat and a few primitive blood cells. This marrow has mass and contributes to the weight of the bone, but is of no structural consequence. Red marrow exists in the proximal ends of the humerus and femur. (It can also be found in the

FIGURE **1.8** The general form of a long bone.

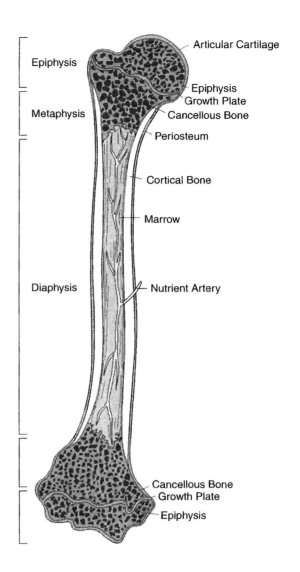

short and flat bones and in the central portions of vertebral bodies.) Red marrow is associated with cancellous bone tissue and is where red blood cells are made.

The outer, or periosteal, surface of the bone is covered by a fibrous membrane called the periosteum. This membrane covers the bone, except at the flared ends where the bone is covered by articular cartilage. The inner surface of the bone is called the endosteal surface.

The bone gets its rich blood supply through two sets of arteries. The periosteal arteries are associated with a dense network of vessels in the periosteum. The medullary or nutrient artery usually enters the bone somewhere close to midshaft through a canal that is oblique to the long axis of the bone. The epiphyseal regions of the bone usually have additional blood supply from other arteries.

Finally, it is interesting to note that a case can be made that the various bones are optimally suited for the functions they must perform. For example, the shafts of long bones have wall thicknesses optimal for a structure that has minimum mass if the mass of the marrow is included and appropriate constraints for strength or stiffness are applied. It can also be argued that the enlarged ends of long bones are optimal for transmitting large joint loads without high contact pressure. The enlarged ends distribute the load over a large area, and the cancellous bone transmits the load progressively to the dense cortical bone of the diaphysis, which has a relatively small cross-sectional area. The design of these remarkable structures, whose form is so well suited to their function, is indeed impressive and a topic of continuing study.

1.4 | Joints of the Body

There are two ways to classify joints: functionally and structurally. The functional classification is based on the amount of relative motion permitted by the joint. One that allows essentially no relative motion between the bones is called a synarthrosis. If the joint allows slight motion, it is called an amphiarthrosis. Finally, a joint that allows large relative motions is called a diarthrosis or a diarthrodial joint.

When considering the mechanics of various types of joints, it is often more useful to employ the structural classifications. Fibrous joints and cartilaginous joints are held together by fibrous connective tissue or cartilage, as their names imply. For analysis of most human motion and the design of total joint replacements, the joints of most interest are the synovial joints, a subset of diarthrodial joints (Figure 1.9). The bones forming a synovial joint are stabilized and constrained by a fibrous joint capsule, which may contain connective ligaments. The articulating surfaces of the bones are covered with a thin layer of articular cartilage, and the joint contains highly viscous synovial fluid, which is secreted by a thin layer of synovial cells (the synovium) that lines the inside of the joint capsule and

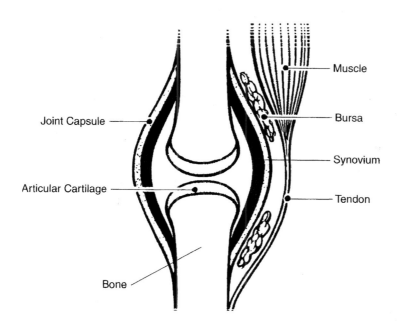

FIGURE 1.9 The structure of synovial joints.

TABLE 1.1

Coefficients of Friction for Some Human (cadaver) Joints and Common Bearing Materials[†]		
Joint/Materials	Coefficient of Friction	Investigator
Human knee	0.005–0.02	J. Charnley (1960)
Human hip	0.01–0.04	A. Unsworth (1975)
Brake material on cast iron	0.4	
Steel on steel	0.6–0.8	
Brass on steel	0.35	
Graphite on steel	0.1	
Teflon on steel	0.04–0.2	
Polyethylene on steel	0.2–0.4	

[†] Unless noted, from Table 8.4 of "Introduction to the Biomechanics of Joints and Joint Replacement" D Dowson and V Wright, editors. MEP, London, 1981.

helps provide joint lubrication. Human synovial joints have extremely low friction because of the lubrication mechanisms that occur in natural joints, which include boundary lubrication and fluid film lubrication between deformable surfaces. When these complex lubrication processes are characterized by a simple coefficient of friction, it is found to be lower than virtually any coefficient of friction for engineered bearing surfaces (Table 1.1).

The synovial joints fall roughly into three groups: ball and socket joints, bicondylar joints, and multiple bone joints. The hip and the shoulder are ball and socket joints. In the hip, the ball (head of the femur) and the socket (acetabulum) are conforming, and the geometry of the joint surfaces provides substantial kinematic constraint. The socket of the shoulder joint (glenoid) does not conform to the head of the humerus, but is nearly flat. Consequently, the shoulder is particularly dependent upon muscle forces and soft tissue structures for stability and constraint.

Bicondylar joints, such as the knee joint (see later section on the knee), have two pairs of articulating surfaces. Two curved condyles articulate against relatively flat surfaces on the mating bone. Consequently, the surface geometry provides little, if any, kinematic constraint, and the joints depend upon soft tissue structures and muscle forces for constraint and stability. Bicondylar joints have a greater range of motion in one plane. For example, the primary motion of the knee joint is flexion or extension in a sagittal plane. Other angular rotations and displacements are small. Each condyle of a bicondylar joint can transmit load. The loads can be unequal, which enables the joint to resist externally applied moments about the joint in a plane perpendicular to the primary plane of motion. This provides a mechanism for resisting moments due to functional loads in that plane without the need for large amounts of muscle or soft tissue.

The joints between the long bones of the hand and foot are harder to classify. They seem to fall somewhere between ball and socket joints and bicondylar joints in most cases—some are approximately cylindrical in extension and bicondylar in flexion. Cylindrical surfaces will have functional characteristics similar to a bicondylar joint like the knee.

The wrist and the ankle are multiple bone joints. The wrist (carpus) is made up of eight small carpal bones, and the ankle (tarsus) is made up of seven tarsal bones. These bones are closely fitted and bound together by ligaments. They do have synovial cavities, and some movement occurs between them. Although the movement between adjacent bones in these joints is small, the combined motion of these bones with respect to each other and with the bones on either side of the joint permits substantial overall motion of the joint.

1.5 | Soft Tissue Structures

Muscles

There are approximately 700 different muscles in the human body, divided into three different types: skeletal, cardiac, and smooth or visceral muscles. Skeletal muscle is voluntary and striated and makes up approximately 36 percent of the total body weight in women and 42 percent in men. The cardiac muscle is also striated but is an involuntary muscle. Smooth muscle tissue is involuntary and is not striated.

We will be concerned almost exclusively with skeletal muscles, and because many common movements are coordinated by muscles acting in groups, we will often consider them as such. For instance, the quadriceps (or more precisely, the quadriceps femoris on the anterior of the thigh) includes the rectus femoris, vastus medialis, vastus lateralis, and vastus intermedius, but they all act together to extend the knee. The main condition for lumping muscles together in this fashion is that they all have a common insertion point on the bone, thereby creating no moment about that point. For example, the quadriceps muscles all come together at the patella, and both the long and short heads of the biceps attach to the radius through a single tendon. A summary of the major muscles or muscle groups is provided in Table 1.2, along with the action that they effect.

TABLE 1.2

Major Muscle Groups and Their Actions on the Knee, Hip, Lumbar Spine, and Elbow		
Joint	Action	Muscles/Muscle Groups
Knee	Flexion	Hamstrings, gastrocnemeus*
	Extension	Quadriceps femoris**
Hip	Flexion	Iliacus, psoas major
	Extension	Hamstrings*, gluteus maximus
	Abduction	Abductors (gluteus minimus, gluteus medius, etc.)
	Adduction	Adductors (adductor magnus, adductor longus, etc.)
Lumbar Spine	Flexion	Rectus abdominis, internal and external obliques
	Extension	Erector spinae
Elbow	Flexion	Brachialis, biceps brachii
	Extension	Triceps brachii

*The hamstrings consist of three different muscles, the semitendinosus, semimembranosus, and biceps femoris.

**The quadriceps consists of four different muscles, the rectus femoris, vastus lateralis, vastus medialis, and vastus intermedius.

The muscles activate, position, and stabilize the skeleton. Active contraction of the muscles produces motion of one bone with respect to another. Because the moment arms of the muscles with respect to the joints are small, large motions of the bones can be produced quickly for small amounts of contraction. Contraction without a change in length of the muscle creates (along with the associated tendon) a spring. These springs are an important part of the energy exchanges that take place in activities such as running. Co-contraction of agonist and antagonist muscles around a joint provides joint stability. A good example is the contraction of the hamstrings and quadriceps to stiffen and stabilize the knee joint in flexion–extension. Thus, the muscles not only position and move the skeleton, but they provide infinitely varying stiffnesses at the joints as well.

Tendons and Ligaments

Tendons connect muscle to bone; ligaments connect bone to bone. For example, the quadriceps tendon connects the quadriceps muscle to the patella, and the patellar ligament connects the patella to the proximal tibia at the tibial tuberosity. At one level, tendons and ligaments can be considered to be simple cables. Such simple models are often useful in describing the overall behavior of the musculoskeletal system. To describe the behavior of these structural elements in more detail, one must consider their constituents. A closer look reveals that these cables are themselves structures consisting of fibers. In some cases—for example, long tendons—the tendon consists of a bundle of parallel fibers. In others—for example, the anterior cruciate ligament in the knee—the fibers are of substantially different lengths and have a complex twisting orientation with respect to the "axis" of the "cable." At a microscopic level, we find that the fibers themselves are made of fibrils and more than one type of collagen, but primarily type I, from which tendons and ligaments (and bone) get their strength.

Articular Cartilage

Articular cartilage is also a complex structure consisting of an elastic matrix (itself a structure consisting of fibers), water, large molecules, and other elements. It is typically 2–4 mm thick in hip and knee joints and has no blood or nerve supply, which makes it difficult to detect and repair damage. It can be modeled in various ways, depending upon the questions being asked. For structural analyses of joints, it is sometimes appropriate to think of it as a single-phase elastic continuum. If its time-dependent behavior is to be studied, it may be considered to be biphasic or triphasic material. Others have established the overall behavior of cartilage by using micromechanics to model the detailed structural interactions of fibers, proteoglycan molecules, and other constituents.

1.6 | The Hip, Knee, and Spine

Three major joint systems of interest to us in later chapters are the hip, the knee, and the spinal motion segment. They are of primary importance to normal activities of daily living and are also sources of some of the major clinical problems in musculoskeletal medicine. Their failure to function properly has major consequences. They are also prototypical of three distinct kinds of joints that bring unique considerations in analysis and design of devices for treatment of associated disease or injury. Thus, we give them special consideration in the sections that follow.

The Hip

Both the hip and knee joints are synovial joints. The hip joint is a relatively simple ball and socket joint in which the head of the femur rotates relative to the acetabulum in the pelvis (Figure 1.10). Because the hip joint is a ball–socket joint, contact can be modeled by a single force that acts through the center of the joint. Obviously, this is not quite right, because there is a small, but finite, friction force and possibly some forces generated by the joint capsular tissues that keep it from being an ideally frictionless joint. We are, however, often able to analyze the mechanics of the hip joint and the femur by using relatively simple models to determine the forces and their effects. For example, the femoral diaphysis can often be approximated by a

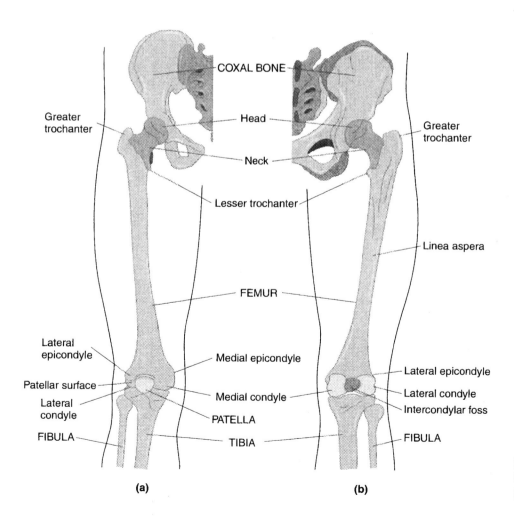

(a)   **(b)**

FIGURE 1.10 The right femur: (a) anterior view; (b) posterior view.

hollow circular beam. The metaphysis (the region where the shaft starts to expand—remember, "meta" means "change") is more difficult to analyze since the load transfer to the surrounding bone is more complicated, and we must often resort to finite element studies. Also important to the load distribution and overall mechanical analysis are the ephiphysis and the linea aspera. The ephiphyses (one at each end of the bone) contain spongy trabecular bone and are two of the principal sites for hematopoiesis. During growth, bones lengthen by adding bone at the epiphyseal plate, a soft cartilaginous tissue that eventually fuses and turns into bone. Fractures across the epiphyseal plate in children are therefore dangerous since they can interrupt or even terminate bone growth. The linea aspera is a raised bony ridge on the posterior side of the femur to which many of the muscle groups attach. The greater and lesser trochanters on the proximal femur are additional examples of specialized muscle attachment points (Figure 1.10). Biomechanically, ridges, trochanters, and other raised structures on bones create an increased moment arm for the muscles with respect to the joint center.

The Knee

The knee joint (Figure 1.11) is a bicondylar joint that allows the femur and tibia to rotate, twist, and slide relative to one another. Each type of motion is important to the stability of the joint and must be reproduced in an artificial knee replacement. Otherwise, abnormal forces can develop on the cartilage or in the ligaments, which can lead to their deterioration. This intimate relationship between the kinematics and loads is a characteristic of most synovial joints. Among the most important structures in the knee are the medial collateral ligament (MCL), the lateral collateral ligament (LCL), quadriceps tendon, patellar ligament, anterior cruciate ligament (ACL), and posterior cruciate ligament (PCL). Athletes, especially football players and gymnasts, are well acquainted with the MCL, LCL, ACL, and the pain associated with injuries to these structures. The ACL and PCL lie within the joint capsule; the other ligaments are outside the capsule (LCL) or are part of the capsule (MCL). The cruciate ligaments pass through the notch between the femoral condyles (Figure 11.1b). The ACL attaches at the anterior side of the tibial plateau

FIGURE 1.11 (a) Side and (b) anterior views of the knee joint. Note that the fibular collateral ligament is also known as the lateral collateral ligament and runs along the lateral aspect of the joint. (Tortora, G.J., *Principles of Human Anatomy*. Harper and Row, New York, 1983.)

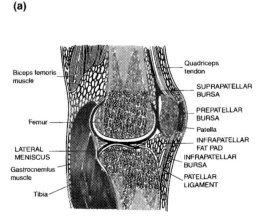

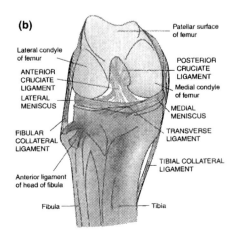

Loads and Motion in the Musculoskeletal System

Adopting the view of the musculoskeletal system as a mechanism or a machine lets us use common tools of mechanics to analyze the mechanical behavior of the system. The analyses generally fall into one of two categories, those where we are interested in the motion of elements of the system, or those where we are interested in the deformations and stresses in the elements of the system. For the first problem, we view the musculoskeletal system as a mechanism consisting of rigid links, actuators, and constraint elements and use the dynamics or statics methods of rigid body mechanics to analyze the behavior. The stress analysis problems usually require that rigid body analyses precede or accompany them to define the loads that are necessary for boundary conditions. Therefore, regardless of whether our interest is in the rigid body dynamics problems themselves or stress analysis problems, the rigid body mechanics problem will probably have to be addressed.

In applications of rigid body mechanics to study the mechanical function of the musculoskeletal system, the common ingredients are (1) the description of the elements of the system in mechanical terms; (2) the description of the external constraints on the system; and (3) the application of the laws of motion. The elements of the musculoskeletal system range from bones to nerves, and their corresponding analogs in the model vary from rigid links to active force generators and controllers (Table 2.1). The elements to be included in the model and the complexity of their descriptions in the model are the first choices to be made in rigid body analyses.

The literature that addresses issues regarding the elements listed in Table 2.1 is extensive. Much of it is relevant to biomechanics, including the biological processes involved in the formation, growth, aging, disease, and repair of each anatomical element. Because our goals are limited primarily to describing the skeleton as a mechanism or machine, we will forgo consideration of many of these issues. However, because the goals of any individual analysis may impinge directly on some biological behavior or some more detailed issue of mechanical behavior, it may be necessary to incorporate them in a particular analysis. Here we briefly consider some of the primary musculoskeletal characteristics that enter into rigid body analyses.

TABLE 2.1

Rigid Body Model Elements	
Anatomic Element	Model Element
Bones or limb segments	Rigid links
Joints	Standard joints: spherical, revolute, cardan, etc.
	Rigid contact surfaces (kinematic constraints)
	Deformable contact surfaces (force constraints)
Muscles + tendons	Actuators
Nerves	Actuators + elastic + viscous elements
Ligaments + joint capsules	Controllers
	Elastic or viscoelastic springs

2.1 | Basic Concepts

Bones

In this chapter, we regard body segments as individual rigid links with dimensions and mass properties determined by the combination of tissues that make up the segments. Bones are organs that primarily make it possible to take such an approach, being relatively rigid frameworks to which all the other tissues are directly or indirectly attached. Obviously, bones are not rigid, and in fact we will be very much interested in the way they act as deformable structures when we address their structural behavior. The mechanical properties of bone tissue as a structural material will be addressed at that point. However, for the present problem of describing forces in the skeletal system, we need not be concerned with the deformability of bone.

Joints

Joints are also discussed in more detail subsequently. From the perspective of a dynamics problem, the joints represent kinematic constraints. The two basic categories of skeletal joints are articulating joints, found at most appendicular skeletal joints, and deformable joints, particularly the intervertebral discs between adjacent vertebral bodies in the spine. Anatomists might add joints such as the pubic symphysis, which is essentially a fibrous tissue union. For our purposes, we need not deal with such joints, since the relative motion is well within our allowance for defining rigid bodies.

Some anatomical joints are readily modeled in dynamic or static analyses as simple joints, particularly spherical (ball–socket) or revolute (hinge). The hip joint and the scapulo-humeral joint at the shoulder are examples of the former, and the humero-ulnar joint at the elbow is an example of the latter. However, most joints are not so simply defined. For example, the wrist is a complex joint, and supination–pronation motion of the hand involves the relative rotation of the radius about the ulna. The shoulder complex involves motion of the scapula with respect to the rib cage, as well as motion of the humerus with respect to the scapula. Even the knee, which is often regarded as having a cam-like, planar motion, is in fact three-dimensional. One of the major issues in developing appropriate kinematic models for link dynamics problems in musculoskeletal motion is defining appropriate kinematics at the joints.

The direct measurement of motion of individual links in theory allows the consideration of each element as an unconstrained rigid link. In this case, the nature of the joint can be inferred by the methods of kinematics. A number of studies have been carried out for such joints as the knee and the wrist to establish the characteristics of the joints. These provide some guidance in making choices about the nature of the model for the joint in a given application. A recurring theme in this book is matching the choice of the model with the nature of the question being asked.

Treating joints as kinematic constraints (where the relative motion is prescribed in some sense) ignores any deformations and determines contact forces. The reality, of course, is that even the articulating joints are not rigid connections. Articulating surfaces are covered with hyaline cartilage, which distributes the contact forces and provides remarkably low-friction bearings. In many problems of interest, it can be assumed that contact is frictionless and cartilage deformations are negligible. However, the detailed mechanics of the joints are often of interest, and this will be addressed in more detail later.

Muscles and Tendons

In works focusing on biomechanics of tissues, it is customary to consider the properties of tendons along with those of ligaments because of their similarities in structure and load-carrying function. However, for our purposes, it is better to consider tendons and muscles in combination. The crucial feature of muscle–tendon units as organs is their ability to actively convert chemical energy to mechanical work. This is accomplished by a process initiated by a neural input at the cellular level. The generation of an active force involves complex dynamics in both the activation and contraction processes. The total muscle force is the combination of the active force generation and the viscoelastic behaviors of the tendon and the passive muscle tissues. A simple representation of a muscle is shown in Figure 2.1. The force generated by the active element is a function of the level of activation, the length of the muscle, and the speed of contraction or lengthening. The general nature of these functions can be represented mathematically, but the model parameters are muscle specific. The passive elements in the force model are also muscle specific, but can be much more easily estimated experimentally.

In order to incorporate such a model into a musculoskeletal dynamics problem, it would be necessary to include some representation of the activation–contraction dynamics. A commonly used alternative is to apply the link dynamics equations to

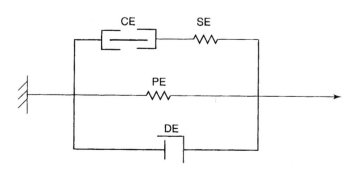

FIGURE 2.1 One model of a skeletal muscle as an actuator includes four components: a contractile element that generates a force based on a neural stimulus through an activation and contraction dynamic process; an elastic element in series with the contractile element; a parallel elastic element; and a parallel viscous element. The passive elements represent the combined elastic and viscous effects of the muscle and the tendon.

determine the muscle actions that must necessarily be generated. While this avoids the explicit incorporation of muscle dynamics, it must also be recognized as an idealization that may lead to errors.

In order to incorporate muscle forces into models, it is necessary to know their lines of action. The simplest approach is to assume that the muscles act along straight lines from their origin to their insertions. Many muscles have broad attachments, particularly at their origins, or have multiple heads. This may necessitate representing the muscles as several subunits in order to accurately represent the muscle action. Further, most muscles do not really act along straight lines, since they lie over deeper structures that restrict their tendency to straighten under tension. Nonetheless, useful results have been obtained with the use of straight-line models of muscles.

Ligaments and Joint Capsules

In addition to the actions of muscles, the ligaments that cross any joint may carry loads. In some cases, such as for the collateral and cruciate ligaments at the knee, the ligaments are quite discrete. In other cases, a complex array of ligaments surrounds the joint, which is intimately integrated with the joint capsule. The hip joint and the posterior capsule of the knee are examples.

Ligamentous structures may be modeled as nonlinear springs that have a low stiffness over some length range (the toe region) and then substantially increased stiffness upon further lengthening (Figure 2.2). This behavior limits the range of motion of the joint. Because the stiffness remains quite low over a normal range of motion for many ligaments, they are often omitted from models. In some cases, they are included as single spring elements. However, this is inadequate for many ligaments that have sufficiently large cross sections. For example, different portions of the anterior cruciate ligament are tightened (reach the stiffer portion of the force–length curve) at different lengths. If ligament behavior is important to the model, it may be necessary to represent a particular ligament as an assembly of ligamentous structures.

If the length–force curve for a ligamentous structure is known, and the coordinates of the attachments are known in each corresponding bone, then the forces in the ligaments can be predicted from knowledge of the joint motions. That is, if the position of one bone is known with respect to the other, the ligament lengths can be calculated and the length–force curve used to calculate the forces. In this way, the

FIGURE 2.2 The typical force–length curve for a ligament tested to failure shows a region of relatively low force and then a region where the forces increase substantially. In addition to the nonlinear elasticity, there can be significant rate effects due to viscosity at sufficiently high speeds.

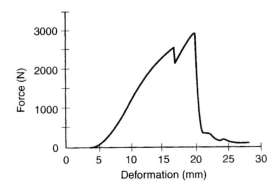

ligaments can be incorporated into the link dynamics models of the musculoskeletal system without conceptual difficulty.

Link Dynamics Models

For modeling of any engineering system, the choices we make about elements in the model should reflect the goals of the analysis. For example, if the purpose of the analysis is to estimate the steady-state maximum bending moment that occurs in the mid-diaphysis of the femur during single-legged stance, then it is not necessary to include details in the model such as ligament deformation or muscle activation–contraction dynamics since they are unlikely to significantly influence the solution. By contrast, if the goal is to estimate the forces in the knee ligaments due to a lateral impact force, ligament models with load versus deformation behavior would certainly be required.

The external boundary conditions on the system are the external forces and kinematic constraints. Again, the choices we make in modeling these boundary conditions should be determined by the goals of our analysis. For example, it may be acceptable in one situation to describe the interaction of the foot with the floor as a kinematic constraint, while it may be better in another situation to model the contact as a force constraint and describe it as though there are springs between the foot and floor.

There are also a number of choices to be made within the context of applying Newton's three laws. In the absence of motion, the problem reduces from a dynamics problem to a static problem. In addition, there is the so-called quasi-static problem, where the system does not maintain a fixed configuration (the statics problem), but the accelerations are small enough that the inertial terms in the equations of motion can be ignored. This is a fairly common circumstance in skeletal motion problems, and in this case the analysis is effectively a statics problem with variable geometry. In addition to incorporating the changing geometry of the problem, this approach can capture relevant dynamic effects, since it can reflect the dynamic nature of the external loads acting on the system for each static analysis. For example, in a quasi-static analysis of gait, the ground reaction forces acting on the foot include dynamic effects generated by the impact forces that develop at the foot on contact.

In this chapter we present the application of rigid body mechanics to analyze forces and motion of the skeletal system. Our goal is to develop modeling approaches that permit us to characterize the internal forces in the system—the forces acting on individual bones, ligaments, and tendons due to external loads and motion. We will see that it is relatively straightforward to arrive at the resultant forces and moments that represent the combined actions of all the load-carrying elements across individual joints. However, we will find that it is not even possible for us to arrive at the forces in the individual elements by using only the equations of dynamics or statics for the general circumstance. We will explore some ways to deal with this dilemma. We will also examine the problem of determining the kinematic input often required for these problems. Our most important goal is to present ways of thinking about such problems, not to catalog specific methods of solution. The latter task would be huge indeed, given the large and ever-growing literature on these methods.

2.2 | Static Analysis of the Skeletal System

Static Analysis

In general terms, the problem of interest is the prediction of the forces that are internal to the musculoskeletal system when supporting some external loads. For example, lifting or carrying an object involves the generation of muscle forces, joint contact forces, and, possibly, passive soft tissue forces throughout the upper limbs, the appendicular skeleton, and the lower limbs. In many problems of this type, we can assume that inertial effects are insignificant. Starting with the description of a musculoskeletal subsystem (some assembly of musculoskeletal elements) as a set of connected links, we write the equilibrium equations for each link. Keep in mind that the statics problem can be regarded as the special case of the dynamics problem in which the acceleration terms are all set to zero. The general form of the equations for the statics problem in vector form is

$$\sum_j \mathbf{F}_{ij} = 0$$

$$\sum_j \mathbf{r}_{ij} \times \mathbf{F}_{ij} + \sum_k \mathbf{M}_{ik} = 0$$

where

i indicates the link number,

j and k indicate the force or moment acting on link i,

$\mathbf{F}_{ij}$ is force number j acting on segment number i,

$\mathbf{r}_{ij} \times \mathbf{F}_{ij}$ is the moment of force $\mathbf{F}_{ij}$ with respect to a reference point on segment i, and

$\mathbf{M}_{ik}$ is a pure moment (force couple) acting on link i.

The force couples, $\mathbf{M}_{ik}$, rarely arise in biomechanics, but are generally included in mechanics texts. These two vector equations represent 6 scalar equations for the three-dimensional case. The reference point for each moment equation can be chosen arbitrarily for the statics problem and is usually chosen for convenience in solving the equations.

Many problems can be treated as though there are only forces and moments acting in one plane. For the planar problem, the equations reduce to

$$\sum_j (F_x)_{ij} = 0$$

$$\sum_j (F_y)_{ij} = 0$$

$$\sum_j (F_{ij} d_{ij}) + \sum_k M_{ik} = 0$$

Hence, for a skeletal subsystem consisting of n elements, we can write $6n$ independent equations of equilibrium for the three-dimensional case, or $3n$ equations for the planar case.

EXAMPLE 2.1 2-D Static Analysis of Shoulder Abduction

Question   Slow shoulder abduction in the frontal plane with a weight in the hand is a common exercise to strengthen the deltoids. What are the forces required to sustain a weight held in the hand at an abduction angle of 90 degrees (Figure 2.3a)?

Solution   We will treat the model as planar, so we can use a 2-D analysis. We now must decide what details to include in our analysis. Since we are interested in only the forces at the shoulder, we can leave the entire arm plus the weight as a single segment. The specified external forces are the weight of each anatomic segment—upper arm, forearm, and hand—plus the free weight. We will assume in this problem that the entire arm weighs 30 N and its center of mass is 30 cm from the center of the scapulo-humeral joint along a line from the center of the shoulder joint to the center of the of the wrist. We will also assume that the free weight is 60 N and is along the same line at a distance of 50 cm from the scapulo-humeral joint.

   We begin by isolating the segment from the shoulder and drawing a free-body diagram of the arm plus weight (Figure 2.3b). The full free-body diagram would include a number of force-carrying elements across the shoulder joint. In fact, it would be necessary to decide the extent of the shoulder joint—does it include only the scapulo-humeral joint? If we assume that it does, then we would "cut" the following muscles across the joint: the deltoid, the pectoralis major, the supraspinatus, the infraspinatus, the teres minor, the teres major, the subscapularis, the latissimus dorsi, the biceps brachii, and the triceps brachii.

   If we regard each of these muscles as single vectors, each represents two unknown scalar quantities. We will now make another common assumption,

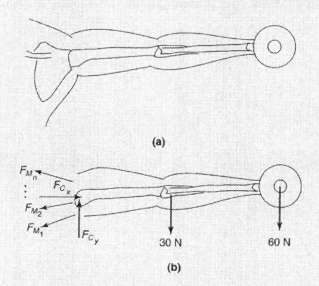

(a)

(b)

FIGURE 2.3   (a) Supporting a weight with the arm horizontal. (b) Free-body diagram of the arm and weight as a single segment.

namely, that we know the line of action of each muscle force from knowledge of the anatomy. We thereby reduce each muscle force to a single unknown magnitude. We can also assume that the joint contact force acts through a known point, the center humeral head. We cannot assume anything about the direction of the contact force, so it represents two unknowns in this problem. In addition, there are ligamentous and capsular forces. Another reasonable assumption might be that the shoulder is not at its limits of the range of motion, and as a result, the ligaments do not develop significant forces. Accepting all these assumptions reduces the unknowns to 10 muscle force magnitudes and 2 components of the unknown contact force. We can express the equations of equilibrium in terms of horizontal (x direction) forces, vertical (y direction) forces, and a moment equation taken about the shoulder as follows:

$$\sum_{i=1}^{10} F_{M_i} \cos(\theta_i) + F_{J_x} = 0$$

$$\sum_{i=1}^{10} F_{M_i} \sin(\theta_i) + F_{J_y} - 60 - 30 = 0$$

$$\sum_{i=1}^{10} F_{M_i} d_i - (60)(50) - (30)(30) = 0$$

Here, i refers to the muscle number, F_{M_i} refers to the muscle force magnitude, θ_i refers to the (known) angle between the x axis and the direction of the muscle force, and d_i refers to the (known) moment arm of the muscle with respect to the shoulder. Obviously, with 12 unknowns and only three equations, we cannot solve for individual muscle forces and the joint contact force. The most we can do is express their relationship to the external forces and moments; that is,

$$\sum_{i=1}^{10} F_{M_i} \cos(\theta_i) + F_{J_x} = 0$$

$$\sum_{i=1}^{10} F_{M_i} \sin(\theta_i) + F_{J_y} = 90$$

$$\sum_{i=1}^{10} F_{M_i} d_i = 3900$$

It is evident that the equations of statics alone are insufficient to determine individual muscle forces and the joint contact force, even given several major assumptions. In fact, to reduce the equations to a determinate set, we would have to limit the action to only one muscle. If, for example, we chose to consider only the deltoid to be active, the equations would become

$$F_M \cos \theta + F_{J_x} = 0$$
$$F_M \sin \theta + F_{J_y} = 90$$
$$F_M d = 3900$$

Obviously, this problem is now solvable for the deltoid muscle force and the two components of the joint contact force once we specify the geometric parameters d and θ that define the line of action of the deltoid. If, for example, the muscle acts at an angle of $\theta = 175°$ (i.e., 5° above horizontal in the medial direction) and with a moment arm $d = 3$ cm, the equations yield

$$F_M = 1300 \text{ N}$$
$$F_{jx} = +1295 \text{ N}$$
$$F_{jy} = -23 \text{ N}$$

Note that the results are very sensitive to uncertainties in the values of d and θ.

The preceding example illustrates the typical musculoskeletal statics problem, which can be stated as follows: Given a set of external forces and a configuration for a skeletal subsystem, what are the internal forces in the load-carrying elements of the musculoskeletal system? Specifically, what are the muscle forces, what are the joint contact forces between the limb segments or other elements, and what are the passive constraint forces in the system? We can rewrite the general statics equations to reflect these questions by separating internal forces and external forces:

$$\sum (\mathbf{F}_i)_{\text{int}} = -\sum (\mathbf{F}_i)_{\text{ext}}$$
$$\sum (\mathbf{M}_i)_{\text{int}} = -\sum (\mathbf{M}_i)_{\text{ext}}$$

On the right-hand side of the equations are the external forces due to gravity and contact with external surfaces, which are known or estimated. The sums on the left-hand side represent the joint contact forces, muscle forces, ligament forces, and other soft tissue forces. (Note that, for convenience, we have included the moments of all forces plus the force couples in each term of the second equation.) For each identified body segment, there are only six independent equations (three if the problem is posed as a planar problem).

As illustrated in the shoulder joint example, the foregoing set of equations typically is well short of the number of unknowns. As another example, consider the lower limb isolated and analyzed as three connected links (foot, shank, and thigh segments, Figure 2.4). There are $3 \times 6 = 18$ equilibrium equations, which are sufficient to yield the values of the six vector unknowns (18 scalar unknowns) representing the resultants at the ankle, hip, and knee. Since there are more than 40 muscles, plus a number of ligaments, that can act across the three joints, there are many more than 18 unknowns if all these internal forces are included in the left-hand terms.

This problem of indeterminacy of forces, sometimes called the *muscle redundancy problem*, is a mathematical problem, not a physiological problem. The muscle set may be redundant in terms of satisfying the statics (or dynamics) equations for a specific situation. However, a little thought reveals that muscles of no value to one action are necessary for another. Looking at it another way, the muscle redundancy problem is merely a manifestation of the physiological ability to do isometric muscle contractions without any external loading (agonist–antagonist muscle

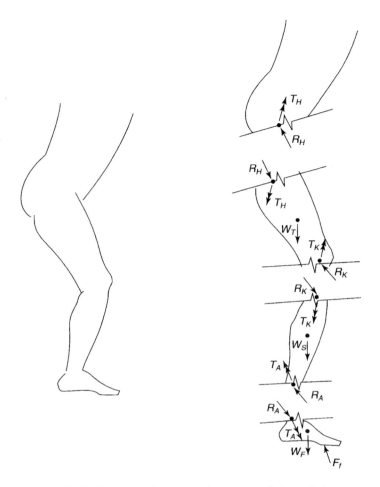

FIGURE 2.4 Free-body diagrams for a simple system of three links representing the lower leg. The external forces are the weights of each link, the contact force on the foot. The unknowns are represented as the resultant forces and torques acting across the ankle, knee, and hip joints. The hip joint force and torque are actually external to the system, but correspond to our definition of internal musculoskeletal forces.

action). It is also clear that, while the equations of mechanics do not reveal the distribution of muscle forces, the musculoskeletal system, under the control of the central nervous system, does indeed generate a specific set of muscle actions to provide the desired action. Finally, it is evident that in the mechanics analysis we can lump the unknowns together and represent the net effects of all the internal forces acting across each joint as a *resultant intersegmental force vector* $\mathbf{R}_i$ and a *resultant intersegmental moment vector* $\mathbf{T}_i$. That is, we can rewrite the preceding equations as follows:

$$\mathbf{R}_i = -\sum (\mathbf{F}_i)_{\text{ext}}$$
$$\mathbf{T}_i = -\sum (\mathbf{M}_i)_{\text{ext}}$$

For the three-segment lower limb example just discussed, the number of unknown resultant forces and moments is 18 (three force components and three moment components at each of the three joints; see Figure 2.4). For the earlier planar problem of the shoulder, we would arrive at three scalar unknowns representing the net torque at the shoulder and the resultant intersegmental force—that is, the vector sum of the muscle forces and the joint contact force. These then can be regarded as solvable problems, where the number of unknowns is reduced to match the number of available equations. In general, we can use the equations of statics or dynamics to arrive at a single force vector and a single moment vector representing the interactions across joints between adjacent segments or at any cross section in the skeleton.

A number of studies in musculoskeletal dynamics report resultant forces and moments. Resultant force and moment data certainly can be of interest, and they can be determined for the typical musculoskeletal motion problem as previously discussed. However, in stress analysis and design analysis problems, we are more often interested in specific forces, not the resultant of all the forces. For example, when analyzing the stresses on the neck of a hip prosthesis, the only force causing stresses on the neck is the joint contact force at the hip, not the resultant force, which includes action of all passive soft tissues and muscles, as well as the (required) joint contact force. So, some means must be devised to form a problem solvable for the individual forces when they are required. As we will see, this is not a trivial problem.

Quasi-Static Analysis

The quasi-static problem differs from the statics problem only in that the configuration of the system is not fixed. The accelerations are small enough, however, that the inertia terms in the dynamics equations can be ignored, compared with the applied external loads and other forces. Thus, we can use the equilibrium equations as we did for the statics problem, but since the geometry is not constant, the geometric parameters in the statics equations are variables—the statics equations are solved for a sequence of positions representing the motion of the system. The dynamics of the system are not necessarily ignored, since the external loads may contain dynamic effects.

EXAMPLE 2.2 2-D Quasi-Static Analysis of Physical Therapy of the Quadriceps

Question   A common exercise to strengthen quadriceps muscles is to place a weight on a patient's foot and require the patient to extend and flex the lower leg between the vertical position and the horizontal position. What are the intersegmental resultant force and moment components as a function of flexion angle?

Solution   We are going to examine this maneuver by using quasi-static analysis, under the assumption that the motion is sufficiently slow that the inertial effects are small compared with the gravitational load. To conduct the analysis, the obvious free body is the lower leg, plus foot, plus weight, isolated at the knee.

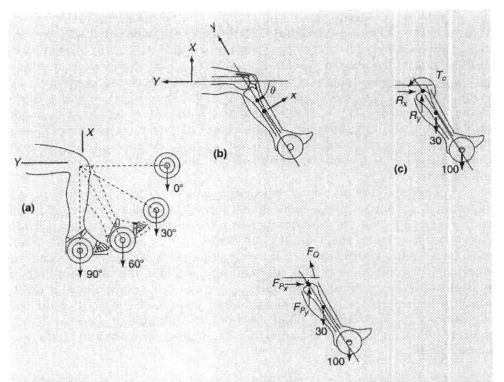

FIGURE 2.5 (a) Schematic of the lower limb during a gravity-based strengthening exercise for the quadriceps; (b) the model shown with the leg at an angle θ (bottom left); (c) the corresponding free-body diagram.

A detailed free-body diagram of the lower leg isolated at the tibial–femoral joint would include the muscle and soft tissue forces, along with the joint contact force. Following the earlier notion of first defining the resultants, we represent the free-body diagram as in Figure 2.5b. Here, we are confronted with a common problem in skeletal mechanics—namely, that the knee joint is kinematically complex; the knee is not a simple revolute or hinge joint, but involves sliding between noncylindrical surfaces. It is reasonable, however, to assume for our problem that there is only one degree of freedom at the knee, that the upper leg is stationary, and that the fundamental motion at the knee is extension–flexion. The orientation of the lower leg with respect to the upper leg is then specified by one coordinate—for example, the orientation of the nominal long axis of the lower leg with respect to the nominal long axis of the upper leg.

The forces and moments on the free-body diagram include the weight of the lower leg and the intersegmental resultant force and torque at the knee. Although it is not necessary for this simple example, we will use a routine that is often helpful or necessary and define reference frames imbedded in each rigid body segment. Since our free-body diagram includes the foot and lower leg, we will use a single segment reference frame located at the combined mass center for the leg and foot (assumed to be known). Additionally, we will attach an external reference frame to the upper leg. The position of the lower leg with respect to the upper leg can now be defined as the angle θ between the Y axis on the femur and the y axis on the lower leg.

In order to write the equations of equilibrium corresponding to the free-body diagram, we need to define the reference point for the resultant force and moment. If we have enough anatomical information to define the surface contact location on the femur and on the tibia, we could use it as the reference point. It has the obvious convenience of excluding the contact force from the resultant intersegmental torque. (Note another implicit assumption in this approach—namely, that the distributed contact force can be regarded as a single vector acting through a theoretical single contact point.) Alternatively, we can use a more easily identified reference point as the intersection of the femoral Y axis and the tibial y axis. Having made the choice of a reference point (which in general will be a function of θ), we can write the corresponding vector equation.

We will choose as the reference point the point on the tibia at coordinates $x = 0$, $y = 20$ cm. If the weight of the lower leg and foot is 30 N, acting at $x = 0$, $y = 0$, and the free weight of 100 N acts at $x = 8$ cm, $y = -20$ cm, the equations for the intersegmental resultants are

$$R_X = 0$$
$$R_Y = -(-30 - 100) = 130 \text{ N}$$
$$T_C = -[-20 \cdot 30 \cdot \cos(\theta) - 40 \cdot 100 \cdot \cos(\theta) - 8 \cdot 100 \cdot \sin(\theta)]$$
$$= 4600 \cos(\theta) + 800 \sin(\theta)$$

The Joint Force Distribution Problem

In the preceding example, the analysis almost certainly yielded less information than we would usually desire. For example, the question really might be, What weight can be safely used for exercising a reconstructed quadriceps tendon? If so, we are left with limited information. We now consider some ways of dealing with the basic difficulty, namely, that rigid body mechanics analysis is typically insufficient to determine all of the internal forces in the musculoskeletal system.

Numerous schemes have been devised to distribute the resultant intersegmental force and moment acting across a joint among the muscles, other soft tissues, and the joint contact force. The methods that have been employed make use of general or specific information about the behavior of the neuromusculoskeletal system, and they can be divided into two classes. The first is the addition of auxiliary information about the load-carrying elements in the form of added constraint conditions sufficient to provide an equal number of unknowns and equations.

The second approach is to use some added performance criterion, which, when met, specifies a unique set of forces among the load carrying elements. This approach is based on a general, teleological argument that the physiological system performs in such a way that some behavior is optimized. This concept allows us to use mathematical optimization techniques to find a solution that satisfies equilibrium, while maximizing or minimizing some performance criteria like energy expenditure or joint contact force. The optimization approach easily permits the inclusion of the auxiliary conditions from the first approach, as well as others, such as the requirement that muscle or ligament forces cannot be compressive or that joint contact forces cannot be tensile.

Auxiliary Conditions

• *Force Reduction.* In this approach, a sufficient number of relationships among the forces in individual elements are defined to make the number of unknowns match the number of equations. The simplest case is just setting enough individual forces to zero to reduce the number of unknowns to match the number of independent equilibrium (or dynamics) equations. For a single joint, if the joint contact force is to be regarded as an unknown vector, only three additional unknowns (only one for the planar problem) can be determined from the mechanics equations. This would correspond to three muscle forces—or for the planar problem, one—if the muscle lines of action are known. This approach is often used when one muscle dominates the behavior. Or, if multiple muscles meet at a single point, their combined action can be replaced by the action of a single resultant force, since they will not create any moment about their coincident point of action. This situation is common in musculoskeletal problems. The four muscles of the quadriceps insert together at the patella to extend the knee; the anterior and posterior aspects of the deltoid insert together in the proximal humerus for sagittal abduction; and the two muscles of the hip abductors insert together at the greater trochanter on the proximal femur. This is the case in Examples 2.2 and 2.3 for planar models of the shoulder and knee.

EXAMPLE 2.3 Estimation of Quadriceps Force for Physical Therapy Exercise

Question For the exercise to strengthen quadriceps muscles in the previous example, what is the required quadriceps force as a function of the knee flexion angle?

Solution The exclusion of all muscles other than the quadriceps is a reasonable assumption, since we expect it to be a dominant force. In particular, if we focus on the tibia, the patellar tendon is the load-carrying element that transfers the quadriceps muscle force. (Note that this is not necessarily the force in the quadriceps tendon; to estimate the error in this assumption, we would have to analyze the patella.) We will estimate the location of the patellar tendon insertion in the tibial reference frame as $x = 2$ cm, $y = 10$ cm, and assume that the line of action of the patellar tendon is 20 degrees anterior to the y axis of the tibia and is a constant value (Figure 2.6). We will assume that the femoral–tibial contact point lies at the previously chosen location in the tibial reference frame with coordinates $x = 0$ cm, $y = 20$ cm. With this set of assumptions, we can now estimate the quadriceps tendon force during the maneuver, using the previous results. The relationship between the intersegmental resultant moment and force and the internal forces (patellar tendon force magnitude, two components of joint contact force) is

$$10 \cdot F_Q \cdot \sin(25°) + 2 \cdot F_Q \cdot \cos(25°_P) = 4600 \cos(\theta) + 800 \sin(\theta)$$
$$F_{P_X} = R_X - F_Q \cdot \cos(25° - \theta) = -F_Q \cos(25° - \theta)$$
$$F_{P_Y} = R_Y - F_Q \cdot \sin(25° - \theta) = 130 - F_Q \sin(25° - \theta)$$

From these three equations, the quadriceps force as well as the joint contact force for any flexion angle θ can be determined.

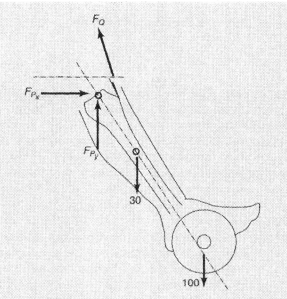

FIGURE 2.6 The free-body diagram of the lower limb with the explicit assignment of a single nonzero muscle force, F_Q. The reference point P is usually chosen to have some physical meaning such as the estimated location of the contact force.

Sometimes, other auxiliary information, such as EMG measurements, is available. If some muscles lack evident EMG activity, they are obvious candidates for setting their values to zero. Also, they can be combined into groups on the basis of synchronous activity in a particular action. Unfortunately, no means is yet available to use EMG in a quantitative way to estimate muscle forces directly, except in extremely restricted circumstances. Obviously, this ability would obviate the problem of force redundancy.

This simple approach of reducing the number of active muscles to permit solving for a unique set of forces is very common and useful in many circumstances to estimate the magnitude of forces. The challenge to the analyst is to have some reasonable idea of the relative accuracy of the results in light of numerous assumptions. As is always the case in developing models for engineering analysis, the model needs to match the question.

• *Muscle scaling.* One particularly interesting aspect of muscle mechanics is that the maximum stress that can be sustained by virtually all skeletal muscle tissue—regardless of its anatomic site or species—is approximately constant at a value of about 0.2 MPa. Thus, the stress in each muscle will be constant if all muscles during an activity are activated to their maximum value. This implies that the ratio of force to muscle cross-sectional area is constant, which allows all the muscle forces F_i to be expressed in terms of just one of the muscle forces, F_1:

$$F_i = \left(\frac{A_i}{A_1}\right)F_1$$

This results in an extra equation for every muscle in the model beyond the reference muscle F_1, and the problem can be solved by one of the previous methods.

The most obvious limitation of this approach is that several muscles are assumed to be equally active. Often this is not the case, although using this information in combination with the auxiliary information from EMG activity may permit realistic scaling among active subgroups. Another limitation with this approach is that data on muscle cross-sectional areas are troublesome. Measuring muscle cross-sectional area is not trivial, since artifacts can arise from a number of sources. The cross-sectional area varies along the length of the muscle, so it is not clear which section should be used for measurement. If data are taken from cadavers, there can be dehydration effects that reduce the size of the muscle; and data for young subjects are difficult to obtain. If data are taken by noninvasive scans of live subjects, it is difficult to ensure that the muscle geometry matches that for the activity under analysis, and it is difficult to avoid projection errors. For this reason, muscle cross-sectional area is usually given as the ratio of its volume (which in fact does not change under contraction) to its length (the distance between the ends of the muscle belly), a measure that is known as the physiological cross-sectional area.

• *Use of soft tissue force–deformation relations.* Often it is necessary to include passive elements such as ligaments in the model. If the force–deformation relations are known for these tissues (either elastic or viscoelastic; linear or nonlinear), then it is possible to calculate their forces from their deformations. The force in each soft tissue element can be calculated independent of the equations of equilibrium if the kinematic information is available that defines the deformations of the elements as a function of position. Note that this method could be used for passive (ligament and joint capsule) or active (muscle) soft tissues as long as the appropriate constitutive equations are employed. For muscles, however, the force is dependent not only upon passive properties, but upon an active component generated from an external neural input as well, which is unknown in the general circumstance.

EXAMPLE 2.4 Forces in the Collateral Ligaments

Question The collateral and cruciate knee ligaments plus the joint capsule have important functions in knee motion stability. Particularly under extreme loading conditions, it is necessary to include the ligaments in the analysis. If the knee is loaded with a varus–valgus moment, the joint tends to open medially or laterally. Consider the knee joint that is opened on its lateral aspect due to the application of a large medial force distally (Figure 2.7a). What information about the ligament is required to be able to determine the joint force?

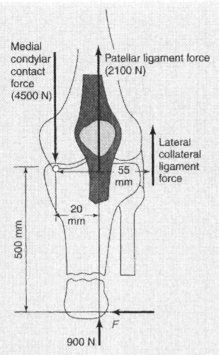

FIGURE 2.7 Frontal view of the knee joint, showing opening on the lateral aspect due to application of a medi-ally directed force distally. (Adapted from Burstein and Wright, *Fundamentals of Orthopaedic Biomechanics*, page 82).

Solution   Because the joint is opened, there is contact in the frontal plane only on the medial condyle, but there is also a force generated in the lateral collateral ligament as it is stretched. Assuming that the quadriceps are the dominant muscle force for this problem and that all other soft tissue forces are negligible, then there are four unknowns in this problem (the magnitudes of the ligament and muscle forces, and the two components of the joint contact force), but only three equations of equilibrium (for this two-dimensional analysis). However, from the kinematics of the problem at the particular instant of interest, the deformation in the lateral collateral ligament is 10 mm; and from its force–deformation curve (Figure 2.2), the corresponding tensile force in this soft tissue element is about 1000 N. This reduces the number of unknowns to three, and the problem can be solved. Note that, with this approach, both the kinematics and the anatomy of the joint must be known to determine the magnitude and direction of the soft tissue forces.

Optimization Technique.   The goal of the foregoing options is to equalize the number of unknowns and equations, thereby producing a statically determinate system. In contrast, the optimization approach is a method that finds a unique "best" solution among the infinite number of solutions of the statically indeterminate problem. The rationale for this approach is that the neural system arrives at a solution somehow, and in some sense this is a best choice. This optimal solution may depend on the specific activity. For example, the body may try to maximize the rate of muscle contraction when speed is needed or minimize the stress on the cartilage for habitual ambulatory activities.

With these ideas, an optimization problem can be formulated in which some mathematical measure of performance is minimized or maximized. The general form of any optimization problem consists of an objective (or "cost") function that will be minimized or maximized, a set of equality or inequality constraints that must be satisfied, and identification of the design variables that can be varied to arrive at a unique solution. When the problem is properly formulated, the tools of mathematical optimization are available to find solutions. Most software packages for optimization are written in terms of minimization, because a maximization problem can always be recast as the minimization problem.

The force distribution problem formulated as an optimization problem is as follows: Choose a set of muscle, soft tissue, and joint contact forces (design variables) such that some measure of performance is optimized (objective function), subject to a number of constraints. The equations of equilibrium function mathematically in this formulation as a set of equality constraint equations. We can also impose some obvious inequality constraints, such as requiring that muscle and ligament forces be tensile and joint contact forces be compressive. We might also impose the more complex constraint that friction at the joint surface should be minimal—that is, the joint contact force should be perpendicular to the joint surface.

We write the general problem in the following way:

Minimize $f(\mathbf{x})$
  subject to

$$h_i(\mathbf{x}) = 0$$
$$h_i(\mathbf{x}) = 0, i = 1, 2, \ldots, m$$
$$g_j(\mathbf{x}) \leq 0, j = 1, 2, \ldots, p$$

where

  $f(\mathbf{x})$ is the objective function
  $\mathbf{x}, (x_1, x_2, \ldots, x_n)$ is a vector of decision or design variables (the unknown forces)
  $h_i(\mathbf{x}) = 0$ are the equality constraints (equilibrium conditions, constitutive equations)
  $g_j(\mathbf{x}) \leq 0$ are the inequality constraints (restrictions on forces, etc.)

The objective function is a mathematical representation of the performance criterion, which depends explicitly or implicitly on the unknown forces. The constraint conditions represent the necessary conditions to be met by any candidate solution and are independent of the performance criterion.

Linear Programming Problems   One simple choice for an objective function to minimize is the sum of the muscle forces or muscle stresses, which may be written

$$f(\mathbf{x}) = a_1x_1 + a_2x_2 + \cdots + a_Nx_N$$

where the a_i are constants. If the constraints are also linear combinations of the unknowns, that is,

$$h_i(\mathbf{x}) = b_{i1}x_1 + b_{i2}x_2 + \cdots + b_{iN}x_N - d_i = 0$$
$$g_j(\mathbf{x}) = c_{j1}x_1 + c_{j2}x_2 + \cdots + c_{jN}x_N - e_j \leq 0$$

where $b_{i1}, b_{i2}, \ldots b_{iN}, d_i, c_{j1}, c_{j2}, \ldots c_{jN}, e_j$ are constants, a linear programming problem results. This formulation has been used by a number of investigators to compute force distributions. There are well-established methods for solving linear programming problems, which can be used to (a) show whether or not any set exists that satisfies all the constraint conditions—a feasible solution, (b) show whether a unique optimum solution exists, and (c) find that solution. If a solution to the muscle force (or stress) problem exists, it is guaranteed that the number of nonzero forces will equal the number of independent constraints. In other words, this is equivalent to the force-reduction approach, with the added advantage that a set of nonzero forces is chosen to minimize an objective function.

Consider the following linear programming problem:

Choose $\mathbf{x} = x_1, x_2, \ldots, x_{10}, x_i \geq 0$
to minimize $f(\mathbf{x}) = a_1x_1 + a_2x_2 + \cdots + a_{10}x_{10}$
subject to
$$h_i(\mathbf{x}) = 0 \quad i = 1, 2, 3$$
$$g_j(\mathbf{x}) \leq 0 \quad j = 1, 2, \ldots, 20$$

This general formulation could be applied to the shoulder problem in Example 2.1, where $h_i = 0$ represent the three equilibrium equations and $g_j \leq 0$ are the upper and lower bounds on the muscle forces. The equality constraints are three linear equations, which could be used to eliminate three of the twelve unknown forces, leaving nine to be determined. As a result, the problem could be written as follows:

Choose $\mathbf{x} = x_1, x_2, \ldots, x_7$
to minimize $f(\mathbf{x})$
subject to $g_j(\mathbf{x}) \leq 0 \quad j = 1, 2, \ldots, 14$

In this case, as many as nine independent constraints could be active at the solution.

EXAMPLE 2.5 Optimization Solution for Wrist-Tendon Forces

Question   What are the muscle forces acting across the wrist when a weight is held in the hand and the hand forearm is at an arbitrary pronation–supination angle?

Solution   We will consider that the forearm and hand are horizontal, so the hand is at a neutral position with respect to both dorsi–palmer flexion and radial–ulnar deviation. The wrist is a kinematically complex joint, actually involving relative motion at a number of articulating joints. The overall motion at the wrist is roughly the motion achieved in a cardan or universal joint, with rotations about transverse axes corresponding to flexion–extension and radial–ulnar deviation. There are a number of tendons that cross the wrist, with their lines of action roughly parallel along the forearm axis. To estimate the forces in the muscles necessary to maintain equilibrium about the two transverse axes, we will consider the free-body diagram of the hand with the cutting plane perpendicular to the axis of the forearm and to the muscles crossing the wrist. We will assume that the locations of the tendons crossing the wrist are known. We will assume that the location of the effective joint contact force is known and coincides with the origin of the axes. We can then write three equilibrium equations that involve the muscle forces, the moment equations about the x-axis and y-axis and the force equation in the z direction:

$$F_1 + F_2 + \cdots + F_7 - F_c = R_z = 0$$
$$b_{11}F_1 + b_{12}F_2 + \cdots + b_{17}F_7 = M_x$$
$$b_{21}F_1 + b_{22}F_2 + \cdots + b_{27}F_7 = -M_y$$

The coefficients b_{11}, etc., are the moment arms about the x and y axes through the assumed contact point (Figure 2.8). To arrive at a set of muscle forces, we will use an optimization approach, taking as an objective function the sum of the muscle forces; that is, the objective is to minimize the total muscle action. This simple idea has some intuitive appeal as a physiologically meaningful performance criterion. Since the two moment equations do not involve the z direction contact force at the wrist, we can write the optimization problem as the following:

$$\text{Minimize } f(F_1, F_2, \ldots, F_7) = F_1 + F_2 + \cdots + F_7$$

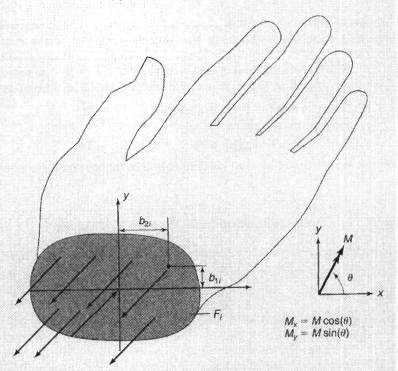

FIGURE 2.8 A free-body diagram of the hand. The seven tendons crossing the wrist are assumed to be acting perpendicular to the cutting (x, y) plane. Their moment arms with respect to the reference point $(x = 0, y = 0)$ are also assumed to be known. The applied external moment $\mathbf{M}$ is oriented at an arbitrary angle θ from the positive x axis in the x, y plane.

subject to

$$b_{11}F_1 + b_{12}F_2 + \cdots + b_{17}F_7 = M_x$$
$$b_{21}F_1 + b_{22}F_2 + \cdots + b_{27}F_7 = -M_y$$
$$F_j \geq 0; j = 1, 2, \ldots, 7$$

The inequality constraint conditions represent the requirement that the muscle forces all be tensile (positive). The foregoing problem formulation fits the requirements for a linear programming problem. Note that the force equilibrium equation has been omitted from the set of constraints. It could be included, and the contact force F_c could be included in the set of variables to be determined. However, if the contact force just equals the sum of the muscle forces, it can be calculated post-hoc. The optimization problem can be solved for an arbitrarily oriented unit moment $M_x = \cos(\theta)$, $M_y = \sin(\theta)$, to see what muscles are chosen as a function of the orientation angle θ. Figure 2.9 shows the results for the solution of this linear programming problem for a unit moment as a function of the angle of orientation, and for the numerical values of the moment arms listed in Table 2.2. The results (Figure 2.9) show that the solution for any orientation of the moment θ produces only two nonzero forces, which matches the number of equilibrium equations. This is a result that is expected from the linear programming formulation. In effect, the solution procedure has chosen the pair of muscles for any position with the most efficient combination of moment arms to sustain the applied moment.

Some other fairly easy modifications of the problem can perhaps lead to more realistic solutions. One is to use muscle stress rather than muscle force. In this case, the new objective function becomes

$$f(F_1, F_2, \ldots, F_N) = \frac{F_1}{A_1} + \frac{F_2}{A_2} + \cdots + \frac{F_7}{A_7}$$

Another objective function that might be reasonable is to minimize the contact force. In this particular problem, we see from the previous force equilibrium equation

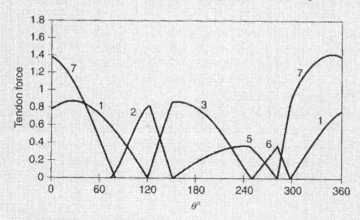

FIGURE 2.9 The results for the optimization solution as a function of the orientation of the unit moment. It can be seen that, typically, only two muscles are active in this solution for the minimum muscle action. The unique points where only one muscle is active correspond to the orientation where a single muscle is positioned to generate a moment parallel to the applied moment.

TABLE 2.2

Moment Arms for the Wrist Example[1]

Muscle #	x Moment Arm, b_{1i}	y Moment Arm, b_{2i}
1	0.4 cm	1.8 cm
2	−0.6 cm	1.0 cm
3	−1.0 cm	0.6 cm
4	−0.7 cm	−1.0 cm
5	−1.0 cm	−2.5 cm
6	0.5 cm	−2.6 cm
7	0.5 cm	−1.0 cm

[1] The muscle numbers correspond to Figure 2.8. The coefficients b_{ij} are used in the preceding equilibrium constraint conditions.

that the contact force equals the sum of the muscle forces. Hence, this formulation would produce the same result as minimizing the sum of the muscle forces.

Nonlinear programming problems   A number of other, more complex objective functions have been proposed on the basis of various arguments from physical grounds. One is to minimize some nonlinear measure of performance, as in

$$\text{Minimize} \quad \left[\sum_i \sum_j |w_{ij}(\mathbf{F}_{ij})_{\text{int}}|^n \right]^{1/n}$$

where w_{ij} is a weighting function. If w_{ij} is the inverse of the cross-sectional area of the muscle, it converts force to stress. One choice that has been suggested for the parameter n is 3, because there is some evidence that this value corresponds to the effect of muscle stress on fatigue rate.

It is often possible to combine the optimization approach with the more empirically based approach by using experimental knowledge of active muscles. For example, the constraint conditions for the problem can include the requirement that the muscle is known to be active based on EMG information. If EMG measurements show a muscle is inactive at a particular phase of motion, it can be excluded from the set. In addition, if the physiological force limits of the muscles, soft tissues, and bones are known, these limits can be incorporated in the problem as inequality constraints on the allowable forces.

The big issue with the optimization approach is whether the objective function is appropriate. Unfortunately, there is no simple answer; the results vary with the choice of objective function. Consequently, there is always inherent uncertainty concerning the magnitudes of the *in vivo* forces in muscles, bones, and ligaments, regardless of the sophistication of the model used for their calculation.

2.3 | The Musculoskeletal Dynamics Problem

Fundamental Concepts

We now turn our attention to the problem where inertial effects due to accelerations cannot be ignored. For the general musculoskeletal dynamics problem, we can state the governing equations of motion (Newton's second law) as

$$\sum_j \mathbf{F}_{ij} = m_i\ddot{\mathbf{r}}_i$$

$$\sum_j \mathbf{r}_{ij} \times \mathbf{F}_{ij} + \sum_k \mathbf{M}_{ik} = \dot{\mathbf{H}}_i$$

where

$\mathbf{F}_{ij}$ is force number j acting on segment number i,

$\mathbf{r}_{ij} \times \mathbf{F}_{ij}$ is the moment of force $\mathbf{F}_{ij}$ about the mass center of segment i,

$\mathbf{M}_{ik}$ is pure moment (i.e., force couple) number k acting on segment i,

$\ddot{\mathbf{r}}_i$ is the acceleration of the mass center of segment i (the double dot indicates the second time derivative),

m_i is the mass of segment i ($m_i\ddot{\mathbf{r}}_i$ is the rate of change of linear momentum),

$\dot{\mathbf{H}}_i$ is the rate of change of angular momentum of segment i about its mass center (the single dot indicates the first time derivative),

the sums on j are over all forces, and

the sum on k is over all force couples acting on segment i when it is isolated from adjacent segments.

Note that the moment equation in this simple form also holds about a point other than the mass center only if it is a nonaccelerating point. For an accelerating point other than the mass center, a more complicated expression for the angular inertia must be written. This situation is considered subsequently.

For the case of motion in three-dimensional space, these two vector equations represent six independent equations for each segment. The angular momentum involves angular velocities, and its derivative $\dot{\mathbf{H}}_i$ involves angular accelerations as well as angular velocities. In the three-dimensional case, the expression for angular momentum can be complicated. For the case of planar motion, which is adequate for a number of problems, the set reduces to two force equations and one moment equation. In this case, the rate of change of angular momentum is simplified to a product of the moment of inertia and angular acceleration. The equations of motion for each segment can be written as the following three scalar equations:

$$\sum_j (F_x)_{ij} = m_i\ddot{x}_i$$

$$\sum_j (F_y)_{ij} = m_i\ddot{y}_i$$

$$\sum_j (F_{ij}d_{ij}) = I_i\alpha_i$$

Here, the x and y subscripts indicate two convenient perpendicular directions in the plane of motion, $\ddot{x}_i$ and $\ddot{y}_i$ are the accelerations of the mass center of the ith segment, α is the angular acceleration of that segment, F_{ij} is the magnitude, d_{ij} is the moment arm of force $\mathbf{F}_{ij}$, and I_i is the mass moment of inertia of the ith segment about an axis through its mass center and perpendicular to the plane of motion. The dynamics problem equations, like the statics equations, can be recast in terms of internal $\mathbf{F}_{int}$ and external $\mathbf{F}_{ext}$ forces:

$$\sum (\mathbf{F}_i)_{ext} + \sum (\mathbf{F}_i)_{int} = m_i\ddot{\mathbf{r}}_i$$

$$\sum (\mathbf{M}_i)_{ext} + \sum (\mathbf{M}_i)_{int} = \dot{\mathbf{H}}_i$$

Here, the goal is most often to calculate the internal forces acting on the bones, muscles, or soft tissue. Obvious examples of activities when a dynamics approach is required for analysis of skeletal forces include high-speed motion, such as sprinting, and high-speed collisions in sports injuries or car accidents. However, there are a number of examples (e.g., rapid gait) where it is not clear whether or not a dynamic analysis is required, and in these cases it may be necessary to perform a preliminary dynamic analysis to justify the assumption of a static or quasi-static analysis.

In general, dynamics problems in biomechanics are formulated in one of two ways. The first is the *direct or forward problem,* in which all the forces on the left-hand side of the foregoing equations are known, and the unknowns are the motion histories of the segments. In the direct dynamics problem, the number of unknowns equals the number of equations, so a solution for the unknown motion can always be obtained. The unknown displacements and velocities must be solved by integrating the differential equations of motion, usually by numerical methods. This approach is not common in musculoskeletal biomechanics problems, since it is rare that all internal forces and moments are known *a priori.*

The second kind of dynamics problem—which is by far the most common in musculoskeletal biomechanics and which was illustrated in the last example—is the *inverse dynamics problem* in which the motion history and the external forces are known, but the internal forces are unknown. For the inverse dynamics problem, just as in the statics problem, we are confronted with the redundancy problem, where the number of unknowns (muscle, ligament, joint contact forces, etc.) exceeds the number of available dynamics equations. Hence, a unique solution for the history of these forces cannot be determined from the dynamics equations alone. Unfortunately, this is very often the case for problems of real interest in musculoskeletal dynamics. What can be observed and measured is the motion history of the skeletal segments and the external forces; what cannot be measured are the forces internal to the moving system. As we did for the statics problem, we rewrite the dynamics equations in the following form:

$$\mathbf{R}_i = \sum (\mathbf{F}_i)_{\text{int}} = m_i \ddot{\mathbf{r}}_i - \sum (\mathbf{F}_i)_{\text{ext}}$$
$$\mathbf{T}_i = \sum (\mathbf{M}_i)_{\text{int}} = \dot{\mathbf{H}}_i - \sum (\mathbf{M}_i)_{\text{ext}}$$

The first term on the right-hand side represents the inertial effects. The second term represents the external forces such as gravitational and ground contact forces that occur during gait, which can be measured by using a six-degree-of-freedom force plate. As with the statics problem, to distribute the resultant intersegmental force and moment among the internal load-carrying structures, one of the strategies outlined previously for the statics force distribution problem must be used, where the dynamics equations are substituted for the statics equations.

For problems involving movement about human joints, it is often more convenient to take moments about some other point rather than the mass center. For example, we could take moments about the joint contact point, which will eliminate the unknown resultant joint force from the moment equation. However, the moment of the inertia vector acting through the mass center must now be taken into account. This notion can be visualized in the following way: Consider the schematic form of the dynamics equation shown in Figure 2.10.

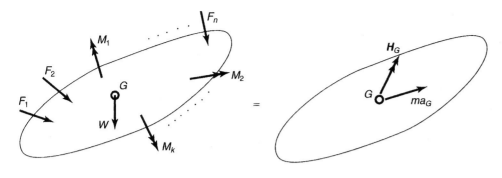

FIGURE 2.10 A "cartoon" version of Newton's second law for a rigid body. The figure on the left of the equals sign is the typical free-body diagram, with forces F_i, $i = 1, 2, \ldots, n$ and force couples M_j, $j = 1, 2, \ldots, m$ acting on the rigid body shown. The figure on the right shows the two inertial vectors, the rate of linear momentum change (mass × acceleration) and the rate of angular momentum change.

The left-hand side is the usual free-body diagram. The right-hand side shows the vectors corresponding to the rates of change of linear and angular momentum. For the set of vectors on the left-hand side to equal the set of vectors on the right-hand side, the sums of the vectors must be equal *and* the moments of all the vectors about any arbitrary point must be equal. If we choose the mass center as the reference point, the earlier set of equations results. If we choose another point P as the point of reference, then a force acting through that point is omitted from the moment equation but the (mass × acceleration) vector on the right-hand side does have a moment about the non-mass-center reference—that is,

$$\sum r_i \times F_{i/P} + \sum M_j = \dot{H}_G + r_{G/P} \times ma_G$$

The reader can readily verify by example that if P is an accelerating point, then in general the inertial terms do not equal the rate of change of angular momentum about point P—that is, $\dot{H}_G + r_{G/P} \times ma_G \neq \dot{H}_P$.

Many problems are well approximated with a two-dimensional analysis since the motion about the joint is mainly planar. For planar motion, the preceding moment equation becomes

$$\sum_j (F_{ji}d_{ji}) = I_{cm}\alpha + |\mathbf{d} \times m\ddot{\mathbf{r}}|$$

We note that another form of the moment equation can be utilized which actually uses the moment of inertia about the arbitrary accelerating point P. Specifically, we can write

$$\sum_{i=1}^{n}\mathbf{r}_{i/P} \times \mathbf{F}_i + \sum_{j=1}^{k}\mathbf{M}_j = (\dot{\mathbf{H}}_P)_{rel} + \mathbf{r}_{G/P} \times m\mathbf{a}_P$$

where $(\dot{\mathbf{H}}_P)_{rel}$ is the rate of change of relative angular momentum about the point P. (This latter equation can be derived from the earlier form by using the relation for the momentum of point P relative to point G—that is, $(\mathbf{H}_P)_{rel} = \mathbf{H}_G + \mathbf{r}_{G/P} \times m\mathbf{v}_{G/P}$.)

The approaches just described put no restrictions on the reference point P. In fact, the idea holds for any two sets of vectors that are equivalent. It is a useful technique for simplifying the moment equation by eliminating the explicit appearance of unknown forces acting at P. For the special case when the point P is fixed (not moving) at the center of rotation, the motion is fully circular about point P and the foregoing equation of motion is further simplified to

$$\sum M_P = I_P \alpha$$

where $I_P = I_{cm} + m|\mathbf{d}|^2$ by the parallel axis theorem. Besides the cases for the mass center and the fixed point, it can be seen that there is a third situation where the general forms of the equations reduce to the simple form, specifically when $\vec{r}_{G/P}$ and $m\vec{v}_{G/P}$ are parallel to each other. The bottom line of this discussion is that, in developing link dynamics equations for the musculoskeletal system, you have to be careful. Sometimes it is handier to write the moment equation about a general accelerating point, but the form of the equation is more complicated than when the mass center or a nonaccelerating point on the body is used as the reference point.

Measurement of Body Segment Mass and Geometric Properties

The rigid body analyses require a number of physical properties to be specified for each anatomical segment in the models. These include the masses of the segments and the locations of the mass centers for the static or quasi-static problem. Dynamics problems typically require the moments of inertia for the segments. If muscle forces or ligament forces are included in the model, the geometric parameters describing their lines of actions are needed. These lines of action are often described by locating the origins and insertions of the muscle or ligament. In order to arrive at useful parameters for our problems, we can rely on empirical data alone, or on empirical information plus analytical models.

Empirical data for mass properties   A number of investigators have measured segment mass properties for living subjects or cadavers. Mass distribution among anatomical segments, locations of mass centers, and mass moments of inertia have been cataloged with this approach. These have been used to develop empirical formulae for estimating body segment parameters for a given subject on the basis of easily obtained information such as weight and height. Table 2.3 was assembled by Winter to summarize some results from various studies.

To use the tabulated results, it is necessary to know segment lengths. Some average values for segment lengths were assembled by Drillis and Contini and are summarized in a figure by Winter. (See Figure 2.11.)

The values in the table and figure are only averages from small populations of subjects. There are numerous papers in the literature describing various attempts to determine the best empirical formulas for scaling the data for individual subjects. It's important to recognize that when you use these numbers, there is a reasonable amount of uncertainty and the results of your model have a corresponding level of uncertainty (a point to always keep in mind for biomechanics models). If you are really concerned about the results, the reasonable thing to do is to get answers for several values of the parameters to get an idea of how much the uncertainties can affect your results.

TABLE 2.3

Anthropometric Data

Segment	Definition	Segment Weight/ Total Body Weight	Center of Mass/ Segment Length		Radius of Gyration/ Segment Length			Density
			Proximal	Distal	C of G	Proximal	Distal	
Hand	Wrist axis/knuckle II middle finger	0.006 M	0.506	0.494 P	0.297	0.587	0.577 M	1.16
Forearm	Elbow axis/ulnar styloid	0.016 M	0.430	0.570 P	0.303	0.526	0.647 M	1.13
Upper arm	Glenohumeral axis/elbow axis	0.028 M	0.436	0.564 P	0.322	0.542	0.645 M	1.07
Forearm and hand	Elbow axis/ulnar styloid	0.022 M	0.682	0.318 P	0.468	0.827	0.565 P	1.14
Total arm	Glenohumeral joint/ulnar styloid	0.050 M	0.530	0.470 P	0.368	0.645	0.596 P	1.11
Foot	Lateral malleolus/head metatarsal II	0.0145 M	0.50	0.50 P	0.475	0.690	0.690 P	1.10
Leg	Femoral condyles/medial malleolus	0.0465 M	0.433	0.567 P	0.302	0.528	0.643 M	1.09
Thigh	Greater trochanter/ femoral condyles	0.100 M	0.433	0.567 P	0.323	0.540	0.653 M	1.05
Foot and leg	Femoral condyles/medial malleolus	0.061 M	0.606	0.394 P	0.416	0.735	0.572 P	1.09
Total leg	Greater trochanter/ medial malleolus	0.161 M	0.447	0.553 P	0.326	0.560	0.650 P	1.06
Head and neck	C7–T1 and 1st rib/ ear canal	0.081 M	1.000	— PC	0.495	1.116	— PC	1.11
Shoulder mass	Sternoclavicular joint/ glenohumeral axis	—	0.712	0.288	—	—	—	1.04
Thorax	C7–T1/T12–L1 and diaphragm*	0.216 PC	0.82	0.18	—	—	—	0.92
Abdomen	T12–L1/L4–L5*	0.139 LC	0.44	0.56	—	—	—	—
Pelvis	L4–L5/greater trochanter*	0.142 LC	0.105	0.895	—	—	—	—
Thorax and abdomen	C7–T1/L4–L5*	0.355 LC	0.63	0.37	—	—	—	—
Abdomen and pelvis	T12–L1/greater trochanter*	0.281 PC	0.27	0.73	—	—	—	1.01
Trunk	Greater trochanter/ glenohumeral joint*	0.497 M	0.50	0.50	—	—	—	1.03
Trunk head neck	Greater trochanter/ glenohumeral joint*	0.578 MC	0.66	0.34 P	0.503	0.830	0.607 M	—
HAT	Greater trochanter/ glenohumeral joint*	0.678 MC	0.626	0.374 PC	0.496	0.798	0.621 PC	—
HAT	Greater trochanter/ mid rib	0.678	1.142	—	0.903	1.456	—	—

*NOTE: These segments are presented relative to the length between the greater trochanter and the glenohumeral joint.

Source: Table 3.1 from Winter, D.A., *Biomechanics and Motor Control of Human Movement*. Wiley Interscience, New York, 1990.

Source codes: M, Dempster via Miller and Nelson; *Biomechanics of Sport*, Lea and Febiger, Philadelphia, 1973. P, Dempster via Plagenhoef; *Patterns of Human Motion*, Prentice-Hall, Inc., Englewood Cliffs, N.J., 1971. L, Dempster via Plagenhoef from living subjects; *Patterns of Human Motion*, Prentice-Hall, Inc., Englewood Cliffs, N.J., 1971. C, Calculated.

FIGURE 2.11 Average segment lengths as a function of height. (Figure 3.1 from Winter, D.A., *Biomechanics and Motor Control of Human Movement*. Wiley Interscience, New York, 1990.)

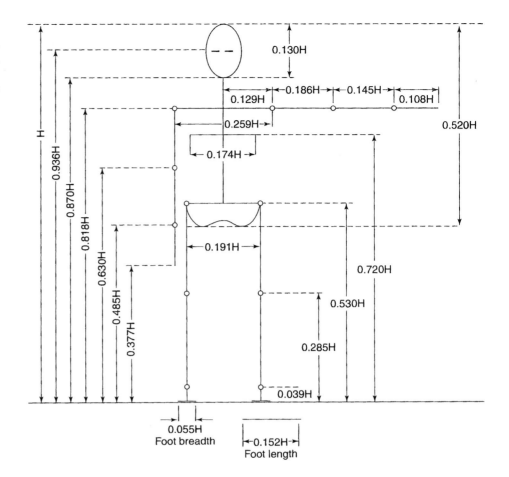

Mathematical models for mass properties By assuming that the major body segments correspond roughly to some common shapes, standard formulae for simple shapes can be combined with anatomical measurements and known density information to predict mass properties. Various models have been proposed that use ellipsoids, truncated cones, or ellipsoidal cylinders (Figure 2.12).

Estimates of individual segment parameters can be obtained from estimates of average density and measured lengths and diameters. Obviously, the model could be refined by defining more complex solid shapes to model the segments. For example, truncated ellipsoidal cones, instead of truncated circular cones, could be used for the limb segments. For the trunk segments, an alternative is to use a composite volume, such as a stadium solid, defined as a solid with cross sections composed of rectangles completed with semicircles on each end. The mathematical approach represents a significant idealization, but it can easily be programmed, and it can readily handle three-dimensional problems, whereas most of the experimental data is limited to the sagittal plane.

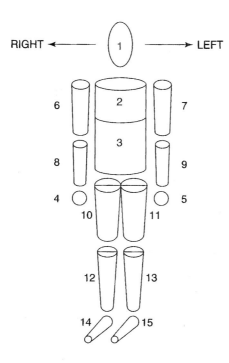

RIGHT ←——— LEFT

FIGURE 2.12 The Mathematical Model From Hanavan, AMRL-TR-64-102, or from Miller and Morrison (1975) *Med and Sci in Sports* 7 (3): 207.

EXAMPLE 2.6   Vehicle Occupant Deceleration

Question   Consider an individual whose height and weight are 1.7 m and 75 kg, who is riding in a vehicle, facing forward and restrained by a lap belt. What is the initial angular acceleration of the upper body due to a sudden deceleration of 10 g's?

Solution   To solve the problem, we will assume that the body rotates about the hip, and the entire upper body—i.e., the head, arms, and trunk (HAT)—moves as a single unit. A free-body diagram for the problem is shown in Figure 2.13.

We will also assume, as indicated in Figure 2.13, that the intersegmental resultant forces act at the hip joint and that there are no restraining moments due to internal forces and no external restraints such as a shoulder belt or air bag. This means that the upper body rotates unrestrained about the hip. Also, we will assume for convenience that the weight force for the combined HAT acts through the hip joint center. This allows us to skip writing the initial force equations. If we then use the previous equation for angular acceleration about the hip joint J, the only unknown will be the angular acceleration. To define the appropriate body segment parameters, we will use Figure 2.11 and Table 2.3.

With the aforementioned assumption, the previous equation for moment about the hip joint (which is an accelerating point) is

$$\sum_j (F_j d_j) = I_{cm}\alpha + |\mathbf{d} \times m\ddot{\mathbf{r}}| = 0$$

The hip joint J acceleration is $\mathbf{a}_j = 10(9.81) = 98.1$ m/s^2 to the left. The acceleration of the mass center can be written in vector terms as $\ddot{\mathbf{r}} = \mathbf{a}_G = \mathbf{a}_j +$

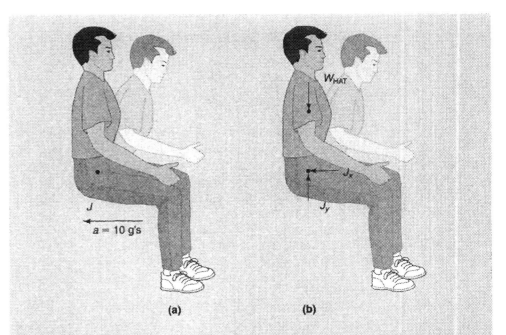

FIGURE 2.13   Inertial effects due to sudden deceleration. (a) Hip joint J is decelerated at a rate of 10 g's. The upper torso is assumed to rotate as a rigid body about point J. (b) Forces in the free-body diagram include only the weight force (assumed to act initially through the hip joint) and the hip joint forces. The restraining moment about the hip is assumed to be zero.

$(\mathbf{a}_{G/J})_{\text{normal}} + (\mathbf{a}_{G/J})_{\text{tangential}}$. For this planar problem, $(\mathbf{a}_{G/J})_{\text{normal}} = h\omega^2$ directed from G toward J, where ω is the angular velocity, which we assume is initially zero. The tangential component is given by $(\mathbf{a}_{G/J})_{\text{tangential}} = h\alpha$. Using this information, we can write that $\ddot{\mathbf{r}} = \mathbf{a}_G = (-98.1 + h\alpha)\hat{\mathbf{i}}$, and $\mathbf{d} \times m\ddot{\mathbf{r}} = h\hat{\mathbf{j}} \times m(-98.1 + h\alpha)\hat{\mathbf{i}} = -(-98.1mh + mh^2\alpha)\hat{\mathbf{k}}$. (Here we have done the vector math carefully to illustrate the formal approach that can get us through much more complicated problems.) Putting this result into the above equation yields our answer in parametric form:

$$I_{cm}\alpha + mh^2\alpha - 98.1mh = 0 \quad \Rightarrow \alpha = \frac{98.1mh}{(I_{cm} + mh^2)}$$

From Table 2.3, the mass for the HAT is $m = .678(75) = 50.8$ kg. From Figure 2.11, the length of the trunk from hip (greater trochanter) to shoulder (glenohumeral joint) is given by $L_{HAT} = (.870 - .530)(1.7\text{m}) = .578$ m. From Table 2.3, the center of mass is then located at $h = .626(.578) = .362$ m. The corresponding moment of inertia is $I_{cm} = m(k^2) = 50.8(.287)^2 = 4.18$ kg-m^2. Substituting these values into the foregoing equation yields the result $\alpha = 166$ radians/s^2.

Muscle and ligament forces   To model muscle forces, the minimum requirement is often to define lines of action for the muscles. Quantitative muscle and soft tissue anatomy have been developed using three-dimensional reconstructions of anatomy from cadaveric specimens. Modern imaging techniques also allow for some measurements on living subjects. The simplest models are based on the idea that muscles can be regarded as strings or groups of strings transmitting force in straight lines between their origins on one segment and their insertion on another segment. In other cases, it is necessary to account for the fact that the muscles lie along some restraining surface like deeper muscles, or that tendons wrap around the ends of bones, as the patellar tendon does at the knee. In some problems, this will be accurate enough for approximating forces. In some circumstances, more attention must be given to the fact that muscles are complex, and that parts of muscles can be activated independently.

Since muscles cross joints, the effect of joint position on the muscle lines of action usually must be taken into account. If the muscle or muscle compartment can be idealized by a line of action between two points, this is not so hard to do. It requires that the origin be located on the proximal segment, the insertion be located on the distal segment, and the relative position of the distal segment with respect to the proximal segment be specified. Then the line of action can be calculated in both segment reference frames.

EXAMPLE 2.7 Determining Muscle Force Lines of Action

Question   The locations of the origin and insertion of several of the primary hip muscles are known in their local pelvic and femoral reference frames respectively (Table 2.4). What are the muscle force lines of action in each reference frame when the hip is flexed at 45°?

Solution   The origin of the pelvic reference frame is defined as the midpoint between the anterior superior iliac crests, and the origin of the femoral reference frame is taken as the center of the femoral head. Pelvic reference axes are x = anterior, y = medial lateral (right toward left from right hip joint), and z = superior. The location of the center of the femoral head in the pelvic reference

TABLE 2.4

Locations of Muscle Origins and Insertions[1]

Muscle	x_{origin}	y_{origin}	z_{origin}	$x_{insertion}$	$y_{insertion}$	$z_{insertion}$
Abductor medius	−.0829	−.0874	.0284	−.0262	−.0533	−.0074
Abductor minimus	−.0645	−.0968	−.0069	−.0101	.0557	−.0097
Tensor fascia latae	−.0311	−.1241	.0214	.0294	−.0597	−.0995
Rectus femoris	−.0295	−.0968	−.0311	−.043	.0373	.0019
Femoral head	−.707	−.0835	−.0661			

[1] All locations for origins are in the pelvic reference frame, and all values for the insertions are in the femoral reference frame. Dimensions are in meters.

frame is listed in the table. When the leg is in full extension, the femoral and pelvic reference frames are aligned. The hip is assumed to be 45 degrees in flexion, and we want to determine the line of action of the abductor in each reference frame.

To express the vector from origin to insertion in the pelvic reference frame, we transform the insertion point to the pelvic reference frame. This can be done with simple trigonometric construction:

$$x_i^p = x_i^f \cos(45) + z_i^f \sin(45) + x^{f/p}$$

$$y_i^p = y_i^f$$

$$z_i^p = -x_i^f \sin(45) + z_i^f \cos(45) + z^{f/p}$$

Note that the subscript i indicates the insertion, and the superscript p or f indicates the pelvic or femoral reference frame. The last terms add the shift from the femoral reference frame origin (the femoral head) to the pelvic reference frame origin. If we wanted to write this in a more general form that would correspond to the full three-dimensional problem, we would write

$$\begin{Bmatrix} x_i^p \\ y_i^p \\ z_i^p \end{Bmatrix} = \begin{bmatrix} \cos(45) & 0 & \sin(45) \\ 0 & 1 & 0 \\ -\sin(45) & 0 & \cos(45) \end{bmatrix} \begin{Bmatrix} x_i^f \\ y_i^f \\ z_i^f \end{Bmatrix} + \begin{Bmatrix} x^{f/p} \\ y^{f/p} \\ z^{f/p} \end{Bmatrix}$$

Then, each element of the 3×3 matrix corresponds to a direction cosine between the corresponding pairs of axes. This expression reminds us that the y value is unchanged by the rotation about the y-axis. To calculate the line of action, we can just write the vector difference between the two points in the now common pelvic reference frame:

$$x_{i/o}^p = x_i^p - x_o^p$$

$$y_{i/o}^p = y_i^p - y_o^p$$

$$z_{i/o}^p = z_i^p - z_o^p$$

Since we are interested only in the direction and not the magnitude of this vector, we would usually write it as a unit vector:

$$l_{i/o}^p = (x_i^p - x_o^p)/\sqrt{(x_i^p - x_o^p)^2 + (y_i^p - y_o^p)^2 + (z_i^p - z_o^p)^2}$$

$$m_{i/o}^p = (y_i^p - y_o^p)/\sqrt{(x_i^p - x_o^p)^2 + (y_i^p - y_o^p)^2 + (z_i^p - z_o^p)^2}$$

$$n_{i/o}^p = (z_i^p - z_o^p)/\sqrt{(x_i^p - x_o^p)^2 + (y_i^p - y_o^p)^2 + (z_i^p - z_o^p)^2}$$

To determine the line of action in the femoral reference frame, we could transform the origin from the pelvic to the femoral reference frame and repeat the previous calculation. However, it is simpler to just do the vector transformation of the unit vector:

$$\begin{Bmatrix} l_{i/o}^f \\ m_{i/o}^f \\ n_{i/o}^f \end{Bmatrix} = \begin{bmatrix} \cos(45) & 0 & -\sin(45) \\ 0 & 1 & 0 \\ \sin(45) & 0 & \cos(45) \end{bmatrix} \begin{Bmatrix} l_{i/o}^p \\ m_{i/o}^p \\ n_{i/o}^p \end{Bmatrix}$$

The numerical values in Table 2.4 can be substituted to obtain the direction cosines of each muscle line of action in each reference frame. This is left as an exercise for the reader.

A second geometric property of muscles that is sometimes incorporated into dynamics problems is the size of the muscle. It has been proposed that muscles might be recruited on the basis of their efficiency in a particular effort. This is in part determined by the moment arm for the given activity, but also by the size of the muscle. Furthermore, it has been suggested that muscle capabilities are determined by a maximum stress level that is approximately constant over all muscles. Consequently, if the effective load-carrying (generating) area of the muscle is known, something more can be said about its potential role in a given action. It has been demonstrated that muscles stay very near the same total volume over their physiological length changes. This fact can be used to estimate an effective cross-sectional area on the basis of a measured length. Obviously, the length of the muscle plus any tendon is easily generated from the calculation in the previous example as the length of the vector:

$$L_{M+T} = \sqrt{(x_i^p - x_o^p)^2 + (y_i^p - y_o^p)^2 + (z_i^p - z_o^p)^2}$$

So, if the volume of the muscle and the tendon length can be estimated, an effective muscle area is easily calculated as $A = $ (volume)/(total length − tendon length).

For ligaments, the length as a function of joint position can be calculated in a similar way as for the muscle on the basis of the locations of the attachments in the local segmental coordinate systems. If the length–force relationship is available for the ligament, you can then calculate the force in the ligament directly and include it in the known forces for your particular joint force problem. The problem is complicated for many ligaments by the fact that the areas of attachment can be fairly broad, particularly compared with the length. So, a given change in joint position may change the effective length differently across the breadth of the ligament. This is not a difficult problem to handle conceptually, but it requires a lot of effort. It is made even more complicated because we often do not have a good way of knowing where the "zero" point (i.e., the free length of each ligament component) really is. Fortunately, for many problems of interest, ligaments do not generate substantial force. However, as is obvious from examples elsewhere in this book, in some cases it is the forces in the ligaments that play a major role in joint stability.

Kinematics and Motion Analysis

The kinematic data required for the inverse dynamics problem include position and orientation data, velocity data, and acceleration data for each body segment as a function of time. In the most general approach, each segment can be regarded as an independent rigid body requiring three independent location coordinates (two in planar motion) and three independent orientation coordinates (one in planar motion). Each degree of freedom requires an independent measure. The independent measure may be an actual coordinate of a point, or it may be some other measure like an angle. In dynamics, all measures that can independently describe degrees of freedom are called *generalized coordinates*. If a joint between segments can be represented mathematically—for example, as a revolute joint, a ball and socket joint, or in terms of some other surface-to-surface constraint—the number of degrees of freedom is reduced, and correspondingly some of the generalized coordinates can be related by *kinematic constraint conditions*. As an example, if the elbow is regarded as a hinge, the forearm is located with respect to the upper arm by one angular coordinate. If the wrist is regarded as a universal joint, the hand is located with respect to the forearm with two angular coordinates. If the hip is regarded as a ball and socket joint, the thigh segment is located with respect to the pelvis with three angular coordinates.

Many choices are available for generalized coordinates that describe position and orientation. A number of alternatives are presented in the literature devoted to the experimental measurement of musculoskeletal kinematics. One of the most straightforward approaches is to define the motion of a reference point (such as the mass center) and the orientation of a set of mutually perpendicular reference axes that are attached to the reference point. To make the data meaningful for the orientation of the segment reference frames, they are usually constructed with reference to particular anatomical reference points. For example, a reference frame for the upper leg might be constructed from the following three points: (1) the center of the head of the femur, (2) the medial epicondyle, and (3) the lateral epicondyle. By defining an axis perpendicular to the plane of the three points and a second axis within the plane—for example, the line from the center of the femoral head through the midpoint between the condyles—an internal reference frame is defined. Unfortunately, there is no universal agreement on the definition of segment reference frames, and numerous alternative choices are found in the literature.

The inverse dynamics problem requires establishing the history of a set of generalized coordinates and their first and second time derivatives to determine the derivative terms $\ddot{\mathbf{r}}_i$ and $\dot{\mathbf{H}}_i$ in the dynamics equations. The most common approach is to measure displacement histories for the limb segments and then determine time derivatives from the displacement data. This can be done in a variety of ways, but often a stereo-photogrammetric approach is used, where cameras record the motion of reflective or lighted markers that are attached to the moving segments. The angular velocity and angular acceleration of a segment can be readily determined for the planar motion problem. In that case, the magnitude of the angular velocity is determined by magnitude of the relative velocity of two points divided by the distance between them, and the angular acceleration is determined by rate of change of the angular velocity. For three-dimensional motion, the problem requires using velocities and accelerations of at least three points per segment.

The determination of segment angular velocities and accelerations can be done with arbitrarily placed markers on the moving segments. However, for the inverse dynamics problem, the mass center position history is required. Also, it is necessary to establish appropriate anatomical reference frames to define segment moments of inertia and possibly other information such as approximate joint centers, joint contact surface shapes, and muscle attachments. This can be accomplished with the following three steps: (1) setting up a reference frame associated with the external markers; (2) defining the internal reference frame with respect to identifiable anatomical landmarks; and (3) locating the anatomical landmarks in the external reference frame. Then a transformation can be constructed defining the location and orientation of the internal reference frame on the basis of the location and orientation of the external reference frame. Any point whose location is specified in the internal reference frame can then be located in space. For example, for planar motion of the lower limb, a pair of markers on each segment could be located with respect to identifiable anatomical points such as the lateral epicondyle and lateral maleolus. For problems requiring the description of three-dimensional motion, the use of biplanar radiographs or other special techniques may be required to relate external markers to anatomical landmarks.

There are alternative approaches to the measurement of kinematics. One is to use a goniometer to measure the relative orientation of adjacent segments directly. In planar motion, a single angle of rotation is generally sufficient. The motion of a reference point on one segment and the relative orientations of each pair of connected segments could be combined with dimensional information to locate and orient each segment. This approach has been used for three-dimensional motion as well, but a fairly complex, multi-degree-of-freedom goniometer is necessary for the general joint. Usually, this approach is used only when the kinematics of relative motion of two segments about a particular joint (e.g., the knee) is the issue of interest.

The determination of velocities and accelerations from displacement data requires a computational procedure for calculating the first and second time derivatives for the displacement data. In the biomechanics literature, there are many descriptions of numerical schemes for doing this with various levels of accuracy. Because a derivative involves the ratio of a change in a dependent variable and a change in independent variable, it is inherently a noisy process. That is, errors in measurement can be amplified. Consider, for example, when an approximate speed is calculated by the simple difference ratio $v = \Delta x/\Delta t$. A small variation in Δt creates a larger variation in the first derivative and an even larger variation in the second derivative $a = (\Delta v/\Delta t)$. For this reason, curve fitting and smoothing techniques are almost always a part of determining velocity and acceleration data from displacement data.

Dynamic Simulation of Musculoskeletal Motion

The equations of motion for the inverse dynamics problem can be used to predict the resultant force and moment that must act across each joint. The methods of force distribution previously described for the static force distribution problem, such as muscle grouping and optimization models, can also be used to predict muscle and joint contact forces in dynamic problems. An alternative to the inverse dynamics approach to musculoskeletal motion problems is the use of dynamic simulation. The forward dynamics problem is solved in an iterative manner, varying the inputs until the predicted outcome matches the observed outcome within some acceptable tolerance. This is a particularly useful approach in motion analysis where performance is to be optimized, but can be used as an alternative to the inverse dynamics approach for any dynamics problem. The inputs for a given simulation can be at several levels. They can be the torque histories due to the muscles acting across the joints, muscle force histories, or even neural control histories for the muscles. In the latter case, the model can even include the muscle stimulation and activation dynamics. In general, the redundant muscle systems require that some strategy, such as an optimal control approach, be used to estimate the inputs required to generate an observed motion. For example, we can pose the problem such that a set of muscle inputs is determined that minimizes the error between observed and predicted motion and also minimizes metabolic energy. While such a sophisticated method may prove to be the most powerful way to approach modeling of musculoskeletal motion, it may not be necessary for the problem of defining loads on skeletal structures.

2.4 | Joint Stability

So far, we have looked at the forces and moments that occur at joints, as well as the motions of the skeleton during various activities. One important issue in understanding normal function and the etiology of various joint diseases is the relationship between the loads on a joint and its motion. This is critical in design of total joint replacements, since historical perspective has shown the importance of reproducing the normal relationship between loads and motion to avoid premature loosening of the components or damage to articulating surfaces. We will see in this section that there is a strong relationship between the two: The body appears to be conditioned to apply specific muscle forces about a joint for specific kinematic tasks. If the joint cannot move in its expected path in response to these loads because of some geometric changes in the system (for example, a damaged meniscus at the knee), the resulting motion may be erratic. Conversely, if the expected loads are not supplied for a given kinematic task due to a disruption of the load bearing tissues such as tendons or ligaments about the joint, it may not be possible to complete the task. In either case, pain can result and function is impaired. We use the concept of joint stability to describe these conditions.

Joint stability can be defined as the ability of a joint to maintain an appropriate functional position throughout its range of motion. A stable joint can move through a normal range of motion while carrying functional loads while producing joint contact forces of normal intensity between the articular surfaces. The characteristics of stable synovial joints are as follows:

1. Joint contact occurs between surfaces, both of which are covered with articular cartilage.
2. Peripheral (edge) loading doesn't seem to occur.
3. There exists a unique position of equilibrium for any loading.
4. Small changes in either the magnitude or direction of the functional load do not lead to large changes in the position of joint contact.

There are three main mechanisms for providing synovial joint stability. The first and perhaps most important is *contact at the articular surfaces*. This is the primary mechanism of stability, and it is a passive mechanism, since it is based on contact. It is present to varying extents in all articulating diarthrodial joints. For example, the hip joint (ball and socket) is very stable due to the geometric constraints imposed by the articulating surfaces. The same is true, but to a lesser extent, at other ball and socket joints such as the shoulder, where there is less socket coverage than in the hip and therefore less stability provided by the contact mechanism. For healthy human joints, the articulations are almost frictionless. Consequently, the joint contact forces are essentially perpendicular to the articulating surface.

The variable curvature of the articulating surface therefore enables joint contact forces of different orientations to develop if the point of contact varies throughout a kinematic task (Figure 2.14). Thus, stability is achieved when the contact point is at a position $\mathbf{x}$, where the surface normal vector $\mathbf{n(x)}$ and the force $\mathbf{J}$ are aligned. This mechanism requires relative motion (mostly translation) between the two articulating surfaces. Learning to walk, for example, represents a trial-and-error process whereby the body determines a unique set of muscle force (and, less so, ligament and other soft tissue force) magnitudes that results in a position of the joint contact force that produces a stable joint for that activity. Conceptually, the problem is unchanged if there are multiple muscles acting about a joint, so long as their action (magnitude and direction) is known.

The issue then arises as to how the position $\mathbf{x}$ of the contact force is determined at a joint for a specific task. Some insight into this can be gained by using the three-force model of a joint discussed previously. In the example where we assumed that only a single muscle with known line of action acted, a statically determinate system resulted. If it is also assumed—and this is critical to this discussion—that the position of joint contact is known, the problem can be solved for the contact force. If the contact position is not assumed to be known, then the system is again indeterminate. If the magnitude of the muscle force is known from independent measures, however, the problem can be solved for the contact position (Figure 2.14). The solution in this case specifies the magnitude and line of action of the joint contact force, and these variables will change with the magnitude (and orientation) of the known muscle force, along with the external loads. Since there is minimal friction at the joint, however, the geometry of the articulating surface at the point of contact must be perpendicular to the orientation of the joint contact force for that particular instant. Thus, there must be an intimate relationship between the geometry of the articulating surface and the associated muscle action and external loads. This is the basic mechanism by which the kinematics and loads at joints are mutually dependent.

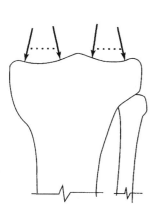

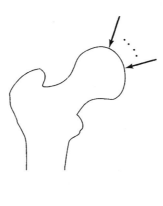

FIGURE 2.14 The range of possible orientations of the joint contact force depends on the orientation of the articulating surface, since the low friction nature of the articulation constrains the effective joint contact force to be perpendicular to the joint surface.

EXAMPLE 2.8 Contact Points and Joint Loading

Question   The location of the contact force within the joint has a profound effect on the magnitude of the resulting joint contact and muscle forces. To better understand this, use the three-force vector triangle approach to analyze the effects of changing the location of the joint contact force from points 1 to 2 in Figure 2.15. Assume that the ground reaction force is unchanged, and that the orientation of the muscle force (the quadriceps) is also unchanged. Discuss also this result in the context of design of artificial joints.

Solution   Since there are only three forces and no moments acting on the lower leg (we'll ignore the weight of the lower leg since it is small compared to the other

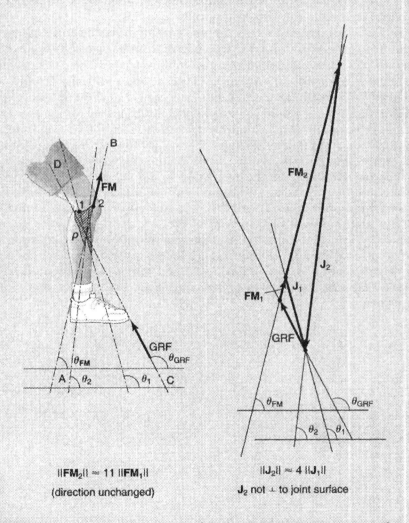

$$\|\mathbf{FM_2}\| \approx 11 \, \|\mathbf{FM_1}\|$$
(direction unchanged)

$$\|\mathbf{J_2}\| \approx 4 \, \|\mathbf{J_1}\|$$
$\mathbf{J_2}$ not $\perp$ to joint surface

FIGURE 2.15   Left: Free-body diagram of the lower leg during gait, using a three-force model. Right: Vector force diagram corresponding to the three-force model of the leg shown on the left.

forces acting on the segment), all three forces must be concurrent (i.e., go through a single point). This point p is found by the intersection of the lines of action of the ground reaction and muscle forces (GRF and FM, respectively). The orientation of the joint contact force (J) is found for points 1 and 2 by passing its line of action through point p and respectively points 1 and 2. It is seen that the angles of this force to the horizontal at points 1 and 2 are θ_1 and θ_2, respectively (Figure 2.15). Construction of the vector force triangle starts with placement of vector for the known GRF at an angle θ_{GRF}. We don't know the magnitude of the muscle force but do know its orientation, θ_{FM}. Thus, we construct a line at this angle that intersects with the head of the GRF vector. Similarly, we also don't know the magnitude of the joint contact force but do know its orientation, θ_1 (or θ_2). To complete the closed vector force triangle, we construct a line with orientation θ_1 intersecting with the tail of the GRF vector. This is done separately for the two orientations of the joint contact forces. It is readily seen then that the magnitude of the joint contact force is much greater when it acts at point 2 than at point 1, as is the magnitude of the muscle force. In particular, the joint contact and muscle forces are increased by about a factor 4 and 11, respectively, when the location of the joint contact force moves from point 1 to point 2.

This strong association between the location of the joint contact force and the magnitude of the muscle force is a key attribute that needs to be incorporated into design of artificial joints. As we learn to walk and run, etc., our muscles become programmed to provide the precise force to provide equilibrium at the joint for the specific activity. The body becomes accustomed to these requirements, and over the years the muscles and soft tissues adapt accordingly in their size and load capacity. If the required muscle force is suddenly substantially altered—as it could be if the contact point moved from point 1 to point 2 upon implantation of an artificial knee joint—then the patient could have difficulty in performing certain tasks since the required force on the muscle may be too high. Development of large joint contact forces with nonideal placement of the location of the joint contact force could also accelerate wear of the artificial joint. For these reasons, it is critical to reproduce as much as possible the natural kinematics when designing artificial joints. While this is relatively trivial for stable ball and socket joints such as the hip, it is quite challenging for more complex joints such as the knee.

A related contact mechanism is specific to bicondylar joints, where the joint contact force can be distributed unevenly between the two condyles to produce a resultant moment about the joint center that can counteract some externally applied moment (Figure 2.16). This results in more of the joint contact force being applied to one of the condyles. Eventually, if the external load is high enough, the contact will be lost on one of the condyles and the joint will begin to open up on that side. In that event, any ligaments on that side of the joint will be stretched to enhance stability in the absence of muscle co-contraction. This important contact mechanism is described in more detail in one of the examples that follow. The important concept here is that of a *multi-condylar joint*, which allows for forces to be moved in part or fully from one condyle to another.

One of the secondary mechanisms of stability is muscle action, which is an active mechanism because it can be voluntarily induced by muscle contraction. As illustrated

FIGURE 2.16 Distribution of the joint contact force unevenly across the condyles of a bicondylar joint produces a net moment about the joint center that can resist externally applied loads. In this way, a moment is created at the joint without the need to generate tensile forces in the surrounding soft tissues.

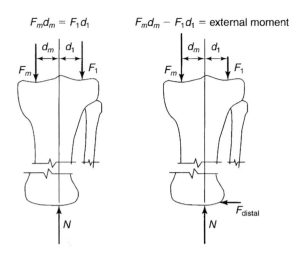

in the last example, if the magnitude of the muscle force can be controlled (and therefore changed), the orientation of the equilibrating joint contact force will change, as will the point of contact. Thus, equilibrium can be achieved and the point of contact controlled by control of the muscle forces that act around the joint.

Co-contraction of agonists and antagonists about a joint can also increase stability by resulting in an increase in the compression across the joint (by increasing the magnitude of the joint contact force), thereby keeping the two articulating surfaces of the joint in contact. As will be illustrated shortly, this mechanism is particularly important at the knee for stability in the frontal plane. However, it should be noted that it takes at least 20 milliseconds for a muscle to generate any force, even after it has been signaled to do so neurologically. Thus, this active mechanism can protect the joint only if there is ample time to generate adequate muscle force. This may not be possible in traumatic situations where unexpected loads can be applied to the skeleton in a few milliseconds.

Another secondary stability mechanism, which is passive in nature and which was mentioned above, is stretching of ligaments and capsule individually or in combination. The main mechanical role of the ligament is to limit the range of the joint contact to lie within the articular cartilage surfaces. When the joint opens or slides beyond its normal range of motion, ligaments are stretched, therefore producing restoring forces that limit subsequent motion of the joint. The direction of the force produced by the ligament is along the line of action of the ligament.

For habitual activities in healthy joints, the ligaments can allow relative motion (sliding and rolling) of joints without developing significant forces, although it is unknown to what extent this occurs *in vivo*. This initial low force resistance by the ligaments is possible because the ligament has a slack region over which it develops minimal force as it is stretched. Because of its nonlinear force–deformation behavior, significant forces only develop when the ligament is stretched beyond its slack region. Thus, there is an important balance between laxity of the ligament and allowable joint motion. This balance can be upset by trauma to the ligament, by diseases such as rheumatoid arthritis, by congenital disorders, or by replacement of the joint with an artificial joint that leaves the ligaments too taut or too slack. Depending upon the circumstances, the ligaments may allow either too much motion of the joint or too little; both can affect the stability of the joint.

As illustrated next, ligaments also contribute to joint stability when nonhabitual functional loads are encountered during the normal range of activity. The ligament in this situation provides a component to the reaction force that cannot be supplied by the joint contact force, due to the constraint placed on its orientation by the geometry of the articulating surface. Again, if a ligament is damaged, the joint may become unstable if it encounters certain nonhabitual functional loads. Conversely, if the functional load is too large, the ligament may be damaged.

The extent to which ligaments provide stability depends on the activity. For example, individuals with torn or lost anterior cruciate ligaments often have trouble running and twisting, indicating that this ligament is perhaps a primary stability mechanism for these activities. It is important in analysis of stability mechanisms to consider the response to forces and moments over the full range of anticipated loadings.

Stability is an extremely important part of the design of total joint replacements, because a weak link in terms of stability may jeopardize the integrity of the arthroplasty. Thus, it is important for the surgeon to ensure correct alignment of the bones after the arthroplasty.

The stability mechanisms previously discussed are well illustrated by considering the stability of the knee joint in the frontal plane in response to a medially directed force applied at the foot. Such forces occur during the gait cycle and can be very large during sports activities such as a side-step, when full body weight is supported by a single foot used to brake the body or quickly change direction. Thus, it is necessary to consider knee stability in response to the medially directed force and to the "varus–valgus" moment that this force creates about the knee joint.

The mechanism that provides stability under the action of a medially directed force component is a combination of contact and ligament stretch. The medial distal force moves the tibia medially with respect to the femur at the knee joint, resulting in contact of the lateral aspect of medial femoral condyle against the curved medial surface of the medial plateau of the tibia (Figure 2.17a). Because of the curvature of this articulating surface, the resulting medial joint contact force will have a laterally directed component, which equilibrates in part the distal medially directed force on the foot. Stretching of the collateral and cruciate ligaments can also produce laterally directed components of the joint reaction force (Figure 2.17b).

The primary stability mechanism in response to the varus moment is contact, but is based primarily on the ability of the contact force to be distributed unevenly across the two condyles. For a medially directed distal force typical of gait, contact forces will be larger on the medial condyle. Consistent with this mechanism, there are more clinical problems at the knee joint on the medial side, compared with the lateral side. As the magnitude of the medially directed foot force increases, the force on the lateral condyle may become zero, after which further increases in the medially directed foot force will cause the joint to open on the lateral side. At this point, the secondary stability mechanisms become active. Note that the action of the knee extensors (the quadriceps via the patellar ligament) creates no varus or valgus moment about the joint center, although these forces can contribute indirectly to varus–valgus stability.

The secondary stability mechanisms are muscle co-contraction and ligament stretch. For muscle co-contraction, the force in the quadriceps increases, as does the force in the previously inactive hamstrings. (These muscles act in such a way as to create no additional moments in the sagittal plane so as not to affect sagittal stability.)

FIGURE 2.17 (a) Medial translation of the tibia with respect to the femur produces contact at a point where the joint reaction force has the appropriate laterally directed component required for static equilibrium. (b) If the contact mechanism cannot produce sufficient stability, ligament stretch can also counteract the distal medial force.

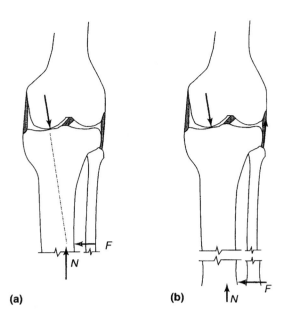

(a)   (b)

This increases the net compressive force across the joint, thereby closing any gaps. This mechanism works in conjunction with the primary contact mechanism, since equilibrium of the varus–valgus moment is still obtained by medialization of the joint contact force.

Note that the "cost" of this secondary stability mechanism is increased compression on the medial tibial plateau. For a medially directed foot force of 200 N, over five times body-weight is transmitted through the medial condyle. Recall also that, since muscles take up to 20 msec to start generating force once activated by nerves, muscle co-contraction cannot work in situations where there are traumatic impact functional loads. In this situation, the ligaments provide another secondary mechanism. As the joint opens, collateral ligaments are stretched beyond their slack region and therefore generate forces that can resist the varus bending moment.

2.5 | Summary

The musculoskeletal system can be modeled as a mechanism, or a machine, which lets us use common tools of mechanics to analyze the mechanical behavior of the system. We can view the musculoskeletal system as a mechanism consisting of rigid links, actuators, and constraint elements and use the dynamics or statics methods of rigid body mechanics to analyze the behavior. In applications of rigid body mechanics to study the mechanical function of the musculoskeletal system, the common ingredients are (1) the description of the elements of the system in mechanical terms; (2) the description of the external constraints on the system; and (3) the application of the laws of motion.

If accelerations cannot be neglected, the full dynamic version of Newton's laws must be applied. In the absence of motion, the problem reduces from a dynamics problem to a statics problem. When the system does not maintain a fixed configuration (the statics problem), but the accelerations are small enough that the inertial terms in the equations of motion can be ignored, the problem is quasi-static. This is a fairly common circumstance in skeletal motion problems, and in this case the analysis is effectively a statics problem with variable geometry. This approach captures some dynamic effects for the system, if the external loads have been determined from dynamic experimental or theoretical analyses.

Static, quasi-static, and dynamic analyses based on Newton's laws can always be used to compute the resultant forces and torques at the joints, but in human and animal joints there are always more structures than the minimum needed for equilibrium. Therefore, the distribution of forces among anatomical structures is statically indeterminate. The distribution problem can be reduced to a determinate problem if the number of unknowns is reduced by using force reduction, muscle scaling, soft tissue force–deformation relations, or some combination of these approaches. The indeterminate problem can be solved directly by using optimization methods that minimize or maximize some mathematical measure of performance.

Dynamic and inverse dynamic problems can be formulated. The kinematic data required for the inverse dynamics problem include position and orientation data, velocity data, and acceleration data for each body segment as a function of time. These data can be determined from displacement data gathered in a motion analysis laboratory.

Joint stability can be defined as the ability of a joint to maintain an appropriate functional position throughout its range of motion. A stable joint can move through a normal range of motion while carrying functional loads while producing joint contact forces of normal intensity between the articular surfaces. This definition of stability can be translated into a requirement of equilibrium among the various forces in the joint that provide the stability.

2.6 EXERCISES

2.1 Use a vector force diagram to estimate the magnitudes (in terms of body-weight W) of the patellar ligament and knee joint contact forces for the person shown squatting (Figure P 2.1).

2.2 An individual is doing sit-ups from the position shown in Figure P 2.2. If the initial angular acceleration of the head, arms, and trunk (in the starting horizontal position) is 3 rad/sec^2, determine the corresponding resultant moment at the hip. The height and mass of the person are $h = 1.8$ m and $m = 70$ kg. You can assume that the legs do not move and the entire head, arms, and trunk move as a single rigid body. Various mass properties are in the accompanying table. (Note: You can use the single HAT data set for mass, moment of inertia.)

2.3 An individual lying in a supine position executes a straight leg lift (Figure P 2.3). For the thigh: $l_T = 40$ cm, $d_T = 18$ cm, $m_T = 8$ kg, $m_{LL} = 5$ kg, $I_T = 4000$ kg-cm^2 (about the hip joint center). For the lower leg (shank + foot): $d_{LL} = 20$ cm, $(I_{LL})_{GL} = 500$ kg-cm^2 (about the mass center of the shank plus foot, point GL).

What is the initial applied moment at the hip to produce an initial angular acceleration of 2 rad/sec^2? What is the corresponding moment at the knee to keep the leg straight?

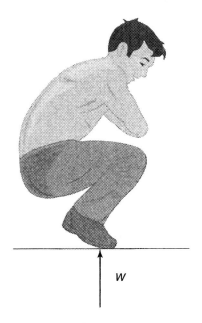

FIGURE P 2.1

2.4 An individual lying in a supine position executes a leg lift (Figure P 2.3). Instead of keeping straight, as in the previous problem, he flexes the hip while keeping the lower leg horizontal. The initial angular acceleration of the thigh is 3 rad/sec. For the thigh: $l_T = 40$ cm, $d_T = 18$ cm, $m_T = 8$ kg, $I_T = 4000$ kg-cm^2 (about the hip joint center). For the lower leg (shank + foot): $d_{LL} = 20$ cm, $m_{LL} = 5$ kg, $(I_{LL})_{GL} = $ 500 kg-cm^2 (about the mass center of the shank plus foot, point GL).

What are the initial applied moments at the hip and the knee?

2.5 A person lifts a 2-kg ball by rotating his shoulder while keeping the elbow and wrist rigid. Initially, the arm is at rest, with the upper arm vertical and the lower arm and hand horizontal.

Determine the initial applied moment at the shoulder and at the elbow if the initial angular acceleration of the arm and hand is 4 rad/sec^2 ccw. Assume that the shoulder E is a fixed hinge and the elbow E also acts as a hinge. Use the following data:

L_U = length of upper arm (shoulder to elbow) = .25 m.

L_L = length of lower arm (elbow to wrist) = .25 m.

d_U = distance from shoulder to mass center for upper arm = 0.12 m.

d_L = distance from elbow to mass center for lower arm = 0.10 m.

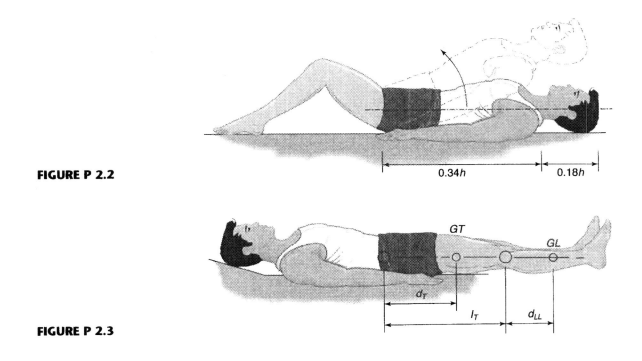

FIGURE P 2.2

FIGURE P 2.3

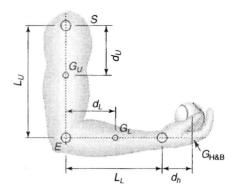

FIGURE P 2.5

d_h = distance from wrist to mass center for hand and ball = 0.06 m.

I_U = mass center moment of inertia of upper arm = .016 kg-m².

I_L = mass center moment of inertia of lower arm = .014 kg-m².

I_h = mass center moment of inertia of hand and ball = negligible.

m_U = mass of upper arm = 3 kg.

m_L = mass of lower arm = 2 kg.

m_h = mass of hand = 0.5 kg.

2.6   An individual stands erect and executes a straight leg kick (Figure P 2.6). The observed initial

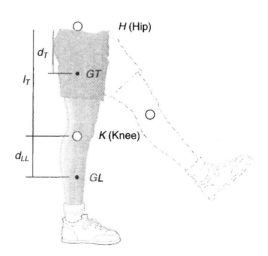

FIGURE P 2.6

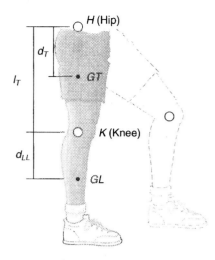

FIGURE P 2.7

angular acceleration for the leg is α = 20 rad/sec². Given the mass distribution properties that follow, what is the initial applied moment at the hip? What is the corresponding moment at the knee to keep the leg straight?

For the thigh: l_T = 18 in, d_T = 8 in, m_T = .045 lb-sec²-in, $(I_T)_O$ = 4.2 lb-sec²-in. (about the hip joint O). For the lower leg: d_{LL} = 8 in, m_{LL} = .025 lb-sec²-in, $(I_{LL})_{GL}$ = 1.4 lb-sec²-in (about the mass center of the thigh plus foot, point GL).

2.7   In the previous problem, the hip and knee moments were calculated for initiating a straight leg kick when the initial angular acceleration for the leg is α = 20 rad/sec². Suppose that, instead, the kick was done with the lower leg kept vertical while the upper leg accelerated at the same rate as before (Figure P 2.7). What is the required initial applied moment at the hip? What moment is required at the knee to keep the lower leg vertical?

For the thigh: l_T = 18 in, d_T = 8 in, m_T = .045 lb-sec²/in, $(I_T)_O$ = 4.2 lb-sec²-in. (about the hip joint O). For the lower leg: d_{LL} = 8 in, m_{LL} = .025 lb-sec²/in, $(I_{LL})_{GL}$ = 1.4 lb-sec²-in (about the mass center of the thigh plus foot, point GL).

2.8   The accompanying table of data consists of coordinates of two markers at the hip and knee for a series of successive time points. Calculate a set of angular speeds and angular accelerations for as many data points as you can.

TABLE P 2.8

t, sec	x_1, cm	y_1, cm	x_2, cm	y_2, cm
.0	131.8	6.1	162.6	6.9
.1	132.6	6.2	160.3	13.7
.2	132.4	5.9	158.2	20.6
.3	131.8	5.2	153.0	27.2
.4	131.4	5.6	147.6	31.3

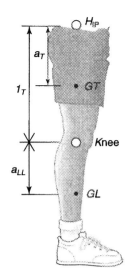

FIGURE P 2.8

2.9 Table P 2.9 of data consists of coordinates of four markers at successive time points. Markers 1 and 2 are attached to the thigh, and markers 3 and 4 are attached to the shank. Write out an algorithm for numerically determining approximate corresponding values for angular velocity of the shank with respect to the thigh. Use it to calculate the approximate angular velocity at $t = 0.1$ and $t = 0.15$.

2.10 Table P 2.10 shows a sequence of position data (x, y) for a set of four markers (Figure P 2.10). Markers 1 and 2 are attached to limb segment A, and markers 3 and 4 are attached to limb segment B. All data are measured at equal time intervals in a common reference frame. Calculate the locations of the average centers of rotation in a coordinate system defined on segment A as shown Figure P 2.10.

2.11 One objective function for the muscle force distribution problem is minimizing the total muscle stress (sum of the muscle stresses) instead of the total muscle force or the contact force magnitude. For the elbow

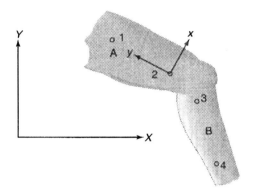

FIGURE P 2.10

TABLE P 2.9

t, sec	x_1, cm	y_1, cm	x_2, cm	y_2, cm	x_3, cm	y_3, cm	x_4, cm	y_4, cm
.05	51.0	85.1	57.0	57.9	57.9	45.8	57.9	10.8
.10	53.6	85.1	60.3	55.9	61.5	46	61.9	11.0
.15	56.3	85.2	63.8	56.1	65.1	46.3	65.8	11.3
.20	58.9	85.2	67.2	56.4	65.7	46.6	69.7	11.6

TABLE P 2.10

Table of coordinate values (all values in millimeters):

i	$X1_i$	$Y1_i$	$X2_i$	$Y2_i$	$X3_i$	$Y3_i$	$X4_i$	$Y4_i$
1	89.5	119.5	110.5	−119.5	112.2	−139.5	136.6	−418.4
2	89.2	128.2	131.8	−108.2	135.4	−131.3	253.6	−384.7
3	88.9	135.9	151.1	−95.9	162.9	−126.1	360.9	−324.1
4	89.0	142.7	171.0	−82.7	197.9	−121.6	451.7	−239.9
5	89.3	148.8	190.7	−88.8	241.7	−113.1	520.7	−137.5

TABLE P 2.11

Muscle	Insertion on Forearm (x, y)	Line of Action (from horizontal axis)	Muscle Area
Biceps	3 cm, 1 cm	120 degrees	4.5 cm^2
Brachialis	5 cm, 1 cm	135 degrees	3.0 cm^2

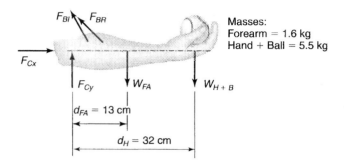

Masses:
Forearm = 1.6 kg
Hand + Ball = 5.5 kg

FIGURE P 2.11

supported by the biceps and brachialis (no triceps force), set up and solve this problem. You can use either equations alone and/or a graphical version of the solution.

2.12 *Fall Mechanics.* Various spring–dashpot models can be used to simulate the contact of the body or foot with a rigid or elastic-viscous surface. Figure P 2.12 shows a number of these models, together with the corresponding ground reaction force vs. time predictions. For example, the mass m_1 may represent the body, k_1 its stiffness; m_2 the foot, k_2 its stiffness and/or the ground stiffness; and c the damping of the foot and/or ground. Write out the equations of motion for each of these four systems.

2.13 If a lateral-to-medial load is applied to the foot, a counteracting moment is produced at the knee joint in a lateral–medial plane, which stretches the lateral collateral ligament and the cruciate ligaments. Estimate the moment produced by cruciate ligaments to that produced by the lateral collateral ligament. Use the force–deflection characteristics of the ligaments in your argument.

2.14 The stick figure shown here of the lower leg plus foot represents the right leg (from the knee down) of a person who is accelerating during single stance phase of normal gait. At the instant shown, the leg is vertical and the foot is flat. Quantify the error in the resultant moment and resultant force at the knee joint when quasi-static analysis is used instead of dynamic analysis.

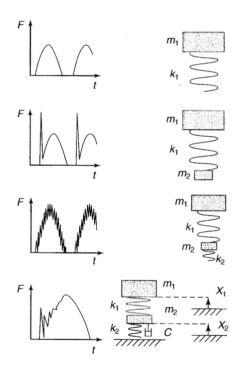

FIGURE P 2.12 Adapted from Alexander et al. (1986) *Journal of Zoology* 209: 405–419.

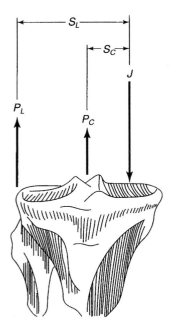

FIGURE P 2.13

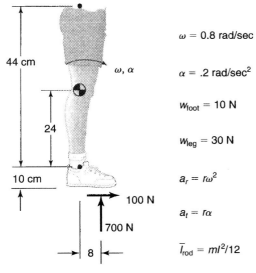

$\omega = 0.8$ rad/sec

$\alpha = .2$ rad/sec^2

$w_{foot} = 10$ N

$w_{leg} = 30$ N

$a_r = r\omega^2$

$a_t = r\alpha$

$\bar{I}_{rod} = ml^2/12$

FIGURE P 2.14

Tissue Mechanics I: Bone

3.1 | Introduction

The material properties of musculoskeletal tissues depend upon their underlying microstructures, which must be known to understand the anatomic site-, age-, and disease-related variations that occur in the tissue and organ level mechanical properties. It is important at the onset to distinguish between material and structural behavior, since terms such as "muscle," "bone," "cartilage," and "tendon" can be used to describe either tissues or organs. The femur, for example, is an organ composed of both cortical and trabecular bone tissues, as well as marrow, blood vessels, periosteum, and nerves, all of which contain a variety of cells. Biomechanically, the organ behaves as a structure, whereas the tissue behaves as a material. Due to the hierarchical composite nature of all biological tissues, at smaller scales the tissue itself can be viewed as a structure. Thus, the real distinction between structures and materials depends upon the geometric scale at which the microstructure becomes blurred and can be considered to be a continuum. When we say "material" behavior, we mean that the tissue can be considered to be a continuum for a particular analysis, but the distinction between material and microstructural behavior is problem specific. For example, in some analyses, trabecular bone can be treated as a continuum; for others, its heterogeneous microstructure must be modeled explicitly.

Material behavior, by definition, is independent of the geometry of the test specimen from which the properties were measured. Material properties are determined from experiments, such as the uniaxial tension test, which are performed on standardized specimens under controlled mechanical and environmental conditions. These tests are designed to eliminate any behavior associated with specimen geometry and to produce uniform states of stress and strain from which the material properties can easily be calculated. One challenge in testing musculoskeletal tissues is measuring deformations, particularly for soft and porous tissues such as tendon and trabecular bone. This, along with inter- and intra-individual heterogeneity, results in considerable variation in the reported material properties for most tissues. These uncertainties must be considered in the development of an appropriate model for the particular analysis at hand.

Since material properties measured from a particular set of mechanical tests are independent of geometry, in principle they can be used to describe the behavior of a small unit of the equivalent tissue anywhere in the skeleton. Thus, we can talk about the material properties of cortical bone tissue, which can be applied to cortical bone in different bones such as the femur, tibia, fibula, humerus, ulna, or radius. Strictly speaking, however, the data are valid only for tissue with the same microstructure and in the same environment as the test specimens.

Because biological tissues are heterogeneous, we usually attempt to relate the measured variations in material properties with corresponding measures of the tissue microstructure and other parameters such as apparent density, mineralization, or organic composition. Whether reported material properties for one anatomic site or individual of a particular age can be extrapolated to other sites or ages depends upon the nature of the analysis objectives and the precision and accuracy required for the material property data in the model.

In contrast to material properties, structural properties describe the overall behavior of the entire (or partial) organ. This behavior includes the combined effects of material and geometric properties:

$$\text{STRUCTURE (ORGAN)} = \text{MATERIAL (TISSUE)} \times \text{GEOMETRY}$$

Further, because of biological heterogeneity, the material properties are generally not uniform throughout the organ, and spatial distribution within the organ is often important. This can complicate determination of the structural properties. For example, the maximum force-carrying capacity of the proximal femur is a structural property that depends upon the material properties of both the cortical bone and the highly heterogeneous trabecular bone within the proximal femur, as well as the relevant geometric properties of the bone, such as its length, cross-sectional area, and area moment of inertia. Thus, structural properties are highly specific to the organ under analysis and rarely can be extrapolated to other anatomic sites, whereas material properties are more generic.

The inter- and intra-individual heterogeneity of various tissues and organs is a fundamental characteristic of biological tissues. Consequently, structural analyses of biological systems differ from many engineered systems for which material properties are often uniform and homogeneous. As a result, stress analysis of the musculoskeletal system is challenging because one has to first determine the appropriate material model to use by answering important questions. Is it necessary to account for heterogeneity, or is it acceptable to assume the simpler case of homogeneous properties? Is linear modeling adequate, or is it necessary to account for complex nonlinear or time-dependent behaviors? To address these issues, we will describe the microstructure of musculoskeletal tissues, describe their material properties, and discuss how these properties are used in different types of biomechanical analyses. We will also address structural analysis of some selected organs as an example of general approaches that can be taken to perform stress analyses of any musculoskeletal structure.

We will also consider briefly in this chapter one characteristic that makes musculoskeletal materials truly unique, which is their ability to adapt to both their biological and mechanical environments. This has been known in general for a long time, but only in recent years have we begun to understand the details of the processes that occur at the cellular and molecular levels. This emerging field of study has come to be known as mechanobiology. It embodies the extremely important concept that, at the cellular and molecular levels, we cannot understand the mechanics without understanding the biology, and we cannot understand the biology without understanding the mechanics.

Although we can learn much about the fundamental mechanics of a bone-implant system at a particular time by using the basic concepts of structural mechanics alone, the mechanobiology of these systems must be included if we are to understand how bone-implant structures change over time in response to altered mechanical and biological environments. Such an approach is the basis of what some have termed "preclinical testing" of implants—the process by which candidate implant designs can be evaluated *in silico* (i.e., by means of computer models) for their long-term effects on bone morphology, long before ever inserting the implant into a patient.

Regarding the adaptive behavior of bone, in the current chapter we have limited ourselves to briefly discussing and illustrating the mechanics of bone adaptation in keeping with the scope and thrust of this book. The description does demonstrate the general concept and illustrates the process by which one can "engineer" adaptive responses to stress into biomechanical analysis and design.

With this background, we can now turn our attention to a description of the major musculoskeletal tissues. In this chapter we focus on bone; in Chapter 4 we consider soft tissues—articular cartilage, meniscus, tendon, ligament, the intervertebral disc, and muscle. The composition and basic structural characteristics of bone tissue will be described first. Then the material properties of cortical and cancellous bone will be presented. Finally, we will address the structural consequences of heterogeneity on tissue behavior.

3.2 | Composition of Bone

From an engineering perspective, bone is a remarkable material having unique material properties and has, like almost all biological tissues, the ability to repair itself and adapt to its mechanical environment by biological remodeling and turnover. As a tissue, it exhibits wide variations in morphology, ranging from the delicate, open-celled architecture of the trabecular physes, to the dense, fiber-reinforced arrangement of the diaphyseal cortex. Bone adjusts to changing environmental conditions by highly organized structural adaptations. For instance, with heavy exercise, whole bones can change both material and geometric properties to provide structures of increased load-bearing capacity. With aging and disuse, bone tissue is resorbed, resulting in substantial losses of tissue stiffness and strength. To compensate, both the periosteal and endosteal diameters of the cortices can expand, thereby maintaining a structure of approximately constant stiffness and strength.

Bone is composed of inorganic and organic phases and, like all biological materials, water. On a weight basis, bone is approximately 60 percent inorganic, 30 percent organic, and 10 percent water. On a volume basis, these proportions are about 40 percent, 35 percent, and 25 percent, respectively. The inorganic phase of bone is a ceramic crystalline type mineral, which is an impure form of naturally occurring calcium phosphate, most often referred to as hydroxyapatite: $Ca_{10}(PO_4)_6(OH)_2$. The apatite crystals are tiny (2–5 nm thick $\times$ 15 nm wide $\times$ 20–50 nm long plates) and contain impurities such as potassium, magnesium, strontium, and sodium (in place of the calcium ions); carbonate (in place of the phosphate ions); and chloride or fluoride (in place of the hydroxyl ions). Thus, bone mineral is best considered as an impure form of hydroxyapatite.

The organic phase of bone consists primarily of type I collagen (90 percent by weight), some other minor collagen types (III and VI), and a variety of noncollagenous proteins (mostly osteocalcin, osteonectin, osteopontin, and bone sialoprotein). The molecular structure of collagen (Figure 3.1), the strongest and most abundant protein in the body, starts with a right-handed triple helix of three left-hand helical polypeptide "alpha" chains. The resulting "tropocollagen" molecule is rod shaped, with a length of about 300 nm and diameter of 1.5 nm. These collagen molecules are then arranged in parallel with each other head to tail, but with a gap or "hole zone" of about 35 nm between each molecule. They are arranged with surrounding collagen molecules in a quarter-staggered fashion. Additional pores exist along the sides of the collagen molecules between neighbors. Mineralization is thought to start within the hole zones and then progress to the pores; the noncollagenous proteins are also found within these spaces. The result of this is the mineralized fibril, which, as we will see next, is arranged in a number of ways to produce the overall composite. Collagen fibrils in bone range from 20–40 nm in diameter, suggesting there are 200–800 collagen molecules in the cross section of a fibril.

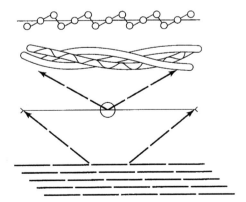

FIGURE 3.1 Diagrammatic representation of the hierarchical molecular structure of collagen. Starting with a single helical protein chain consisting of a variety of amino acids connected by peptide bonds (top), three of these polypeptide chains are combined to form the triple helix tropocollagen molecule (second down), referred to most often as simply the collagen molecule. The different types of collagen have different types of polypeptide chains. The collagen molecules are arranged in parallel in a regular quarter-stagger arrangement to comprise the collagen fibril (bottom).

3.3 | Bone as a Hierarchical Composite Material

Hierarchical Levels

Bone tissue is a hierarchical composite at many levels (Figure 3.2). At the lowest level (≈ 0.1 micron scale), it is a composite of mineralized collagen fibrils. At the next level (≈ 10 micron scale), these fibrils are arranged in two forms, either as stacked thin sheets called lamellae (about 7 microns thick) that contain unidirectional fibrils in alternate angles between layers or as a block of randomly oriented "woven" fibrils. Lamellar bone is most common, although woven bone is found in situations of rapid growth in children and large animals and also during the initial stages of bone fracture healing. Laminar or "plexiform" bone consists of smaller sandwich-type constructions of layered lamellae, arranged around openings for blood vessels. This type of bone is often interspersed with woven bone and is common in large animals, such as cows, that grow rapidly.

Lamellar bone can take various forms at the next hierarchical level (0.5–1.0 mm scale). Primary lamellar bone is new bone that consists of the large concentric rings of lamellae that circle the outer 2–3 mm of the diaphysis, similar to growth rings on a tree. The most common type of cortical bone in adult humans is called osteonal or Haversian bone, where about 10–15 lamellae are arranged in concentric cylinders about a central Haversian canal (a canal about 50 microns in diameter), which contains blood vessel capillaries, nerves, and a variety of bone cells (Figure 3.3). The substructure of concentric lamellae, including the Haversian canal, is termed an osteon, which has a diameter of about 200 microns and lengths of 1–3 mm. Other channels, called Volkmann's canals, about the same diameter as Haversian canals, run perpendicular to the Haversian canals, providing radial paths for blood vessels.

Osteons represent the primary discrete unit of human adult cortical bone, and are continually being torn down and replaced by the various types of bone cells in a biological process called bone remodeling. Over time, the osteon can be completely

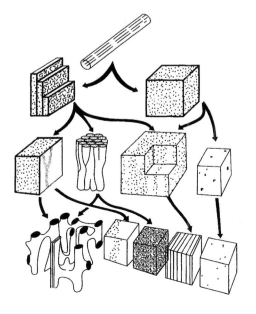

1. Mineralized
   Collagen Fibril
   [0.1 micron]

2. Lamellar
   Woven
   [10 micron]

3. Primary Lamellar
   Haversian
   Laminar
   Woven
   [500 microns]

4. Trabecular
   Cortical
   [>1000 microns]

FIGURE 3.2 The four levels of bone microstructure, from the level of mineralized collagen fibrils to cortical and trabecular bone. It is generally assumed that, at the former level, all bone is equal, although there can be subtle differences in the nature of the lamellar architecture and degree of mineralization between cortical and trabecular bone. (Adapted from Wainwright et al., *Mechanical Design in Organisms*. Halsted Press, New York, 1976.)

FIGURE 3.3 Diagram of a sector of the shaft of a long bone, showing the different types of cortical bone, trabecular bone, and the various channels. The osteons are located between the outer and inner circumferential lamellae. (Tortora, G. J. *Principles of Human Anatomy*. Harper and Ron, New York, 1983.)

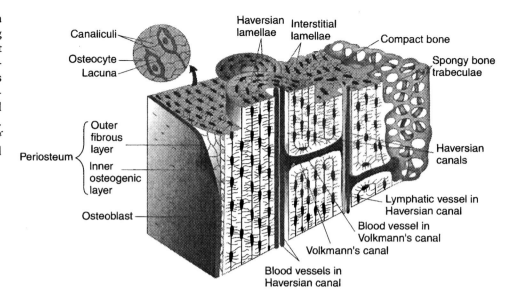

removed, leaving behind a hole (resorption cavity, about 200 microns in diameter), which is then filled in by a new osteon. Typically, there are about 10–15 Haversian canals per mm² cross section of adult human cortical bone. A cement line, which is a thin, low-mineral-content layer of calcified mucopolysaccharides with very little collagen, surrounds each newly formed osteon. The cement line is a weak interface between the osteon and the surrounding interstitial bone. This may actually improve the fatigue properties of cortical bone by providing avenues for dissipating energy during crack propagation.

Since mineralization of a new osteon is a slow process that can take months, the distribution of the degree of mineralization can be large at any time in a particular whole bone cross section. The remodeling process occurs in part to repair the fatigue damage that can occur in bone during strenuous repetitive activities.

Within this structure, there is an underlying level of porosity at the scale of 5–10 microns or less that is associated with the bone cells. Osteocytes, the most common type of bone cell, reside alone, surrounded by a thin layer of extra cellular fluid, in small ellipsoidal holes (about 5 microns minor diameter; 7–8 microns major diameter) called lacunae, of which there are about 25,000 per mm³ in bone tissue (Figures 3.3 and 3.4). The lacunae are generally arranged along the interfaces between lamellae. Each osteocyte has arms or processes that extend from the cell through tiny (≈0.5 micron diameter, 3–7 microns long) channels called canaliculi and meet with the processes of surrounding cells at cellular gap junctions. Gap junctions are arrays of small pores in the cell membrane that make connections between the interiors of neighboring cells, allowing direct passage of small molecules such as ions from one cell to another. There are about 50–100 canaliculi per single lacuna (Figure 3.4) and about one million per mm³ of bone. The resulting intercommunication between osteocytes provides an important mechanism by which bone cells are thought to sense mechanical loading or deformation and transmit signals elsewhere to the osteoclast bone cells that remove bone tissue. In this way, the remodeling

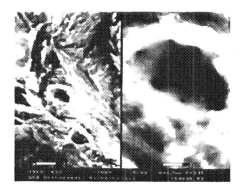

FIGURE 3.4 Environmental scanning electron microscope picture of a fracture surface of a piece of cortical bone, showing a fractured lacuna at low (left) and high (right) magnifications. Note the elliptical shape of the lacuna and the multiple smaller pores. These are the canaliculi, which have a diameter of about 0.5 micron.

sequence is thought to be be initiated when loading becomes too different from some physiological set point or if the bone becomes damaged.

At the highest hierarchical level (1–2 mm), there are two types of bone: (1) cortical bone, which comes as tightly packed lamellar, Haversian, laminar, or woven bone; and (2) trabecular bone, which is a highly porous cellular solid. In the latter, the lamellae are arranged in less well-organized "packets" to form a series of rods and plates, about 200–300 microns thick, interspersed with large marrow spaces (Figure 3.5). Sometimes, when the rods and plates in trabecular bone are very thick, osteons can be found, but this is rare in human bone.

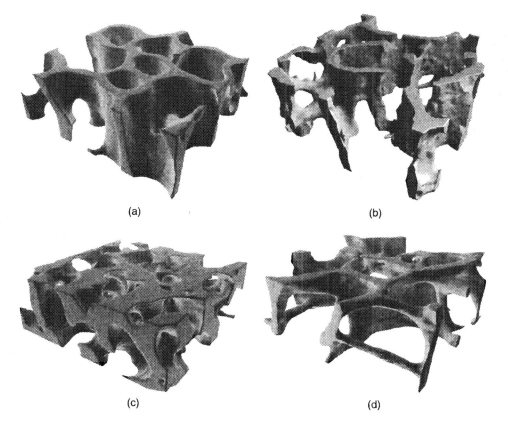

(a) (b)

(c) (d)

FIGURE 3.5 Various architectures of trabecular bone, as demonstrated by small samples $(3 \times 3 \times 1 \text{ mm}^3)$ of trabecular bone from (a) bovine proximal tibia; (b) human proximal tibia; (c) human femoral head; and (d) human vertebral body. In each case, the main trabecular orientation is in the vertical direction. (Keavery et. al., *Annu Rev. Biomed*, Eng. 2001 3:307–333.)

Cortical and Trabecular Bone

The main difference, therefore, between cortical and trabecular bone is the open cellular structure of the latter. The actual bone tissue at the underlying hierarchical level is very similar, being made of lamellar bone arranged as previously described for cortical bone or in the more irregularly shaped packets for trabecular bone. However, one difference does exist. There is more bone remodeling on the free surfaces of the rods and plates within trabecular bone than on the internal surfaces of Haversian canals within the cortical bone, and newly formed bone is less mineralized than older bone. Therefore, trabecular bone tends to be less mineralized than cortical bone, although the difference is subtle. This difference in mineralization and the different arrangements of the lamellar bone are thought to produce slightly lower material properties of the tissue that makes up the struts of trabecular bone—trabecular tissue—compared with the tissue that makes up cortical bone. It is difficult to measure these properties directly due to the small size and irregular shapes of individual trabeculae. The resulting uncertainties in the trabecular tissue-level properties complicate micromechanical analysis of trabecular bone.

Both cortical and trabecular tissues are porous. Cortical bone has a porosity P less than about 30 percent, or equivalently, a volume fraction V_f greater than about 0.70 ($V_f = 1 - P/100$). Volume fraction is the ratio of the volume of actual bone tissue to the bulk volume of the specimen, which includes the volume associated with the vascular pore spaces, but ignores the presence of lacunae and canaliculi. Trabecular bone has a volume fraction rarely greater than about 0.60, so the difference between cortical and trabecular bone is fairly distinct. Porosity of adult human femoral cortical bone, for example, can vary from as low as 5 percent at age 20 up to almost 30 percent at age 80. Porosity of trabecular bone varies from about 50 percent in the young adult femoral head up to about 95 percent in the elderly vertebra.

Volume Fraction and Density

Material properties of bone, particularly stiffness and strength, are strongly dependent on the volume fraction and density. A variety of measures are used to describe bone density, some of which describe the volume fraction, and others of which do not. The terminology can be confusing. The most common measures of bone density are tissue density and apparent density, which can be obtained for hydrated, dehydrated, or deorganified bone. Tissue density, ρ_{tiss}, is defined as the ratio of mass to volume of the actual bone tissue, not including any vascular porosity. It is similar for hydrated cortical and trabecular bone, varies little, and is about 2.0 g/cm^3. The density measures for dehydrated bone, bone that is heated for 1–2 days at 60–70 °C to remove all water, are termed "dry" densities.

Apparent density, ρ_{app}, is defined as the ratio of the mass of bone tissue to the bulk volume of the specimen, including the volume associated with the vascular pore spaces. It is easier to measure than volume fraction, since it does not require use of thin sections or Archimedes' principle; for this reason it is a commonly used indicator of bone porosity. Volume fraction, tissue density, and apparent densities are related as follows:

$$\rho_{app} = \rho_{tiss}V_f$$

The apparent density of hydrated human cortical bone is about 1.85 g/cm^3 and varies little from site to site. In contrast, the average apparent density of trabecular bone depends greatly on anatomic site. It is as low as 0.10 g/cm^3 for the elderly spine, about 0.30 g/cm^3 for the human tibia, and up to about 0.50 g/cm^3 for the load-bearing portions of the proximal femur. After skeletal maturity (around age 25), trabecular bone apparent density decreases with aging at a rate of about 2 percent per decade.

Mineral content (or mineral/organic content ratio) also substantially affects mechanical properties of bone. Ash densities (tissue and apparent) can be obtained when the bone is deorganified by heating it in a furnace for 24 hours at 700 °C, thereby removing all water and organic material. The ratio of ash weight to dry weight is often used to describe the percentage mineralization, or ash content, of bone tissue, regardless of whether it is cortical or trabecular bone. The percent mineralization increases with age during skeletal growth (through age 20–25), but does not appear to change with aging for adults.

The wider variation in density for trabecular than cortical bone results in a much greater heterogeneity in its material properties compared with cortical bone. Given this heterogeneity, it is rarely adequate to discuss the biomechanical properties of trabecular bone without reference to its apparent density (or volume fraction).

Another differentiator between cortical and trabecular bone is the scale of the dominant porosity. Cortical bone is a solid-like structure that contains a series of voids having dimensions about 200 microns or less (Haversian canals, Volkmann's canals, resorption cavities, lacunae, and canaliculi). Trabecular bone is a network of small, interconnected rods and plates, called trabeculae, with relatively large spaces between them. Individual trabeculae contain few of the voids (lacunae and canaliculi—only sometimes do they contain Haversian canals) that are contained in cortical bone. However, typical thicknesses of individual trabeculae are in the range of 100–300 microns, and typical intertrabecular spacing is on the order of 500–1500 microns. Both of these parameters depend heavily upon age and anatomic site (Figure 3.5). Therefore, the porosity of trabecular bone (typically 50 to 95 percent) is dominated by the spaces between individual trabeculae, not the voids within the trabeculae. As the volume fraction increases, the architecture tends to be more plate-like; it is more rod-like at lower volume fractions. The space between trabeculae is filled with marrow *in vivo*, which has a negligible mechanical role, except perhaps in high energy loading.

3.4 | Elastic Anisotropy

There is a preferred orientation in the microstructure of bone. In cortical bone, the preferred orientation is determined by the generally parallel assembly of the osteons, whereas in trabecular bone it is determined by a predominant alignment of the plates and rods. As result of this orientation, bone is an anisotropic material. Like most biological materials—for example, wood—the preferred orientation is called the grain. Anisotropic material properties depend on the direction of loading with respect to the material or grain axes. Common engineered materials such as metals and plastics can often be considered isotropic (their mechanical properties are independent of direction), but even for these materials anisotropy arises in some circumstances. For example, rolled metals have different properties in different directions, and composites are often designed to take advantage of directionality. For musculoskeletal tissues, anisotropy cannot be avoided. Unfortunately, description of the properties for anisotropic materials is much more complex than it is for isotropic materials, since the mathematical description of the anisotropic properties are specific to the coordinate system. We will discuss some overall aspects of anisotropy before we present the general theory in Section 3.7.

Principal Material Coordinate System

The first step in understanding anisotropic material behavior is to describe the degree of anisotropy. Many biological materials are orthotropic, for which the material behavior can be described with reference to three mutually perpendicular material axes (principal material axes) at each point (Figure 3.6). We will restrict our attention to this degree of anisotropy or less.

The description of the principal material coordinate system typically varies from point to point within a structure (Figure 3.7). In many cases, it is convenient to describe such spatial variations by using a curvilinear coordinate system. The latter can be considered as a local coordinate system that accounts for the unique spatial variation in microstructure orientation. If there is symmetry about any one of the principal material coordinate axes, then the other two axes can be interchanged, and isotropy exists in the corresponding plane of these axes. This is called transverse isotropy, since the "transverse" plane is isotropic (Figure 3.8). For isotropic materials, all three axes can be interchanged; there is no preferred orientation.

One important issue in biomechanical analysis of tissues is to decide on the degree of anisotropy. This decision should be made in the context of the analysis objectives and the required accuracy of the solution. Oftentimes, it is necessary to perform a complete orthotropic analysis (see Section 3.8) in order to quantify the error associated with making simplifying assumptions of isotropy. If the error is within the precision of the overall analysis or is otherwise considered to be sufficiently small, then it may be reasonable to ignore the anisotropy in subsequent analyses. The advantage, of course, of assuming isotropy is that analysis is much simpler mathematically, and results are easier to interpret. One example of this is the

FIGURE 3.6 Principal material coordinate system for an orthotropic material. This coordinate system (right) is aligned with the mutually orthogonal "grain" axes of the material's microstructure (left). As a class of anisotropic materials, orthotropic materials have their grain along three mutually perpendicular axes.

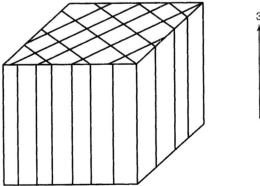
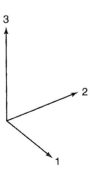

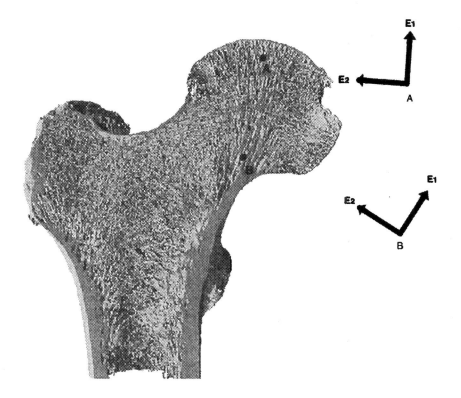

FIGURE 3.7 Spatial variations in the orientation of the principal material coordinate system can occur. In many cases, a local coordinate system in cylindrical coordinates can be used to describe such spatial variations.

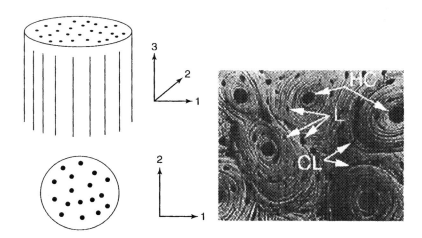

FIGURE 3.8 Transverse isotropy. The 1 and 2 axes in the "transverse" plane can be interchanged. The 3 axis is the stiffest direction and is referred to as the "longitudinal" direction. Adult human cortical bone (bottom right), for example, is often considered to be transversely isotropic, due to the longitudinal orientation of the osteons (surrounded by cement lines, CL) and/or Haversian canals (HC). The lacunae (L) do not have a longitudinal orientation.

trabecular orientation in the proximal femur, which is highly complex, and spatial variations exist in the orientation of the principal material coordinate system (Figure 3.7). The assumption of isotropy may be reasonable for preliminary analyses, but in some cases the elastic and failure behaviors of the structure may depend critically on anisotropic characteristics.

3.5 | Material Properties of Cortical Bone

As a consequence of its composite, osteonal microstructure, the material properties of cortical bone are anisotropic and inhomogeneous (vary with spatial location). These properties depend on loading rate, and when loaded past the yield point, cortical bone shows behavior characteristic of plasticity, damage accumulation, creep, and fatigue. Thus, under typical loading, its behavior is viscoelastic or viscoplastic and can be further modified if damage occurs. For many practical stress analysis applications, however, cortical bone can be regarded as an elastic material over some range of loading.

Anisotropy

Human cortical bone is generally assumed to be transversely isotropic, meaning that it has one primary material axis (the longitudinal direction) and is isotropic in the plane perpendicular to this axis (the transverse plane, Figure 3.8). The longitudinal axis is generally aligned with the diaphyseal axis of long bones. Cortical bone is both stronger and stiffer when loaded in the longitudinal direction, compared with the radial or circumferential directions. This structure efficiently resists the largely uniaxial stresses that develop along the diaphyseal axis during habitual activities such as walking and running.

As shown in Table 3.1, a total of five independent material constants are required to describe the transversely isotropic elastic properties of cortical bone (for example, two Young's modulus values, one shear modulus, and two Poisson's ratios), whereas only two independent material constants are required for isotropic behavior. The longitudinal Young's modulus of human cortical bone is in the range of about 10–22 GPa and is about one-fourth that of aluminum. Its strength properties are also anisotropic (Table 3.2).

In addition to having anisotropic elastic and strength properties, cortical bone also has asymmetric strengths; it is stronger in compression than tension for each principal material direction (Table 3.2). The longitudinal compressive strength of 170–210 MPa far exceeds that of engineering construction materials such as concrete. The strength to modulus ratio for cortical bone is about 1.12 percent and 0.78 percent for longitudinal compression and tension, respectively. Compared with high-performance engineering metal alloys such as Aluminum 6061-T6 and Titanium 6Al-4V, with corresponding ratios of about 0.45 percent and 0.73 percent, respectively, it

TABLE 3.1

Average Anisotropic Elastic Properties of Human Femoral Cortical Bone[1]	
Longitudinal modulus (MPa)	17,000
Transverse modulus (MPa)	11,500
Shear modulus (MPa)	3,300
Longitudinal Poisson's ratio	0.46
Transverse Poisson's ratio	0.58

[1]Note that these properties are referred to the principal material coordinate system.
Source: Reilly and Burstein (1975) *J Biomechanics* 8:393–405.

TABLE 3.2

Average Anisotropic and Asymmetric Ultimate Stress Properties of Human Femoral Cortical Bone[1]		
Longitudinal (MPa)	*Tension*	133
	Compression	193
Transverse (MPa)	*Tension*	51
	Compression	133
Shear (MPa)		68

[1]Note that these properties are referred to the principal material coordinate system.
Source: Reilly and Burstein (1975) *J Biomechanics* 8:393–405.

is seen that cortical bone has a relatively large strength to modulus ratio. In that sense, it is a high-performance material, particularly in compression.

When loaded to failure in a monotonic test, human cortical bone exhibits an initial linear elastic behavior, a marked yield point, and failure at a relatively low strain level (Figure 3.9). Unlike the ultimate stresses, which are higher in compression, ultimate strains are higher in tension for longitudinal loading. These strains can be up to 5 percent in young adults and fall to less than 1 percent in the very elderly; cortical bone becomes more brittle with aging. In contrast to its longitudinal tensile behavior, cortical bone is relatively brittle in tension for transverse loading and brittle in compression for all loading directions. Cortical bone is weakest when loaded transversely in tension and is also weak in shear.

The asymmetry and anisotropy of strength have practical clinical relevance. For example, transverse tension can be generated when large intramedullary implants such as tapered uncemented hip stems are driven too far during surgery into the femoral diaphysis and produce circumferential or hoop stresses. If these stresses become too great, then the bone cracks longitudinally. When this occurs, it is treated by supporting the bone externally with circumferential tensioned wires, and weight bearing is limited until the crack is healed. Development of large transverse tensile stress rarely, if ever, occurs during normal physiological behavior.

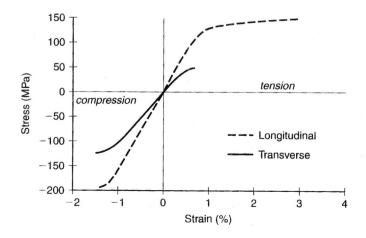

FIGURE 3.9 Typical stress–strain behavior for human cortical bone. The bone is stiffer in the longitudinal direction, indicative of its elastic anisotropy. It is also stronger in compression than tension, indicative of its strength asymmetry (modulus is the same in tension and compression). Cortical bone is relatively ductile for longitudinal tension, but is brittle in all other loading modes.

Because of the complex microstructure of cortical bone, it is clear that simple isotropic and symmetric criteria such as the von Mises criterion cannot describe the anisotropic and asymmetric strength properties of this tissue. The Tsai–Wu criterion, commonly used for fiber-reinforced composite materials, works quite well for cortical bone, although it requires 7–12 constants, depending on the degree of anisotropy assumed (transversely isotropic vs. orthotropic). This criterion takes into account the difference in tensile and compressive strengths, as well as the low shear strength with respect to the tensile strength, and the anisotropy. It is the most suitable criterion available for cortical bone.

For an orthotropic material loaded in its principal material coordinate system, the three-dimensional quadratic Tsai–Wu multiaxial failure criterion can be expressed as

$$F_i \sigma_i + F_{ij} \sigma_i \sigma_j = 1, \, i = 1, 6; \, j = 1, 6 \, (\text{``contracted'' tensor notation})$$

where σ_i are the stress components and F_i and F_{ij} are the experimentally derived Tsai–Wu coefficients. For the principal material coordinate system, the σ_i indices $i = 1$–3 correspond to normal stresses: $\sigma_{11}, \sigma_{22}, \sigma_{33}$, respectively; $i = 4$–6 correspond to shear stresses: $\sigma_{12}, \sigma_{23}, \sigma_{13}$. When the coefficients of odd-power terms in shear are set to zero to ensure sign-independent solutions for shear failure—and realizing the symmetry of the F_{ij} coefficients—this expression is expanded as follows:

$$
\begin{aligned}
&F_1 \sigma_1 + F_2 \sigma_2 + F_3 \sigma_3 \\
&+ F_{11} \sigma_1^2 + F_{22} \sigma_2^2 + F_{33} \sigma_3^2 \\
&+ 2F_{12} \sigma_1 \sigma_2 + 2F_{13} \sigma_1 \sigma_3 + 2F_{23} \sigma_2 \sigma_3 \\
&+ F_{44} \sigma_4^2 + F_{55} \sigma_5^2 + F_{66} \sigma_6^2 = 1
\end{aligned}
$$

Mathematically, this is a quadratic equation, ellipsoidal to be specific. The nine coefficients are found from uniaxial tests (tension, compression, and torsion performed on longitudinally and transversely oriented specimens); and the remaining three "strength interaction" coefficients (F_{12}, F_{13}, and F_{23}) are found from biaxial, triaxial, or off-axis uniaxial tests. Let's derive an expression for the F_1 and F_{11} coefficients.

EXAMPLE 3.1 Tsai–Wu Failure Criterion

Question The coefficients in the Tsai–Wu criterion can be obtained from uniaxial tension and compression tests. What are the expressions for F_1 and F_{11} in terms of the tensile strength σ_1^{TY} and the compressive strength σ_1^{CY}?

Solution In a uniaxial tension test in the 1 direction, failure occurs when the applied stress σ_1 equals the tensile yield strength σ_1^{TY}. Since this is a uniaxial tension test, all other stress components are zero, and the Tsai–Wu equation reduces to

$$F_1 \sigma_1^{TY} + F_{11} (\sigma_1^{TY})^2 = 1$$

Similarly, for a uniaxial compression test to failure along the 1 direction, with a compressive yield strength of σ_1^{CY}, we get

$$F_1\sigma_1^{CY} + F_{11}(\sigma_1^{CY})^2 = 1$$

Solving these two simultaneous equations reveals that

$$F_1 = 1/\sigma_1^{TY} + 1/\sigma_1^{CY} \qquad \text{and} \qquad F_{11} = -1/(\sigma_1^{TY}\sigma_1^{CY})$$

in which compressive strengths should be given negative signs ($F_1 = 0$ if the tensile and compressive strengths are equal, for example). From this, we see that the F_1 term describes the strength asymmetry in the 1 direction. The process can be repeated for the other two directions and applied to pure shear tests also. The strength interaction terms are then found by applying the equation to more complex tests in which controlled multiaxial failure is achieved.

Heterogeneity

While it is often appropriate to assume average properties for cortical bone, as shown in Table 3.1 and Table 3.2, it may be necessary in some cases to account for the heterogeneity that can arise from variations in microstructural parameters such as porosity. For example, for stem stress analysis in bone-implant systems using composite beam theory, since the modulus of the metal is much greater than that of the cortical bone, ±20 percent variations in the modulus of the cortical bone will not affect substantially the calculated stem stresses. However, if there is no implant and the focus is on bone stress—for example, in a study of bone fracture mechanics— errors in the assumed material properties of the bone become more important.

As described earlier, cortical porosity, which is due primarily to the variations in the number, length, and diameter of Haversian and Volkmann's canals, can vary from less than 5 percent to almost 30 percent and is positively correlated with age because the bone becomes more porous with aging. Both modulus and ultimate stress can be reduced by 50 percent when porosity is increased from 5 percent to 30 percent (Figure 3.10). Thus, cortical bone properties for specific individuals depend

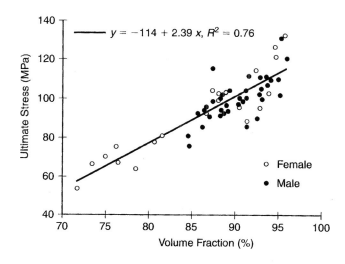

FIGURE 3.10 Dependence of the ultimate tensile stress of human cortical bone on volume fraction (expressed as a percentage). Ages of the specimens were in the range 20–100. Redrawn from McCalden et al. (1993) *J Bone Jt Surg* 75A:1193–1205.

FIGURE 3.11 Modulus vs. calcium content (in mg/g of dehydrated bone tissue) for cortical bone taken from 18 different species. Redrawn from Currey (1988) *J Biomech* 21:131–139.

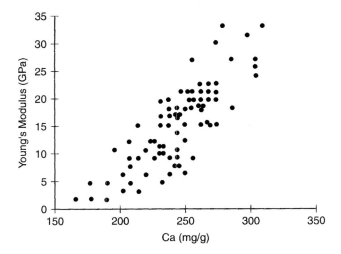

upon porosity. The average values shown in Table 3.1 and Table 3.2 provide reasonable properties for "typical" individuals.

It is well established that, over multiple species in which there is a large variation of mineralization, stiffness and strength increase with increasing mineralization (the ratio of ash to dry weights in Figure 3.11). However, mineralization does not vary much in adult humans, and therefore normal variations in mineralization do not appear to play an important role in modulus or strength of adult human cortical bone. This illustrates an important observation. Even though a tissue constituent can substantially affect material properties over a range of individuals, it may have little effect on the subpopulation of interest.

EXAMPLE 3.2 Effect of Cortical Heterogeneity in a Drug Study

Question   Because of biological heterogeneity, it is necessary to statistically design experiments on bone such that there are sufficient numbers of specimens in a sample to detect any anticipated treatment effects. Consider the following statistical analysis of results from a hypothetical drug study on the treatment of osteoporosis. The hypothesis to be tested is that a new drug will increase cortical bone tensile strength, compared with a placebo control. In the experiment, 30 female animals—rats, dogs, and sheep are common animal models in osteoporosis bone research—were randomly assigned to two groups ($n = 15$ each), one group given the placebo, the other the new drug. All animals were first subjected to an ovariectomy, to simulate the bone loss due to osteoporosis. Then the placebo and drug treatments were assigned. The animals were sacrificed after two years of treatment, and specimens of cortical bone were machined from the femurs and subjected to uniaxial tension testing. Two specimens were lost in each group due to early death of the animals, and an additional specimen was lost in the treated group due to a technical error during mechanical testing. The results for tensile strength were as follows (all expressed in MPa):

	Placebo	Treated
Mean	120	137
SD	23	27
n	13	12

Based on these data, the results suggest that the drug increased mean bone strength by 14 percent. Is this difference statistically significant ($p < 0.05$ level) or is it simply within the range of normal scatter?

Solution   To account for the biological heterogeneity, we need to perform a statistical analysis to determine if the drug is indeed effective. To analyze the data, we use the student's t-test for small ($N < 30$) sample sizes, which relates the t-statistic to the difference in means between the groups ($X_1 - X_2$), the measured standard deviations (s_1 and s_2), and the sample sizes (N_1 and N_2):

$$t = \frac{\overline{X}_1 - \overline{X}_2}{\sigma \sqrt{1/N_1 + 1/N_2}} \quad \text{where } \sigma = \sqrt{\frac{N_1 s_1^2 + N_2 s_2^2}{N_1 + N_2 - 2}}$$

The t-statistic is converted to a p-value with the aid of a standard t-statistic lookup table (found in any statistics book and embedded in all statistics computerized routines), and this mapping depends on the number of degrees of freedom $\nu (= N_1 + N_1 - 2$ for this problem). Inserting our data into this equation, we find that $t = 1.63$, and the corresponding p-value is just greater than 0.10. Since the p-value is greater than 0.05, we conclude that the observed 14 percent increase in strength is *not* statistically significant. The researchers at this junction could give up on the drug; or if they felt the drug was really effective, they could design a follow-up experiment to expand the sample size. A larger sample size would have greater statistical power and thus may be able to show that there is a real effect of the drug. A statistical power analysis can be used to calculate the required sample size to show a significant difference at the observed effect and indeed is a prerequisite to designing any experiments for hypothesis testing in tissue mechanics.

Fatigue, Creep, and Viscoelasticity

Cortical bone also exhibits fatigue (Figure 3.12a) and creep (Figure 3.12b) and has a greater resistance to failure in these modes in compression than tension. Fatigue properties are normally expressed on a traditional S–N curve (stress vs. number of cycles to failure), just as with metals, but stress is usually divided by Young's modulus to minimize interspecimen scatter of the data. Interestingly, for cortical bone, when the fatigue and creep behaviors are expressed as functions of stress/modulus vs. time-to-failure, experimental scatter is reduced, fatigue life is independent of frequency (0.2–2.0 Hz range), and substantial similarities appear between the fatigue and creep behaviors (Figure 3.13). This suggests that levels of strain (=stress/modulus) determine

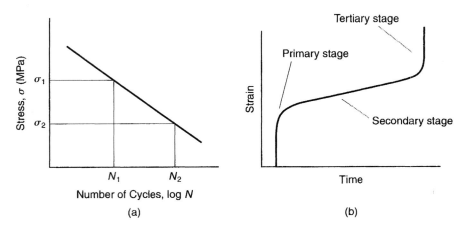

FIGURE 3.12 (a) Typical fatigue *S–N* curve. This is usually plotted with the ordinate on a log scale, where the relationship is linear, but which corresponds to the following type of nonlinear relationship between number of cycles to failure (N_f) and applied constant stress σ: $N_f = A\sigma^B$. According to this model of material behavior, the material will fail at N_i cycles of stress σ_i. (b) Typical creep response showing the three classical stages. First, there is a rapid increase in strain immediately after the constant stress is applied; second, there is a steady rate of increase of strain (an approximately constant "creep rate"); and third, there is a rapid increase in strain just before the specimen fractures.

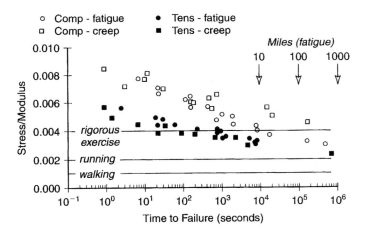

FIGURE 3.13 Fatigue and creep behaviors of human cortical bone vs. time to failure. For fatigue loading, the ordinate on this graph can be converted to number of cycles by multiplying the time to failure by the frequency, which is typically one cycle per second for normal walking. Note that both creep and fatigue resistances are lower in tension, consistent with monotonic behavior. Data from Carter et al. (1981) *Acta Orthop Scand* 52:481–490 and Caler and Carter (1989) *J Biomechanics* 22:625–635.

these failure properties and that the underlying fatigue and creep mechanisms are related.

The fatigue and creep properties shown in Figure 3.13 were obtained from devitalized bone specimens, in which, obviously, no biological healing could occur. Because bone cells repair fatigue damage *in vivo*, these fatigue life values are lower bounds on the *in vivo* fatigue life. Therefore, it is unlikely that high cycle (low stress) fatigue failure occurs *in vivo*, since the resulting fatigue damage would be healed biologically before large enough cracks could develop that would cause overt fracture of the bone. Low cycle fatigue (stress fractures), however, can occur when higher levels of repetitive stress are applied over shorter time intervals, such as in marching military recruits and marathon runners.

When cortical bone is loaded to its monotonic yield point, but not fractured, and is then unloaded, permanent residual strains develop (Figure 3.14) similar to ductile metal behavior. When cortical bone is loaded beyond its yield point, unloaded, and reloaded, its modulus is reduced (Figure 3.14a). This is evidence of damage, something that does not occur in metals where the modulus after plastic yielding is the same as the initial modulus. This complex viscoplastic, damaged material behavior is difficult to account for in stress analyses, but it probably has significant biological consequences. As the surrounding bone matrix permanently deforms and sustains damage, cells may be altered and a biological response may be induced, which prompts the bone cells to repair the damage done to the bone matrix.

Cortical bone is a viscoelastic material (Figure 3.15). Its modulus and strength increase as the rate of loading is increased. Over a six-order-of-magnitude increase in strain rate, modulus only changes by a factor of two, and strength by a factor of three. Thus, for the majority of physiological activities, which tend to occur in a relatively narrow range of strain rates (0.01–1.0 percent strain per second), cortical

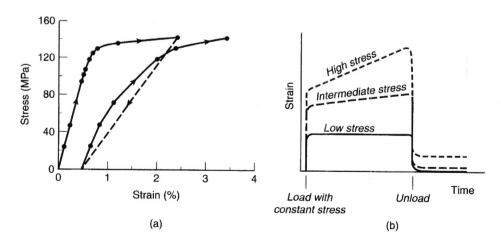

FIGURE 3.14   (a) Damage behavior of cortical bone. Evidence of microstructural damage is seen by the reduction in modulus that occurs when the specimen is reloaded after initial yielding. From MT Fondrk (1989), Ph.D. dissertation, Case Western Reserve University. (b) Viscoplastic behavior of cortical bone. When a low stress is applied to the bone, the strain remains constant over time, and there is no permanent deformation after unloading. As the magnitude of the stress is increased, the rate of creep increases, and a larger permanent deformation exists after unloading. From Fondrk et al. (1988) *J Biomechanics* 21:623–630.

FIGURE 3.15 Strain rate sensitivity of cortical bone for longitudinal tensile loading. This is evidence of viscoelastic behavior, although the effect is not substantial. Typically, modulus and strength increase only by factors two and three, respectively, as the loading rate is increased by six orders of magnitude. From McElhaney (1966) *J Appl Physiol* 21:1231–1236.

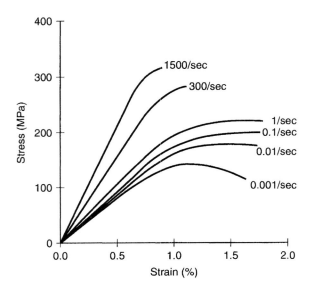

bone can reasonably be assumed to behave elastically. However, the increased stiffness and strength properties and the tendency toward more brittle behavior are important in high strain-rate situations such as high-speed trauma and perhaps during falls. Analysis methods for viscoelastic materials are discussed in Chapter 4.

Aging and Disease

Aging and disease also affect the mechanical properties of cortical bone. Modulus varies little, if at all, with age, but tensile ultimate stress decreases at a rate of approximately 2 percent per decade (Figure 3.16a). Perhaps most importantly, tensile ultimate strain decreases by about 10 percent per decade, from a high of almost 5 percent strain at age 20–30 years to a low of less than 1 percent strain beyond about 80 years (Figure 3.16b). Old bone is more brittle than young bone. Thus, the energy to fracture, given by the total area under the stress–strain curve before fracture, is much less for old bone than for younger bone. Fracture toughness also decreases with aging.

FIGURE 3.16 (a) Reductions of human cortical bone mechanical properties with age. Modulus is not reduced much, if at all, whereas strength is reduced more, at a rate of about 2 percent per decade. From Burstein et al. (1976) *J Bone Jt Surg* 58A: 82–86. (b) Ultimate strain decreases markedly with age, at a rate of about 10 percent of its young value per decade. From McCalden et al. (1993) *J Bone Jt Surg* 75A:1193–1205.

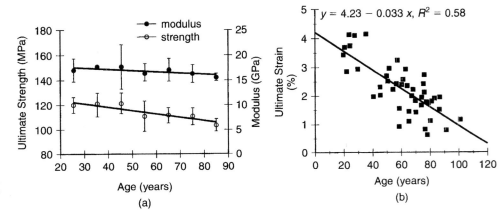

EXAMPLE 3.3 Strain Rate Versus Aging Effects on Bone Strength

Question   When performing any failure analysis of a bone structure, one must use the appropriate strength properties of the bone tissue. These tissue properties depend on both age and loading rate (as well as other factors), and it is important in any failure analysis to account for these factors, since unexpected interactions can sometimes occur. For example, one can compare the strength of cortical bone tissue loaded at a slow loading rate for a young person against that for an elderly person loaded at a high rate. The former might simulate the situation of an impact on the femur in which muscle activity or soft tissue energy absorption can effectively reduce the loading rate. The latter might represent a typical osteoporotic patient who falls unexpectedly without any protective maneuvers and thus loads the bone very rapidly. What are the combined effects of strain rate and age on bone strength of a 90-year-old subject compared with a 20-year-old?

Solution   Here, we combine the effects of aging and loading rate. Let's say the strength of the bone for a 20-year-old at a strain rate of 0.001/sec is S. According to the data shown in Figure 3.16a, by age 90 the strength, on average, will have reduced by about 20 percent to $0.8S$. However, the strain rate effect, going from a slow event at 0.001/sec to a much faster one at, say, 1.0/sec, will increase strength by about 60 percent. Thus, the overall change is $0.8 \times 1.6S = 1.28S$. According to this analysis, the cortical bone strength would be *greater* in the elderly individual by about 25–30 percent—somewhat counterintuitive. Clearly, the key factor in this analysis is the knowledge of the appropriate strain rate for the various injury mechanisms, which is difficult to determine and varies on a case-by-case basis.

3.6 | Material Properties of Trabecular Bone

As discussed earlier, trabecular bone is a highly heterogeneous material, and its material properties vary accordingly. From a biomechanical perspective, the most important microstructural parameter for trabecular bone is its apparent density, in contrast to the tissue density of the individual trabeculae. Similarly, we distinguish between apparent (continuum) and tissue properties of trabecular bone. The continuum properties of trabecular bone primarily depend upon the architecture and, to a lesser extent, on the tissue properties.

To treat trabecular bone as a continuum, its dimensions must be on the order of 5–10 mm or greater. Smaller specimens of trabecular bone may have to be treated as structures for which concepts of material properties such as Young's modulus do not apply, since they depend upon the size of the specimen. This concept of scale and continuum vs. microstructural behavior is critical when analyzing the mechanical behavior of trabecular bone and most other biological tissues. In the discussion that follows, the trabecular bone properties are continuum values, which have been determined with the use of appropriately sized test specimens.

Apparent Density

The compressive stress–strain behavior of trabecular bone (Figure 3.17) is typical of a class of porous materials called cellular solids (recall Figure 3.5). It displays

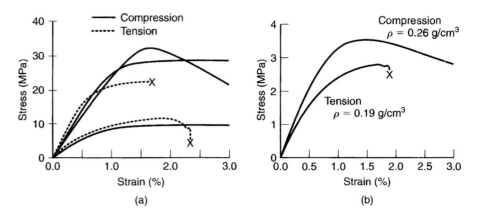

FIGURE 3.17 Stress–strain behavior for compressive and tensile loading of bovine (left) and human vertebral (right) trabecular bone, showing the wide range in strength that is typical for trabecular bone. The bovine bone here is 10 times stronger and stiffer than the human vertebral bone. X indicates tensile fracture. For compression, the curves have been truncated. Left: Keaveny et al. (1994) *J Biomechanics*, 27:1137–1146; and right: Kopperdahl and Keaveny (1998) *J Biomechanics*, 31:601–608.

an approximately linearly elastic region followed by a local peak, and then a strain-softening or plateau region of near constant stress with increasing strain. Tensile behavior is much more brittle, with fracture occurring at relatively low strains. Most importantly, for trabecular bone, the stiffness and strength depend on its apparent density and can vary by two orders of magnitude within the same metaphyseal region.

Because of the large variation in apparent density for trabecular bone, its mechanical properties cannot generally be described by average values. This makes analysis of structural problems with trabecular bone more difficult than those for cortical bone, since it is usually necessary to account for variations in apparent density within a region of trabecular bone. As usual, however, the required accuracy of the properties depends on the precision of the analysis at hand. A two-fold variation in trabecular modulus from 200 to 400 MPa may have little effect on calculated stem stresses in a bone-implant system, but would be crucial in an analysis of osteoporotic spine fracture for which the trabecular bone can be the primary load-bearing component. Regardless, it should be realized that there are substantial variations in the mechanical properties of trabecular bone across anatomic sites, and efforts should be made to use site-specific average values if available. Table 3.3 gives such properties for the tibia, femur, and vertebra.

Depending on the trabecular architecture (the general arrangement, shape, and dimensions of the individual trabeculae for a particular specimen), modulus or strength vary with apparent density by a linear relationship or a power law relationship with an exponent of 1–3. For example, linear relations between strength and volume fraction occur for different sites, the slope typically being lower for the lower density site (Figure 3.18). This is due to underlying differences in architectural structure: The plates for high-density bone are more efficient than the rods of lower density bone. But a squared power law fits the pooled data well (beware statistical artifacts!).

TABLE 3.3

Linear and Power-Law Regressions Between Ultimate Strength (σ in MPa) and Wet Apparent Density (ρ in g/cm^3) for Compressive Loading of Human Trabecular Bone Specimens Loaded at "Low" Strain Rates ($\leq$1.0/sec) and Taken from a Range of Anatomic Sites

Study	Cadavers		Specimens	$\sigma = a\rho + b$			$\sigma = a\rho^b$		
	Number	Age	Number	a	b	r^2	a	b	r^2
Proximal Tibia									
Hvid et al. (1989)*	10	60–83	94	19.2	−1.60	0.78	25.6	1.60	0.82
Linde et al. (1989)**	9	59–82	121	—	—	—	23.7	1.56	0.79
Proximal Femur									
Lotz et al. (1990)‡	4	25–82	49	—	—	—	25.0	1.80	0.93
Lumbar Spine									
Kopperdahl and Keaveny (1998)	11	32–65	22	21.9	−1.46	0.71	33.0	1.50	0.68

‡Proximal specimens only; oriented approximately along the femoral neck axis.
See Table 3.4 for additional legends.

FIGURE 3.18 Dependence of compressive on-axis strength on apparent density for trabecular bone for two different sites: bovine tibial (BPT) and human vertebral (HVB) trabecular bone. The difference in slopes in the linear relations for each site is due to the different architectures, being mainly plate-like in the bovine bone and rod-like in the human vertebral bone. When all the data are pooled, there is a strong squared power law relationship, with $r^2 = 0.94$. (Bone Mechanics Handbook, Editor SC Cowin, CRC Press Boca Raton, 2001.)

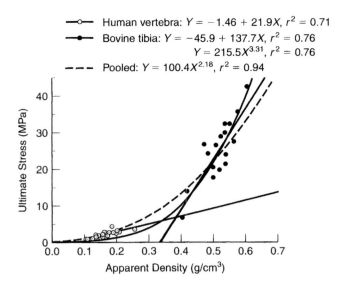

Human vertebra: $Y = -1.46 + 21.9X$, $r^2 = 0.71$
Bovine tibia: $Y = -45.9 + 137.7X$, $r^2 = 0.76$
$Y = 215.5X^{3.31}$, $r^2 = 0.76$
Pooled: $Y = 100.4X^{2.18}$, $r^2 = 0.94$

FIGURE 3.19 Age-related reductions in compressive strength of human femoral and vertebral trabecular bone. Note that for any given age, there remains much scatter in the data; that is, age is not a good determinant of behavior. Data from Mosekilde et al. (1987) *Bone* 8:79–85 and McCalden et al. (1997) *J Bone Jt Surg* 79A:421–427.

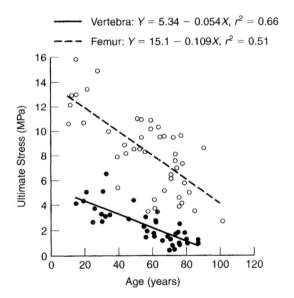

Vertebra: $Y = 5.34 - 0.054X$, $r^2 = 0.66$
Femur: $Y = 15.1 - 0.109X$, $r^2 = 0.51$

Both architecture and apparent density change with aging and disease, resulting in large age–related reductions in strength (Figure 3.19). Table 3.3 gives relationships between strength and density for the tibia, femur, and vertebra. The relationships are slightly different between sites because of the different microstructural architectures of each site, although reasonable performance can be obtained by using relationships for the pooled data.

In general, average modulus values per anatomic site for trabecular bone vary from as low as about 3000 MPa in the elderly spine to over 3000 MPa in the load-bearing portions of the femoral head. Ultimate strength values for individual specimens vary from 0.1–40 MPa, typically being a factor 100 less than modulus (Table 3.4). By contrast, the yield strains are relatively uniform. For higher density trabecular bone,

TABLE 3.4

Average Values of Typical Wet Apparent Densities, Moduli, and Compressive Strengths for Human Trabecular Bone Specimens Taken from a Range of Anatomic Sites[1]

Study	Cadavers		Specimens	Wet Apparent Density (g/cm³)		Modulus (MPa)		Ultimate Strength (MPa)	
	Number	Ages	Number	Mean (SD)	Range	Mean (SD)	Range	Mean (SD)	Range
Proximal Tibia									
Linde et al. (1989)**	9	59–82	121	0.29 (0.10)	0.09–0.66	445 (257)	61–1174	5.33 (2.93)	0.68–14.1
Ashman et al. (1989)†	3	52–67	75	0.26 (0.14)	0.13–0.75	1107 (634)	340–3350	—	—
Femur									
Rohlmann et al. (1980)††**	10	58–83	299‡	0.50 (0.16)	0.14–1.00	389 (270)	44–1531	7.36 (4.00)	0.56–22.9
Lumbar Spine									
Mosekilde et al. (1987)*	42	15–87	40	0.24 (0.07)	0.11–0.47	67 (44)	10–180	2.45 (1.52)	1.00–7.00
Kopperdahl and Keaveny (1998)	11	32–65	22	0.17 (0.04)	0.11–0.26	291 (113)	90–536	2.23 (0.95)	0.70–4.33

[1]Note that modulus values in most studies (shown in italics) have been measured with the use of test techniques that introduce an underestimation systematic "end-artifact" error that has been estimated in the range of 20–40 percent. Thus, it is recommended to attempt to correct for such errors from those studies or use values from alternative studies that were obtained without these errors. Results are more representative of the general population when a higher number of cadavers are used. Caution should be exercised when extrapolating beyond the age range of the tested cadavers.

All mechanical data from tests with specimens oriented in the inferior–superior direction, unless noted.

— Data were not reported.

†Ultrasound was used to measure the elastic properties; strength cannot be measured with ultrasound.

††Proximal and distal femur pooled; proximal specimens oriented approximately along the femoral neck axis.

‡Elastic modulus data for only 122 specimens.

*The ash densities that were originally reported have been converted to wet densities with Y = 1.86X, based on data from Table 1 of Galante et al. (1970).

**The dry densities that were originally reported have been converted to wet densities with Y = 1.25X, based on data from Table 1 of Galante et al. (1970).

FIGURE 3.20 Compressive and tensile yield strains vs. human anatomic site for trabecular bone specimens tested on-axis. Compressive yield strains were always greater than tensile yield strains. Bars denote ±1 SD. The numbers within the bars show the significant ($p < 0.05$) correlation coefficients against apparent density, confirming that in most sites there was no dependence on density, and at most only a weak correlation. From Morgan and Keaveny (2001) *J Biomechanics* 34: 569–577.

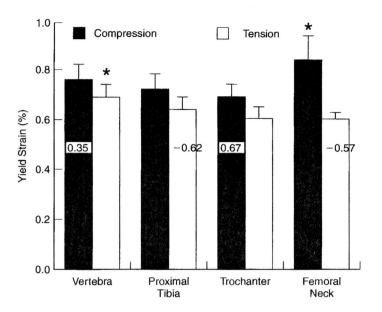

compressive and tensile values are about 0.8 percent and 0.6 percent, respectively (Figure 3.20). For lower density bone, such as in the vertebral body, compressive yield strains are lower at about 0.7 percent, due presumably to underlying large deformation bending or buckling-type failure mechanisms of the individual trabeculae that can occur when the density is low. In this situation, the individual trabecular tend to be longer and thinner than for high-density bone, and according to engineering buckling theory, this may promote buckling as a failure mode, compared with material yielding. Buckling or excessive bending do not appear to occur much for high-density bone (volume fraction > 0.25) and do not occur for tensile loading. It is most interesting, however, that the variation in yield strain within sites is very small and is even small across sites. As seen next, this greatly facilitates statistical analysis of trabecular bone failure properties.

Anisotropy

Like cortical bone, trabecular bone is an anisotropic material. Modulus and strength can vary by as much as eight times, depending on the direction of loading compared with the principal material direction, which coincides with the main trabecular orientation. For some sites, such as the vertebral body of the spine, the general anatomic directions (e.g., the inferior–superior axis) coincide with the main trabecular orientation. However, for most sites this is not the case, and the main trabecular orientation is oblique to the anatomic axes. The classic example of this is in the proximal femur, where the trabecular orientation varies with location and is never aligned with the anatomic axes (recall Figure 3.7). In these cases, a local coordinate system can be used to describe the principal material directions. In the neck region of the proximal femur, for example, the trabecular orientation tends to follow the orientation of the neck axis, but it doesn't do so exactly. Thus, it can be technically challenging to describe the oftentimes spatially varying principal material directions for trabecular bone, and this complicates whole–bone structural analysis. Interestingly

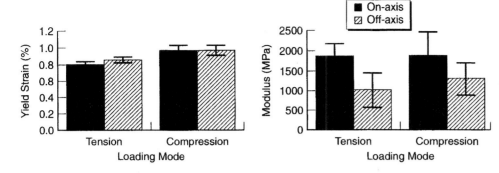

FIGURE 3.21 Dependence of yield strain (left) and Young's modulus (right) on specimen orientation in tension and compression, for dense bovine trabecular bone. For the off-axis orientation, the specimen axes were offset 30–40° from the principal trabecular (on-axis) direction. Error bars show ±1 SD. In contrast to the yield strains, which were isotropic, but asymmetric, elastic modulus and yield stress (not shown) were clearly anisotropic. From Chang et al. (1999) *J Orthop Res* 17:582–585.

enough, the yield strains for trabecular bone appear to be isotropic despite the substantial anisotropy of the elastic and strength properties (Figure 3.21). This can simplify failure analyses, as described below.

Due to the substantial heterogeneity in modulus and strength of trabecular bone, it should now be clear that the question "What is the modulus (or strength) of trabecular bone?" is not easily answered. Details such as anatomic site, species, age, loading direction, and disease state must be specified; in structural analyses of whole bones, one should use average trabecular properties that are appropriate to the specific anatomic site of the patient population under analysis.

Failure, Fatigue, and Creep

The multiaxial failure behavior of trabecular bone is an important aspect of its *in vivo* failure behavior, because failure usually occurs during some type of trauma where loads will be multiaxial or oblique to the principal material direction. Criteria such as von Mises stress failure theory should not be used when shear stresses are high, since these criteria do not account for the relatively low shear strength of trabecular bone, compared with its tensile and compressive strengths. Instead, a criterion based on maximum strains should be used. Such a criterion is advantageous because it is relatively independent of variations in apparent density—at least within an anatomic site—and is also isotropic. The criterion works as follows: Strains for any state of loading are converted into principal strains. When either the maximum or minimum principal strain exceeds the maximum allowable on-axis uniaxial strains, then failure is assumed to occur. The on-axis data shown in Figure 3.20 can be used to estimate the maximum allowable tensile and compressive failure strains for the anatomic site under analysis. Note that, despite this yield strain criterion being both homogeneous and isotropic, strength remains asymmetric, since yield strains are lower in tension than compression.

Like cortical bone, trabecular bone exhibits the phenomena of creep and fatigue (Figure 3.22). Trabecular bone also undergoes modulus and strength reductions if it is loaded beyond its yield point, unloaded, and reloaded (compare Figure 3.23a with

FIGURE 3.22 *S–N* fatigue curve for human vertebral trabecular bone, showing two run-out specimens (marked with X). Applied stress has been divided by Young's modulus to minimize scatter. From Haddock et al. (2004) *J Biomechanics* 37:181–187.

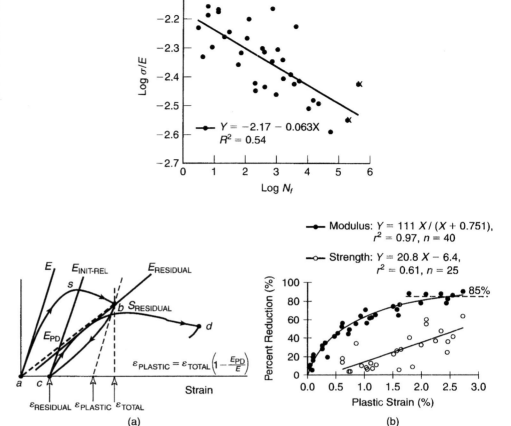

FIGURE 3.23 (a) Typical compressive post-yield behavior of trabecular bone for loading, unloading, and reloading along path a–b–c–d, as shown. The initial modulus upon reloading ($E_{INIT-REL}$) is statistically equal to the Young's modulus E. The reloading curve shows a sharp decrease in modulus, denoted by $E_{RESIDUAL}$. This modulus is similar to the "perfect-damage" modulus (E_{PD}, dashed line), which would occur if the material behaved in a perfectly damaging manner with cracks occurring at yield. (b) Dependence of percent modulus reduction (between E and $E_{RESIDUAL}$) and strength reduction on the plastic strain that develops with overloading. From Keaveny et al. (1999) *J Orthop Res*, 17:346–353.

Figure 3.14a). As in cortical bone, this indicates that some type of microstructural damage is occurring that reduces the modulus and strength. Monotonic yield, post-yield, fatigue, and creep behaviors appear to be dominated by the level of applied strain, regardless of apparent density. Thus, in failure analyses of trabecular bone, once strains are calculated, failure can be predicted in a straightforward manner, despite the large variations in density and architecture typical of trabecular bone. This implies that emphasis should be placed on calculation of correct values of strain, which requires accurate modeling of the elastic behavior of this tissue; care should be taken to use appropriate values per anatomic site and age.

Miner's rule is often used in traditional engineering applications to determine the fatigue life for varied loading conditions. The theory is that the fraction of fatigue life—defined as the applied number of load cycles N_i divided by the fatigue life at that load cycle N_{Fi}—used up at n different load levels sums linearly so that final (fatigue) failure occurs when the sum of fractional fatigue lives equals unity. Thus, if 30 percent of the fatigue life were used up at one stress level, and a further 25 percent were used up at a second stress level, 45 percent would remain for loading at any other stress level. Mathematically, this is expressed as

$$\sum_{i=1}^{n} \frac{N_i}{N_{Fi}} = 1$$

in which the summation is over the n different stress levels. While not validated for bone, Miner's rule remains useful in the absence of any other validated theories. Typically, the number of cycles to fatigue failure N_{Fi} for any stress level σ_i is found by using the empirical S–N power law curve. For use with trabecular (and cortical) bone, we make a modification to this by substituting the quantity σ/E for σ. Doing so enables a single S–N curve to be constructed for specimens spanning wide ranges of porosities (see Figures 3.13 and 3.22). Combining all this provides a direct relation between load level and remaining fatigue life:

$$\sum_{i=1}^{n} \frac{N_i}{A\left(\sigma/E\right)_i^{B}} = 1$$

Here, A and B are empirically found constants.

EXAMPLE 3.4 Miner's Rule

Question   Using the data in Figure 3.22, what is the fatigue life for a specimen of human vertebral trabecular bone subjected to a "high" stress of 0.005 times its Young's modulus for 50 cycles, followed by "moderate" cyclic loading at $\sigma/E = 0.003$ to failure? Based on your results, what is the effect of the 50 cycles of high stress on the fatigue life at moderate stress?

Solution   We first solve for the number of cycles for the second stress level, using the Miner's rule equation for bone:

$$N_2 = \left\{ 1 - \frac{N_1}{A\left(\sigma/E\right)_1^{B}} \right\} A\left(\sigma/E\right)_2^{B}$$

Analysis of the curve fit shown in Figure 3.22 reveals that $A = 3.14 \times 10^{-35}$ and $B = -15.9$. Inserting these values into this equation yields the following value of N_2:

$$N_2 = \left\{ 1 - \frac{50}{3.14 \times 10^{-35}(0.005)^{-15.9}} \right\} 3.14 \times 10^{-35} \times 0.003^{-15.9}$$

$$= 239{,}519 \text{ cycles}$$

If the cyclic loading were at only the moderate level, the fatigue life would have been 408,039 cycles. So the percentage shortening of fatigue life, with the addition of the initial 50 cycles of "high" stress loading, is 41.3 percent.

3.7 | Hierarchical Analysis

Although the focus of this chapter is on mechanics at the tissue level, the study of biomechanics of bone at the microscopic level is also important. At the microstructural level, additional factors come into play, including the local tissue properties and the structure and organization of osteons and trabeculae. The mechanical properties of the trabecular tissue are hard to determine, due in large part to the difficulty of performing accurate mechanical tests on such small specimens. Experimental evidence suggests that the modulus of this tissue is probably 10–20 percent less than the modulus of cortical tissue, and the failure strains are similar to those of cortical bone, being higher in compression than tension. The modulus may be lower for trabecular than cortical tissue, because trabecular tissue tends to be slightly less mineralized than cortical tissue due to its higher turnover rate and due also, perhaps, to subtle differences in the lamellar structure between cortical and trabecular tissue.

Knowledge of these tissue properties is important in micromechanical analysis of trabecular bone. This type of analysis can be used to determine the effects of aging, drug treatment, and disease on the microstructure by and—understanding the structure–function relations for trabecular bone—the continuum-level properties. Analysis of the whole bone at the organ level can then be performed to determine the effects of these apparent properties on whole bone structural behavior. This multistep analysis is an example of a hierarchical, or multiscale, analysis, which is commonly performed in biomechanics in order to determine the underlying causes and mechanisms of clinical problems. This information in turn can be used to improve diagnostics, such as high-resolution imaging. If one knows exactly what one is looking for in terms of biomechanically relevant microstructural changes in a tissue, the diagnostic is more likely to be successful clinically at identifying patients at risk.

Hierarchical analysis can also be used to identify potential treatment strategies for altering microstructural properties that—by design—have a substantial biomechanical impact. For example, on the basis of predicted biomechanical performance hierarchical analysis can help choose between competing strategies and, in that way, help focus drug discovery efforts on where they most likely would have maximum biomechanical significance: at the whole organ level. The corollary is also important. If one has a candidate drug, for example, that can change some property of the microstructure, and it is shown by hierarchical analysis that this property has little biomechanical significance at the organ level, then it may be unwise to proceed with the presumably costly development of this drug. It is mostly for these reasons that understanding the hierarchical structure–function relations for bone, and all biological tissues, is so important clinically.

At the microstructural level, the local mechanical behavior provides the interaction between cell biology and bone mechanical properties, particularly the mechanical stimulus to influence the biology at the local cellular level. In turn, the local cellular activity can alter the amount, composition, and organization of the bone, and therefore the mechanical behavior (Figure 3.24). Armed with sufficient knowledge of the coupling between mechanics and biology of bone, it may be possible to engineer solutions to a variety of clinical problems by control of the appropriate biomechanical behavior. Such principles form the biomechanical basis for the field of tissue engineering, which promises hope in the treatment of various disorders, as well as development of artificial substitutes for biological tissues or their repair.

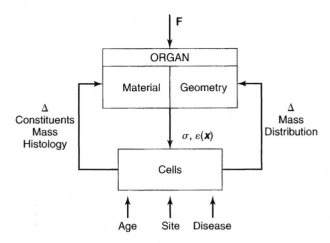

FIGURE 3.24   Flow diagram of the interaction between mechanics and cell biology and possibilities for their "engineering." A force F acts on the whole organ, which is characterized by its material and geometric properties. The organ acts as a mechanical filter, eventually subjecting its cells to position-dependent stresses σ and strains ε. Other factors influence cell behavior, such as age, anatomic site, and disease state (if any). Clearly, numerous physiological parameters not shown also influence and mediate cell behavior. Under all these influences and those of the applied stresses and strains, the cells respond biologically by altering the type of tissue they produce and where they produce it. The type of tissue can be changed by varying the constituents, their amount, and their histological arrangement. These changes will alter the material properties of the tissue within the organ. The mass and spatial distribution of the tissue will also affect the overall geometric properties of the organ. These changes in turn will alter the role of the organ as a mechanical filter and will therefore change the stresses and strains at the cell level, although the force F has not changed. The overall system constitutes a biomechanical feedback control loop, which, if characterized appropriately, might be possible to manipulate in the treatment of disease or damaged tissue.

3.8 | Structural Anisotropy

On-Axis Elastic Behavior

As noted earlier, specific applications, such as fracture analysis of bones, may require detailed modeling of the anisotropy of the tissue. Since most biological tissues are anisotropic, study of structural anisotropy is critical in tissue mechanics. We focus here on the mechanics of anisotropy relevant to elastic constitutive behavior. All constitutive relations should be applied in the principal material coordinate system, the so-called "on-axis" configuration. The general form of the elastic constitutive relation for any coordinate system is

$$\{\sigma\} = [C]\{\varepsilon\}$$

where $\{\sigma\}$ and $\{\varepsilon\}$ are written as one-dimensional arrays and represent the second-order stress and strain tensors, respectively; and $[C]$ is a 6×6 matrix—the *elastic stiffness* matrix, to be more precise—that represents the fourth-order elasticity tensor. The inverse relation reveals the *elastic compliance* matrix $[S]$:

$$\{\varepsilon\} = [C]^{-1}\{\sigma\} = [S]\{\sigma\}$$

For on-axis loading, to avoid ambiguity about the reference coordinate system, the first equation can be written with explicit subscripts to reflect that it refers to the 1–2–3 principal material coordinate axes:

$$\{\sigma\}_{1-2-3} = [C]_{1-2-3}\{\varepsilon\}_{1-2-3}$$

In many cases, such subscripts are not used for convenience. However, it is important in any analysis to explicitly describe the reference coordinate system, since the forms of $[C]$ and $[S]$ for anisotropic materials depend critically on the choice of the coordinate system. For on-axis loading of an orthotropic material, both $[C]$ and $[S]$ are sparse, symmetric matrices. Specifically, there is no coupling between any normal stresses and shear strains. There is also no coupling between any of the shear terms. The expanded general version of the last equation is

$$\begin{Bmatrix} \sigma_{11} \\ \sigma_{22} \\ \sigma_{33} \\ \sigma_{12} \\ \sigma_{23} \\ \sigma_{31} \end{Bmatrix} = \begin{bmatrix} C_{1111} & C_{1122} & C_{1133} & 0 & 0 & 0 \\ C_{2211} & C_{2222} & C_{2233} & 0 & 0 & 0 \\ C_{3311} & C_{3322} & C_{3333} & 0 & 0 & 0 \\ 0 & 0 & 0 & C_{1212} & 0 & 0 \\ 0 & 0 & 0 & 0 & C_{2323} & 0 \\ 0 & 0 & 0 & 0 & 0 & C_{3131} \end{bmatrix} \begin{Bmatrix} \varepsilon_{11} \\ \varepsilon_{22} \\ \varepsilon_{33} \\ \varepsilon_{12} \\ \varepsilon_{23} \\ \varepsilon_{31} \end{Bmatrix}$$

where σ_{11}, σ_{22}, and σ_{33} are the normal stresses; σ_{12}, σ_{23}, and σ_{31} are the shear stresses; and similarly for the strain terms.

The stresses and strains are classified mathematically as tensors, and therefore they rotate according to tensor transformation rules. This is true even though the stresses and strains have been written here in one-dimensional array notation, which is suggestive, but not indicative, of vector quantities. The last equation can also be written in indicial notation, as follows:

$$\sigma_{ij} = C_{ijkl}\,\varepsilon_{kl} \qquad i, j, k, l = 1, 3$$
$$\text{and} \quad C_{ijkl} = 0 \quad \text{if} \quad i = j \text{ and } k \neq l$$
$$i \neq j \text{ and } k = l$$
$$i \neq j \text{ and } (i \neq k \text{ or } j \neq l)$$

Indicial notation can sometimes be very convenient. For example, the symmetry condition can be written simply as

$$C_{ijkl} = C_{klij} \text{ when } i = j \text{ and } k = l$$

We will now derive the on-axis elastic compliance matrix from first principles for an orthotropic material. As will be seen, this is a simple process, but derivation of the elastic stiffness matrix is much more algebraically complex. Consider a cubic specimen loaded sequentially in a uniaxial fashion along each of its principal material coordinate axes (Figure 3.25).

For the first load case, a normal stress σ_{33} is applied, and the resulting normal strains ε_{11}, ε_{22}, and ε_{33} in all three directions are measured. Shear strains will be zero, since there is no coupling between axial and shear behaviors for an orthotropic material when the specimen is loaded in its principal material coordinate system. Thus, the following strains will result:

$$\varepsilon_{11} = -\nu_{31}\varepsilon_{33}$$

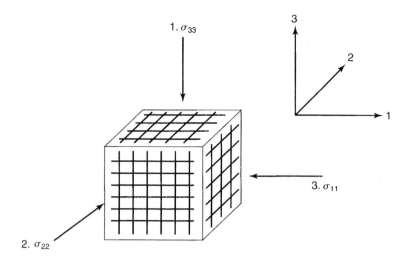

1. σ_{33}

2. σ_{22}

3. σ_{11}

FIGURE 3.25 A cubic specimen is machined in alignment with its principal material coordinate directions (shown by axes 1–3). It is then loaded sequentially and nondestructively three times in a uniaxial fashion as shown, first with σ_{33}, second with σ_{22}, and third with σ_{11}. (The order is not important.) The strains in all three (normal) directions are measured in each case. This is then repeated for pure shear loading in each of the three directions.

$$\varepsilon_{22} = -\nu_{32}\varepsilon_{33}$$

$$\varepsilon_{33} = \frac{1}{E_3}\sigma_{33}$$

Here, ν_{ij} is a Poisson's ratio that is defined as the negative ratio of the strain that occurs in the j direction to the strain that occurs in the i direction when a stress is applied in the i direction; and E_i is the Young's modulus in the i-direction. Note that because of the anisotropy, $\nu_{31} \neq \nu_{32}$. Also, as will be seen next, $\nu_{ij} \neq \nu_{ji}$ for general orthotropy, and it is therefore important to explicitly define the Poisson's ratio notation in all anisotropic analyses.

Substituting the expression for ε_{33} into the first two strain expressions yields the following equation for all the strains in terms of the applied stress:

$$\varepsilon_{11} = \frac{-\nu_{31}}{E_3}\sigma_{33}$$

$$\varepsilon_{22} = \frac{-\nu_{32}}{E_3}\sigma_{33}$$

$$\varepsilon_{33} = \frac{1}{E_3}\sigma_{33}$$

Similarly, the second and third uniaxial loading tests produce the following strains:

Apply σ_{22}:

$$\varepsilon_{11} = \frac{-\nu_{21}}{E_2}\sigma_{22}$$

$$\varepsilon_{22} = \frac{1}{E_2}\sigma_{22}$$

$$\varepsilon_{33} = \frac{-\nu_{23}}{E_2}\sigma_{22}$$

Apply σ_{11}:

$$\varepsilon_{11} = \frac{1}{E_1}\sigma_{11}$$

$$\varepsilon_{22} = \frac{-\nu_{12}}{E_1}\sigma_{11}$$

$$\varepsilon_{33} = \frac{-\nu_{13}}{E_1}\sigma_{11}$$

For shear loading, each shear stress produces just a single shear strain in the direction of loading, since, for an orthotropic material, there is no coupling between the different shear directions or with any of the normal directions. Thus, the shear strains are given as follows:

$$\text{Apply } \sigma_{12}: \quad \varepsilon_{12} = \frac{1}{2G_{12}} \sigma_{12}$$

$$\text{Apply } \sigma_{23}: \quad \varepsilon_{23} = \frac{1}{2G_{23}} \sigma_{23}$$

$$\text{Apply } \sigma_{31}: \quad \varepsilon_{31} = \frac{1}{2G_{31}} \sigma_{31}$$

Note here that the strains are tensor quantities, which explains the factor 2 in the denominator ["engineering" shear strain $\gamma = 2\varepsilon_{ij}(i \neq j)$ and $\sigma_{ij}(i \neq j) = \tau = G\gamma$]. Note also that the shear modulus $G_{ij}(i \neq j)$ is different for each load case since the material is orthotropic. Because $\sigma_{ij} = \sigma_{ji}$ and $\varepsilon_{ij} = \varepsilon_{ji}$ by symmetry of the stress and strain tensors, $G_{ij} = G_{ji}$, so the order of subscripts on the shear modulus is not important—unlike the case for Poisson's ratio.

For the general state of stress in an elastic material, the total strain response for each individual load case is obtained by the linear superposition of the strain responses for each individual load case. Thus, by adding all similar strain terms, the overall constitutive equation is formed:

$$
\begin{Bmatrix} \varepsilon_{11} \\ \varepsilon_{22} \\ \varepsilon_{33} \\ \varepsilon_{12} \\ \varepsilon_{23} \\ \varepsilon_{31} \end{Bmatrix}
=
\begin{bmatrix}
\dfrac{1}{E_1} & \dfrac{-\nu_{21}}{E_2} & \dfrac{-\nu_{31}}{E_3} & 0 & 0 & 0 \\
\dfrac{-\nu_{12}}{E_1} & \dfrac{1}{E_2} & \dfrac{-\nu_{32}}{E_3} & 0 & 0 & 0 \\
\dfrac{-\nu_{13}}{E_1} & \dfrac{-\nu_{23}}{E_2} & \dfrac{1}{E_3} & 0 & 0 & 0 \\
0 & 0 & 0 & \dfrac{1}{2G_{12}} & 0 & 0 \\
0 & 0 & 0 & 0 & \dfrac{1}{2G_{23}} & 0 \\
0 & 0 & 0 & 0 & 0 & \dfrac{1}{2G_{31}}
\end{bmatrix}
\begin{Bmatrix} \sigma_{11} \\ \sigma_{22} \\ \sigma_{33} \\ \sigma_{12} \\ \sigma_{23} \\ \sigma_{31} \end{Bmatrix}
$$

To keep our notation consistent with that previously described for Poisson's ratio, we will define $\sigma_{ij}(i \neq j)$ as the shear stress in the i direction for shear loading of the j plane (i.e., the plane with a normal vector in the j direction) and likewise for shear strains. The elastic compliance matrix $[S]$ is given by the matrix term in this equation. By symmetry of the elastic compliance matrix, it is readily seen that the following constraints exist on the various Young's moduli and Poisson's ratios:

$$\frac{\nu_{ij}}{E_i} = \frac{\nu_{ji}}{E_j} \qquad i, j = 1\text{--}3; \text{ no sum}$$

The equation shown here with the elastic compliance matrix is the simplest mathematical expression of Hooke's law for an elastic orthotropic material in three dimensions. The algebra is much more complex for derivation of the elastic stiffness matrix. Thus, the derivation is not shown here, but the matrix terms are

$$C_{1111} = \frac{1 - \nu_{23}\nu_{32}}{E_2 E_3 \Delta} \qquad C_{1122} = \frac{\nu_{12} + \nu_{13}\nu_{32}}{E_1 E_3 \Delta}$$

$$C_{2222} = \frac{1 - \nu_{13}\nu_{31}}{E_1 E_3 \Delta} \qquad C_{2233} = \frac{\nu_{23} + \nu_{21}\nu_{13}}{E_2 E_1 \Delta}$$

$$C_{3333} = \frac{1 - \nu_{12}\nu_{21}}{E_1 E_2 \Delta} \qquad C_{1133} = \frac{\nu_{13} + \nu_{12}\nu_{23}}{E_1 E_2 \Delta}$$

$$C_{1212} = 2G_{12} \qquad C_{2323} = 2G_{23} \qquad C_{3131} = 2G_{31}$$

where the parameter Δ is given by

$$\Delta = \frac{1 - \nu_{12}\nu_{21} - \nu_{23}\nu_{32} - \nu_{31}\nu_{13} - 2\nu_{21}\nu_{13}\nu_{32}}{E_1 E_2 E_3}$$

By examination of the elastic compliance matrix and its symmetry, it is seen that there are only nine independent elastic constants for an orthotropic material. For a transversely isotropic material, two of the indices on the material constants can be interchanged, resulting in five independent elastic constants. Of course, for an isotropic material, all three indices can be interchanged, and there remain only two independent elastic constants. Indeed, for any plane of isotropy, the following relation holds between the Young's modulus, the shear modulus, and the Poisson's ratio:

$$G = \frac{E}{2(1 + \nu)}$$

Off-Axis Elastic Behavior

So far, we have discussed constitutive behavior only in the principal material coordinate system—"on-axis" behavior. When the applied stresses are applied in a coordinate system other than this, we have so-called "off-axis" behavior. Since the elastic stiffness matrix is not sparse when loading is off-axis, it is difficult to measure the material constants for an anisotropic material unless on-axis loading is used. For this reason, all experiments to determine material constants should be performed in the principal material coordinate system. One technical challenge here is to prepare test specimens with the proper alignment. For some biological materials, specimens oftentimes are machined along general laboratory axes, which usually correspond with anatomical axes (e.g., medial–lateral, anterior–posterior, inferior–superior), but which may not correspond with the principal material axes (Figure 3.26). Knowledge of the mechanics for off-axis loading is important when planning such experiments and when interpreting literature data on material properties derived from specimens that were machined off-axis.

Knowledge of how to deal with off-axis behavior is also important for many structural applications. In the typical stress analysis problem of a biological structure (for example, the proximal femur), the applied stresses may not be aligned with the principal material coordinate system. In that case, it is necessary to extend the constitutive relations from the on-axis configuration to an arbitrary off-axis coordinate system. The overall strategy in these cases involves three steps: (1) rotate the

FIGURE 3.26 Machining of specimens along anatomical axes often leads to "off-axis" specimens that are not aligned with the principal material coordinate system. The schematic here shows an example of this for the proximal femur. By convention, θ is measured positive, as shown, in the counterclockwise direction. The 1–2 axes denote the principal material directions of the excised specimen.

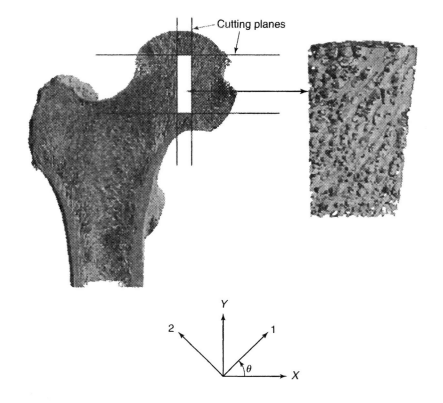

stresses and strains from the off-axis (laboratory) coordinate system into the on-axis principal material system; (2) apply the constitutive relations expressed in the principal material coordinate system—the constitutive model does not have to represent linear elasticity to convert stress to strain, or vice versa; and (3) rotate the stresses and strains back from the on-axis to the off-axis coordinate system. Thus, the key mathematical operations here, besides application of the constitutive model, are those associated with rotation of the stresses and strains between the on- and off-axis configurations. We now describe the mathematics of this whole process for an elastic material. This is done for a two-dimensional problem, for simplicity, although the concepts apply directly to three dimensions.

Let $\{\sigma\}_{1-2}$ and $\{\varepsilon\}_{1-2}$ denote the stresses and strains expressed in the unique on-axis principal material coordinate system, and let $\{\sigma\}_{x-y}$ and $\{\varepsilon\}_{x-y}$ denote these same stresses and strains referred to some off-axis coordinate system:

$$\{\sigma\}_{1-2} = \begin{Bmatrix} \sigma_{11} \\ \sigma_{22} \\ \sigma_{12} \end{Bmatrix}, \quad \{\varepsilon\}_{1-2} = \begin{Bmatrix} \varepsilon_{11} \\ \varepsilon_{22} \\ \varepsilon_{12} \end{Bmatrix}$$

$$\{\sigma\}_{x-y} = \begin{Bmatrix} \sigma_{xx} \\ \sigma_{yy} \\ \sigma_{xy} \end{Bmatrix}, \quad \{\varepsilon\}_{x-y} = \begin{Bmatrix} \varepsilon_{xx} \\ \varepsilon_{yy} \\ \varepsilon_{xy} \end{Bmatrix}$$

Assume that the angle between the 1 and x axes is θ, which is taken as positive in the counterclockwise direction (see Figure 3.26). Following standard rotation transformation rules for second-order tensors such as stress and strain (it is important here to use tensor shear strains; otherwise the equations do not work), the stresses and strains in both coordinate systems are related by

$$\{\sigma\}_{1-2} = [T]\{\sigma\}_{x-y}$$

$$\{\varepsilon\}_{1-2} = [T]\{\varepsilon\}_{x-y}$$

where the rotation matrix for this two-dimensional problem is given by

$$[T] = \begin{bmatrix} \cos^2\theta & \sin^2\theta & 2\sin\theta\cos\theta \\ \sin^2\theta & \cos^2\theta & -2\sin\theta\cos\theta \\ -\sin\theta\cos\theta & \sin\theta\cos\theta & \cos^2\theta - \sin^2\theta \end{bmatrix}$$

and is converted to $[T]^{-1}$ by setting $\theta = -\theta$.

Note that these transformations have nothing to do with constitutive behavior— they are simply mathematical rotations of the coordinate systems that are used to describe the stress and strain components. Constitutive behavior only arises when we try to relate stress to strain.

Let us now derive an expression for the elastic stiffness matrix as written in the off-axis x–y coordinate system, $[C]_{x-y}$. Realizing that we're looking only at the two-dimensional formulation here, in the principal material coordinate system we have the following, in which $[C]_{1-2}$ is a sparse matrix:

$$\{\sigma\}_{1-2} = [C]_{1-2}\{\varepsilon\}_{1-2}$$

Expressing the on-axis stresses and strains in terms of their off-axis values gives

$$[T]\{\sigma\}_{x-y} = [C]_{1-2}[T]\{\varepsilon\}_{x-y}$$

and we therefore get the desired relation in the principal coordinate system:

$$\{\sigma\}_{x-y} = [T]^{-1}[C]_{1-2}[T]\{\varepsilon\}_{x-y}$$

The elastic stiffness matrix in the off-axis system is defined by $\{\sigma\}_{x-y} = [C]_{x-y}\{\varepsilon\}_{x-y}$; $[C]_{x-y}$ is therefore given by

$$[C]_{x-y} = [T]^{-1}[C]_{1-2}[T]$$

Note that $[C]_{x-y}$ is not sparse due to the operators $[T]$ and $[T]^{-1}$ that act on $[C]_{1-2}$.

EXAMPLE 3.5 Off-Axis Elastic Properties

Question Consider the problem of relating the "material properties" in the global x–y coordinate system for loading of a misaligned specimen (Figure 3.26). These are not true material properties, because they depend on the angle of misalignment. Specifically, for an off-axis specimen, what is the relation between "Young's modulus," defined as the ratio of the applied stress σ_{xx} to the measured strain ε_{xx}, to the angle of misalignment θ and the on-axis material properties E_1, E_2, G_{12}, and ν_{12}? For simplicity, consider this only as a 2-D problem.

Solution   The compliance matrix is transformed between the coordinate systems as

$$[S]_{x-y} = [T]^{-1}[S]_{1-2}[T]$$

where, for this planar problem, $[T]$ is as given earlier and $[S]_{1-2}$ is

$$[S]_{1-2} = \begin{bmatrix} \dfrac{1}{E_1} & -\dfrac{\nu_{21}}{E_2} & 0 \\[2ex] -\dfrac{\nu_{12}}{E_1} & \dfrac{1}{E_2} & 0 \\[2ex] 0 & 0 & \dfrac{1}{2G_{12}} \end{bmatrix}$$

Rather than multiply out these matrices, which is cumbersome, we will use engineering indicial notation; to avoid confusion, we write

$$[S]_{x-y} = S_{mn} \text{ and } [S]_{1-2} = U_{op}$$

Then $S_{mn} = T^{-1}_{mo}U_{op}T_{pn}$, in which we sum over any paired indices from 1 to 3. Thus,

$$S_{11} = 1/E_x = T^{-1}_{1o}U_{op}T_{p1}$$
$$= T^{-1}_{11}U_{11}T_{11} + T^{-1}_{11}U_{12}T_{21} + T^{-1}_{11}U_{13}T_{31}$$
$$+ T^{-1}_{12}U_{21}T_{11} + T^{-1}_{12}U_{22}T_{21} + T^{-1}_{12}U_{23}T_{31}$$
$$+ T^{-1}_{13}U_{31}T_{11} + T^{-1}_{13}U_{32}T_{21} + T^{-1}_{13}U_{33}T_{31}.$$

Since $[S]_{1-2}$ is sparse, $U_{13} = U_{31} = U_{23} = U_{32} = 0$; and since $[S]_{1-2}$ is symmetric, $U_{12} = U_{21}$.

Thus, $1/E_x = T^{-1}_{11}U_{11}T_{11} + T^{-1}_{11}U_{21}T_{21} + T^{-1}_{12}U_{21}T_{21} = T^{-1}_{13}U_{33}T_{31}$
$$= c^2U_{11}c^2 + c^2U_{21}s^2 + s^2U_{21}c^2 + s^2U_{22}s^2 + 2scU_{33}sc$$

(where c denotes $\cos\theta$ and s denotes $\sin\theta$)

$$= c^4U_{11} + c^2s^2\{2U_{21} + 2U_{33}\} + s^4U_{22}$$

The final expression is therefore given by

$$\frac{1}{E_x} = \frac{1}{E_1}\cos^4\theta + \left(\frac{1}{G_{12}} - \frac{2\nu_{12}}{E_1}\right)\sin^2\theta\cos^2\theta + \frac{1}{E_2}\sin^4\theta$$

$$\frac{1}{E_y} = \frac{1}{E_1}\sin^4\theta + \left(\frac{1}{G_{12}} - \frac{2\nu_{12}}{E_1}\right)\sin^2\theta\cos^2\theta + \frac{1}{E_2}\cos^4\theta$$

$$\frac{1}{G_{xy}} = 2\left(\frac{2}{E_1} + \frac{2}{E_2} + \frac{4\nu_{12}}{E_1} - \frac{1}{G_{12}}\right)\sin^2\theta\cos^2\theta + \frac{1}{G_{12}}(\sin^4\theta + \cos^4\theta)$$

$$\frac{1}{\nu_{xy}} = E_x \left[\frac{\nu_{12}}{E_1}(\sin^4\theta + \cos^4\theta) - \left(\frac{1}{E_1} + \frac{1}{E_2} - \frac{1}{G_{12}}\right)\sin^2\theta\cos^2\theta \right]$$

Two characteristics of these equations are noteworthy. First, the off-axis moduli (E_x, E_y, G_{xy}) and the off-axis Poisson's ratio (ν_{xy}) all depend on either sine or cosine functions raised to the fourth power. Second, each of these off-axis properties depends on all four of the on-axis material properties $(E_1, E_2, G_{12}, \nu_{12})$. Because of this condition, it is not possible to determine any of the true intrinsic on-axis material properties for an anisotropic material from off-axis loading unless all material properties in the off-axis coordinate system are known (and, of course, the angle of misalignment). Even then, relatively complex mathematical operations need to be performed to solve the four simultaneous equations—which can introduce substantial loss of precision with real experimental data. The measured properties in any off-axis test will have little generality, since they will depend on the angle of misalignment. For these reasons, it should be clear that mechanical testing of anisotropic biological tissues should always be performed in the principal material coordinate system when the objective is to determine the intrinsic anisotropic material properties of the tissue.

3.9 | Biomechanics of Bone Adaptation

We now turn to the consideration of the unique character of bone as an adaptive material. The human skeleton is a remarkable structure in its ability to repair itself after injury. Even more impressive is the ability of bones to adapt to their mechanical environment, thereby producing structures that are optimized for their functional operating conditions. In these regards, bones are truly unique compared with typical engineering structures. The adaptive capability of bone means that it is a structure in which both the geometry and material properties can change in response to mechanical loading. This can be viewed mathematically in terms of a constitutive model that incorporates feedback control. The feedback is provided by the bone cells serving as both the sensors (detecting changes in the mechanical environment) and actuators (causing new bone to be deposited or removed). There is no equivalent of this type of constitutive behavior in traditional engineering materials. Indeed, the mathematics associated with analysis of bone adaptation is very complex. In this section, we will therefore address just the very fundamental aspects of the biomechanics of bone adaptation. Our purpose is to demonstrate the general process by which one can perform engineering analyses to predict changes in bone morphology in response to changes in habitual loading or implantation of a prosthesis. We start our discussion with a look at the different types of cells involved in this remarkable process.

Bone Cells

The growth, repair, and maintenance of bone are ultimately carried out by the four types of cells that inhabit bone tissue: osteoclasts, osteoblasts, osteocytes, and bone lining cells. The osteoclast is a giant multinucleated cell that is formed when precursor monocytes of hematopoietic origin join together for the purpose of dissolving bone tissue. In a sense, the osteoclast is not so much a cell type as it is a state in which the monocytes reside for a short time. The osteoclast attaches itself to an exposed bone surface and forms a tight seal around the periphery of its contact area. It then secretes an acid that dissolves the bone tissue beneath it, and, after ingesting the debris, expels it to the bloodstream. Osteoclasts can be as large as 100 μm in diameter, and their formation is influenced by hormones that act systemically and by local factors, such as proteins secreted by other bone cells.

The osteoblast is responsible for secreting osteoid, the collagenous matrix that is later mineralized to form bone. It is a cuboidal cell approximately 20–30 μm wide and 10 μm tall and sometimes becomes embedded within the bone tissue. The coordinated action of multiple osteoblasts determines which type of bone tissue is developed (woven, lamellar, Haversian, etc).

The osteocyte is the differentiated form of an osteoblast that becomes trapped within the bone matrix after production of new bone tissue. There are over 25,000 osteocytes per mm^3 of bone tissue. The body of the cell inhabits the lacunae, while its processes extend through the half-micron diameter canaliculi and connect to other osteocytes at gap junctions. Osteocytes are never more than about 150 μm from a Haversian canal. It is thought that these cells may sense the strain or some other mechanically induced input signal and transduce it into a chemical signal that then instigates bone remodeling by the osteoclasts and osteoblasts. Osteocytes may also be ideally situated to help control mineral homeostasis, since the surface area per unit volume associated with the canaliculi (about 160 mm^2/mm^3) is over 30 times that associated with lacunae or Haversian canals.

The bone lining cell is a dormant osteoblast. These cells cover 90 percent of the trabecular bone surfaces and line the endosteal and periosteal surfaces of all bones and the Haversian canals. The bone lining cell does not actively produce osteoid, but extends projections that connect it to osteocytes just below the surface of

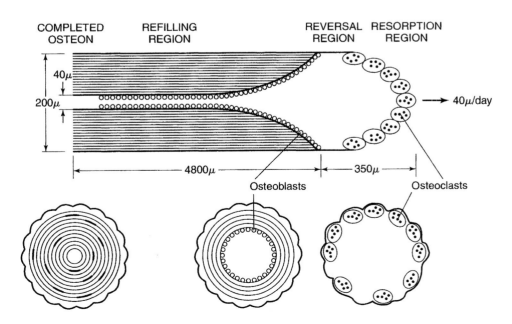

FIGURE 3.27 The coordinated action of a BMU. Cross-sectional views are shown at various stages in the remodeling process.

the bone. These connections may allow the osteocytes to signal the surface cells and somehow attract them toward damaged areas for repair. For example, osteoclasts have cell surface receptors that connect to the proteins OPGL and CSF-1. OPGL (osteoprotegrin ligand) is itself a surface protein on the osteoblast, and CSF-1 (colony stimulating factor-1) is secreted from osteoblasts. Once the osteoclast precursors get exposed to both OPGL and CSF-1, mature osteoclasts are formed, and the bone remodeling cycle is initiated (resorption followed by production of new bone). It is possible that a damage-induced signal, or lack of signal, from the osteocytes to the bone lining cells stimulates production of OPGL and/or CSF-1, which then initiates the remodeling sequence.

Bone Adaptation

Bone constantly experiences the processes of growth, reinforcement, and resorption. It adapts to the mechanical demands placed on it by daily activities (or lack thereof). If one considers the way the heart and other muscles adapt to exercise or atrophy with disuse, it is not hard to imagine that bone goes through a similar process. The adaptation of cortical bone requires both changes in its internal structure as well as its shape, especially its cross-sectional area. The idea that bone adapts to its mechanical environment or damage is not new. As far back as the late 1800s, it was postulated that bone architecture is related to the mechanical loads it experiences, a notion now referred to as Wolff's Law, after its chief postulator. But it is not clear what the bone cells are trying to accomplish. One theory is that the size and shape of the long bones are determined by the need to maintain the maximum compressive strains near 3000 $\mu\varepsilon$. This theory is attractive because many animals experience peak compressive strains between 2000 and 3000 $\mu\varepsilon$, but it does not address the underlying stimulus that actually causes the bone remodeling.

Adaptation of Haversian Bone

Secondary osteons (see Figures 3.3 and 3.8) are formed by the coordinated actions of BMUs (basic multicellular units). Within each BMU, the osteoclasts resorb bone and are followed by osteoblasts, which deposit new bone (Figure 3.27). The BSU (basic structural unit) is the amount of bone that is laid down by each BMU. It includes the bone between the cement lines and the opening of the Haversian canal. Considering the BMU as a single functional unit is a fruitful way of analyzing the remodeling process because it is a predictable biological system. Each BMU goes through the process of activation, resorption and reversal, and formation (the A–R–F sequence).

Activation: The entire process takes about three days. Differentiated, dedicated cells must be recruited. The osteoclasts that do the tunneling may survive for weeks, and it is postulated that the osteocytes play a central role.

Resorption and reversal: Approximately 30 days are required for the resorption and reversal process to pass through a given cross section in human bone. The osteoclasts occupy a half-eggshell region (200 μm in diameter and 300 μm long) that can move 40–50 μm/day. The reversal region is generally quiescent, because the osteoblasts remain a short distance behind the osteoclasts.

Formation: Osteoblasts lay down osteoid, which is a collagenous matrix material that will later calcify and become bone. The average radial closure rate is less than 1 μm/day, taking approximately 90 days to reach completion. As osteoblasts lay down osteoid, some of them become trapped and differentiate into osteocytes. The osteocytes then extend their processes toward the formation front to contact and trap other osteoblasts, and the process continues. Eventually, there will be a network of living cells inhabiting the lamellae of the Haversian canal. Once this is finished, it takes about 10 days before calcium and phosphorus diffuse or convect into the region in sufficient quantities to begin the mineralization process. Once they do, however, 60 percent of the mineralization occurs within 24 hours. The remainder mineralizes over the next six months.

Trabecular Bone Adaptation

Remodeling in trabecular bone is not as organized as it is within Haversian bone. Typically, osteoclasts attach themselves to the surfaces of trabeculae and eat away a small region of bone known as a Howship's lacunae, ordinarily 40–60 microns deep. As long as the osteoclast does not penetrate completely through the trabeculae, osteoblasts will eventually follow and lay down new bone. While trabecular bone does not have the extensive osteocyte array that cortical bone has to act as mechano-sensors, it is still adaptive. It is generally accepted that the architecture represents an optimized state. It is thought that the osteoclasts respond to trabecular damage, as well as to the body's demand for calcium. It may also be that the osteoblasts target areas that are experiencing large deformations.

Modulus Changes and Bone Adaptation

To incorporate bone adaptation into engineering analyses of the skeletal system, it is necessary to include in the model the feedback from the mechanics to the bone adaptation. One practical application of such models is in the design of total joint prostheses, in which the goal is to have a prosthesis that does not change bone stress enough to trigger adverse bone resorption. One strategy in testing candidate designs is to implant the prosthesis in animals and determine after months or years of implantation how the implant has changed the bone morphology. This can be done clinically, too, by radiographic follow-up of patients. Both approaches are expensive in terms of time and money and would raise ethical concerns if *in vivo* performance were worse than the clinical accepted standard. The ability to design a bone response into the implant by using computational methods would clearly speed up the design process and, although never as reliable as true clinical testing, should identify designs that are simply not suitable for clinical testing. In this way, better products can get to the market faster. Sophisticated nonlinear finite element analyses are used for such purposes. We describe here a simple version of a common bone adaptation theory that can be used in such analyses and apply it to a simple structural problem to demonstrate some key features of bone adaptation theory.

In strain-driven bone remodeling theory, a fundamental assumption is made that the bone adaptation process is error driven; that is, the magnitude of the response is based on the difference between the local strain state due to the applied mechanical load and a biological set point (sometimes called an attractor state). Loads well below the set point stimulate bone removal and subsequent reductions in local bone stiffness. Reduced local stiffness leads in turn to increases in local strains until the set point is reached (or approximated) and the bone is adapted to the loading stimulus.

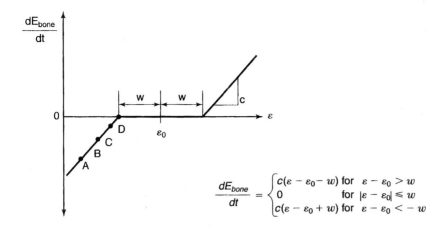

$$\frac{dE_{bone}}{dt} = \begin{cases} c(\varepsilon - \varepsilon_0 - w) & \text{for } \varepsilon - \varepsilon_0 > w \\ 0 & \text{for } |\varepsilon - \varepsilon_0| \leq w \\ c(\varepsilon - \varepsilon_0 + w) & \text{for } \varepsilon - \varepsilon_0 < -w \end{cases}$$

FIGURE 3.28 Relation between rate of change of bone modulus and bone strain. ε_0 is the strain set point, E_0 is the homeostatic elastic modulus at the set point, c describes the magnitude of the response (in GPa/week), and w is half the width of the "dead zone," a range of strain centered on the set point in which no net adaptation occurs. (For simplicity, we are treating compressive strains as positive—tensile strains will not develop in this example.)

The presence of an implant such as a total knee or hip replacement inevitably modifies the local stresses and strains within the bone tissue, stimulating adaptation. The metal in implants is much stiffer than bone and therefore carries much more of the load. A poorly designed implant may reduce the loads locally on the bone tissue so much that the bone tissue supporting the implant is resorbed and the implant fails. Mathematical models of the adaptation process are solved by using the finite element method to determine local stresses and strains to predict bone loss around an implant during the design process. To illustrate the basic idea, consider a much simpler mechanical model that allows us to examine the net effect of an implant on bone stiffness. This simple theory of adaptive strain remodeling is shown in Figure 3.28. The theory assumes that the bone changes its elastic modulus in response to changes in strain from its homeostatic set point. It includes a quiescent zone, over which strain changes do not elicit a remodeling response, and a linearly increasing remodeling rate (modulus change rate) outside that zone.

EXAMPLE 3.6 Bone Adaptation Due to Presence of Prosthesis

Question   Consider an orthopaedic implant with elastic modulus $E_{implant}$ that is placed within the diaphysis of a long bone of modulus E_{bone} so that the bone and implant are loaded in compression as two springs in parallel. As a result of the load sharing between the implant and the bone, there is a reduction in strain on the bone. We will assume that the reduction is enough to move outside the quiescent (or "dead") zone to point A in Figure 3.28. Here, dE_{bone}/dt is negative, indicative of bone loss. If the external functional load applied to the bone-implant system remains constant while the bone elastic modulus is reduced during adaptation, the strain in the bone will be increased to point B, then to point C, and so on. Eventually, this process causes the strain, ε, to reach the dead zone at point D, where $dE_{bone}/dt = 0$, and no further net changes in E_{bone} occur. This is a stable adaptive response.

What is the equation for the change in bone elastic modulus after implantation of the prosthesis? For these purposes, assume that, before implantation, the bone is adapted to the stress σ, so that $\sigma = E_0 \varepsilon_0$. Assume that the cross-sectional area of the bone is A_{bone}, the cross-sectional area of the implant is $A_{implant}$, and the cross-sectional area of the two together is A_{total}.

Solution   If we assume that the addition of the implant reduces the strain so that $\varepsilon < \varepsilon_0 - w$ (you can confirm this assumption later), then the rate of change of the bone elastic modulus is

$$\frac{dE_{bone}}{dt} = c(\varepsilon - \varepsilon_0 + w)$$

Because the bone and implant are loaded as springs in parallel, the strain in each is the same and is given by

$$\varepsilon = \frac{P}{\{E_{bone}A_{bone} + E_{implant}A_{implant}\}} = \frac{A_0 E_0 \varepsilon_0}{\{E_{bone}A_{bone} + E_{implant}A_{implant}\}}$$

Substituting this into the differential equation, we get

$$\frac{dE_{bone}}{dt} = c\left(\frac{A_0 E_0 \varepsilon_0}{\{E_{bone}A_{bone} + E_{implant}A_{implant}\}} - \varepsilon_0 + w\right)$$

Solving this equation numerically, using $c = 2000$ GPa/week, $\varepsilon_0 = 0.005$, $E_0 = 17$ GPa, $E_{implant} = 200$ GPa, $w = 0.4\varepsilon_0$, $A_{bone}/A_{total} = 0.90$ and $A_{implant}/A_{total} = 0.10$ as the values for the constants, and assuming $A_0 = A_{bone}$, indicates that the elastic modulus is approximately at equilibrium after about 20 weeks (Figure 3.29). At this point, the strain in the bone is .003 ($=.005 - .4*.005$).

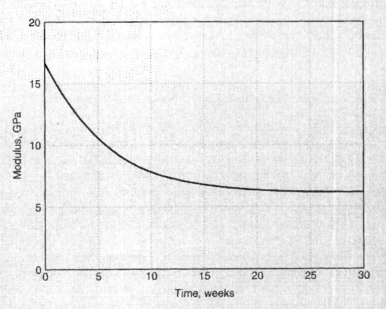

FIGURE 3.29   Numerical solution for Example 3.6. At $t = 0$ weeks, the implant is introduced into the bone and the shared load reduces the strain to outside the dead zone (Figure 3.28). At roughly 20 weeks, a new equilibrium modulus has been obtained that moves the remodeling rate back to zero.

It is often important to calculate the changes in elastic modulus caused by bone adaptation over time, because the applied load may change during the process due to changes in physical activity or changes in neighboring structural elements. The constant c expresses how quickly bone adapts to the new loading situation. For sufficiently small time steps, c does not affect the equilibrium elastic modulus or equilibrium strain. Values for c are determined by calibrating of data from experimental animal studies of mechanical disuse and vary throughout the skeleton.

3.10 | Summary

The mechanical properties of musculoskeletal tissues depend upon their underlying microstructures, which we must know to understand the anatomic site-, age-, and disease-related variations that occur in the tissue and organ level mechanical properties. An important distinction in tissue mechanics is that between material and structural behavior, since terms such as "muscle," "bone," "cartilage," and "tendon" can be used to describe either tissues or organs. Material properties reflect the behavior of only the tissue. Structural properties describe the behavior of the organ and, because they include geometric and material effects, are specific to the particular organ under analysis.

Adult human cortical bone tissue has an osteonal microstructure that results in transversely isotropic material behavior; that is, its material properties depend on the loading direction. For transverse isotropy, one direction has properties different from those in a mutually perpendicular plane. Cortical bone is stronger in compression than tension, and stronger (and stiffer) for longitudinal than for transverse loading. Because of its variable porosity, which tends to increase with age, its elastic modulus and strength can vary almost twofold. Cortical bone exhibits fatigue and creep characteristics consistent with what has been observed in many engineering materials, but quite complex multiaxial failure behavior.

Trabecular bone is much more porous than cortical bone and is classified as a cellular solid material. Its microstructure consists of a number of interconnected rods and plates of irregular geometry. Trabecular bone is also anisotropic, the degree of anisotropy depending on anatomic site. With porosities that vary from about 60–95 percent, trabecular bone is an extremely heterogeneous material. Largely because of this variation in porosity, its modulus and strength can vary by an order of magnitude even within a single anatomic site. Interestingly, the failure strains are relatively constant for trabecular bone and are generally higher for compression than for tension. Like cortical bone, trabecular bone exhibits characteristics of fatigue and creep and also has a complex multiaxial failure behavior. When trabecular bone is overloaded, its mechanical properties are greatly reduced, although the associated physical damage can be visually difficult to detect due to its widespread, but microscopic, nature.

For anisotropic materials such as cortical and trabecular bone, it is essential to apply the constitutive relations in the principal material coordinate system—that is, along the grain of the material. Otherwise, the relations between stress and strain become overly complex due to interactions between the microstructure and the off-axis nature of the loading. Because of this, experimental testing of bone and most biological tissues is quite complex, requiring careful sample preparation for alignment with the principal material coordinate system and tests to measure the many material constants associated with the anisotropy.

Unlike any engineering materials but many biological materials, bone adapts to its mechanical environment and can repair itself when damaged. The mathematics of bone adaptation are complex, in which concepts of non-linear central theory can be used to estimate changes in bone material properties for a given load history. Such theories can be useful to compare implant designs based on patterns of predicted bone loss in the long term.

3.11   EXERCISES

3.1 The various measures of density used to characterize both cortical and trabecular bone can be confusing. The purpose here is to sort out these measures by understanding their nature.

(a) For cortical bone, (hydrated) apparent density, ash density, and ash content are common parameters. Apparent density is defined as the mass of the hydrated bulk specimen divided by its bulk volume; ash density is the same, except that the specimen is first "ashed" in a furnace at about 700 °C for 24 hours to remove all organic material; and ash content has already been described in the text and is the ratio of mass of ashed to dry bone. Let's say that you measured the following respective values for the diameter, length, hydrated mass, dry mass, and ashed mass of a cortical bone specimen: 3 mm, 8 mm, 115 mg, 103 mg, and 70 mg. What are the (hydrated) apparent density, ash density, and ash content of this specimen?

(b) For trabecular bone, density is dominated by the porosity associated with the marrow pore spaces. Archimedes' principle is usually used to measure this porosity, and from this the volume fraction and tissue density (the density of the trabecular tissue that makes up the individual struts of trabecular bone) can be found. In this procedure, the specimen is cleaned of all marrow and weighted in air to find the hydrated, or "wet," mass m_{wet}. Then it is submerged in water and degassed to remove all air bubbles, and the "submerged" mass m_{sub} is measured. Show that the tissue density is given by the expression

$$\rho_{tiss} = \frac{m_{wet}}{m_{wet} - m_{sub}} \rho_{water}$$

and, from that, derive an expression for the volume fraction in terms of these mass measurements and the specimen dimensions.

3.2 Using the cross-sectional population data in Figure 3.10, calculate the percent change of the tensile strength of adult human cortical bone if its porosity is 5 percent vs. 20 percent. Assume now that this change in porosity occurs over time from ages 30 to 80 years. Compare the percent change in strength to the data in Figure 3.16a, and discuss any discrepancies.

The data in Figure 3.10 and Figure 3.16b were taken from the same study. Using these data and any other relevant data you may need, compare the percent change in the energy to failure of the bone for ages 30 vs. 80 years. (Calculate this as the area under the stress–strain curve up to fracture; assume for simplicity that the bone is elastic—perfectly plastic and with its ultimate and yield stresses are the same.)

Based on all the information at your disposal, which aspect of the material properties of adult human cortical bone changes most with aging?

3.3 Tsai–Wu Failure Criterion: Using published average values of the tensile, compressive, and shear strengths for cortical bone (Table 3.2), calculate values for F_1, F_2, F_3, F_{11}, F_{22}, F_{33}, F_{44}, F_{55}, and F_{66} for human cortical bone, assuming it to be transversely isotropic in strength (with the plane of isotropy being the 2–3 plane). If you cannot calculate values for any of these terms, explain what experimental data would be needed to enable you to do so.

Suggest an experiment for measurement of the strength interaction term F_{12}, and show the equations used to determine its value from the experimental data.

3.4 Using the data in Figure 3.13, and assuming that Miner's rule is valid for cortical bone *in vivo*, estimate the total number of cycles to failure if a piece of cortical bone is subjected to tensile compressive of 80 MPa for 100 cycles, 60 MPa for 100,000 cycles, and 40 MPa for the remainder of its life. Compare the life for specimens having a longitudinal Young's modulus of 14 vs. 20 GPa. On the basis of these results, comment on the importance of overloads and bone density in the fatigue life and damage accumulation of cortical bone.

3.5 Cortical bone gets weaker with aging, but it turns out that diaphyseal diameters can also change with aging, particularly in males, such that the safety factor of the diaphysis is approximately constant with aging.

The safety factor *SF* is defined as the failure stress divided by the functional stress for the bone tissue on the periosteal surface of the diaphysis.

If the tissue tensile strength of cortical bone is decreased to 80 percent of its original ("young") value with aging, what is the change in periosteal diameter required to keep the *SF* constant at the periosteal surface?

Assume for simplicity the following:

(i) The diaphysis can be modeled as a hollow circular cylindrical tube.

(ii) The diaphysis is loaded by a pure bending moment *M*, and stresses can be calculated from simple beam theory.

(iii) The endosteal diameter is constant and equal to 15 mm.

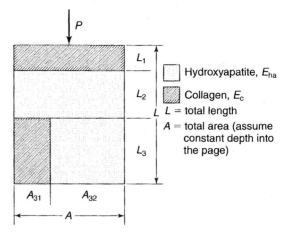

Hint: Analyze the following system of springs:

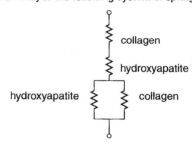

FIGURE P 3.6 Simple spring model of cortical bone constituents.

3.6 (a) Derive the following formula for the modulus of a specimen of cortical bone (E^*) in terms of the moduli of the collagen (E_c) and hydroxyapatite (E_{ha}) for the composite model shown in Figure P 3.6:

$$\frac{1}{E^*} = \frac{1}{E_c}\frac{v(1-\beta)}{(1+v)}$$
$$+ \frac{1}{E_{ha}}\frac{(1-\beta)}{(1+v)} + \frac{(1+v)}{E_c v + E_{ha}}$$

Here,

$$v = \frac{\text{Volume}_{\text{collagen}}}{\text{Volume}_{\text{hydroxyapatite}}} = \frac{L_1}{L_2} = \frac{A_{31}}{A_{32}}, \text{ and } \beta = \frac{L_3}{L}$$

(b) Assuming that $E_{ha} \approx 115$ GPa, $E_c \approx 1$ GPa and that the volume fractions of collagen and hydroxyapatite are equal, what is a typical value of β? Interpret this value (i.e. v 1.0) in terms of whether bone tissue (as a composite) is a constant-stress or a constant-strain type material.

3.7 (a) Using the site-specific relations shown in Table 3.3, compare the on-axis compressive strength of trabecular bone from the human proximal femur, proximal tibia, and vertebral body, for bone specimens having an apparent density of 0.15 and 0.50 g/cm^3. What do you think is the underlying biomechanical cause of any site effects?

(b) Using the data in Figure 3.20, estimate what the corresponding tensile strengths are for these specimens for each site. Compare the degree of strength asymmetry (difference between tensile and compressive strengths) between the high- vs. low-density specimens. Again, what do you think is the underlying biomechanical cause of any density effects on the strength asymmetry?

3.8 (a) Figure P 3.8 shows the multiaxial failure behavior (yield envelope) of trabecular bone when loaded by a combination of on-axis normal stress σ and shear stress τ. The experimental data are shown (filled circles), and some theories are shown to work quite well. Using the fit provided by the cellular solid theory, determine for the given applied normal stresses the magnitude of the simultaneously applied shear stress that would cause failure. Assume that the bone specimen has a Young's modulus of 1000 MPa and a shear modulus of 250 MPa. Positive values of normal stress indicate tension.

   a. $\sigma = 2$ MPa
   b. $\sigma = -2$ MPa
   c. $\sigma = 4$ MPa
   d. $\sigma = -4$ MPa
   e. $\sigma = 8$ MPa
   f. $\sigma = -8$ MPa

(b) How would these values for maximum allowable shear stress change if the shear modulus of the bone were changed ± 25 percent, keeping the Young's modulus constant?

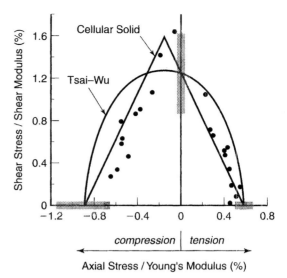

FIGURE P 3.8 Yield envelope for axial-shear loading of (bovine tibial) trabecular bone. The cellular solid criterion fit to the data is $\sigma^* + 0.46\tau^* = 0.0058$, $\sigma^* \geq -0.00155$; $\sigma^* - 0.46\tau^* = -0.0089$, $\sigma^* \geq -0.00155$, where $\sigma^* = \sigma/E$ and $\tau^* = \tau/G$ are the normalized axial and shear apparent stresses, respectively, and have units of strain. From Fenech et al. (1999) *J Biomech Eng* 121:414–422.

(c) On the basis of the preceding results, comment on the limitations of using a simple failure criterion having just one value of yield stress, such as the von Mises, for failure analysis of trabecular bone.

3.9 Indicial Notation and the Lamé Constants. Indicial notation is often used to describe the elastic stress–strain constitutive relations for an *isotropic* material:

$$\varepsilon_{ij} = \frac{1}{E}[(1 + v)\sigma_{ij} - v\delta_{ij}\sigma_{kk}] \quad i, j = 1\text{--}3$$

In this equation, δ_{ij} (the "Kronecker delta") $= 1$ if $i = j$
$= 0$ if $i \neq j$

and a repeated index implies summation ($G_{kk} = G_{11} + G_{22} + G_{33}$).

E, v, and G are often referred to as "engineering" constants. Equivalently, the foregoing equation can be expressed in terms of "Lamé" constants μ, γ, and λ:

$$\varepsilon_{ij} = \frac{1}{2\mu}\sigma_{ij} - \frac{\lambda}{2\mu(2\mu + 3\gamma)}\delta_{ij}\sigma_{kk} \qquad i, j = 1\text{–}3$$

Starting with the expression for the compliance matrix for an orthotropic material, reduce that to one for an isotropic material and show that

$$\mu = G = \frac{E}{2(1 + \nu)} \qquad E = \frac{\mu(2\mu + 3\gamma)}{\mu + \gamma}$$

$$\gamma = \frac{\nu E}{(1 + \nu)(1 - 2\nu)} \qquad \nu = \frac{\lambda}{2(\mu + \gamma)}$$

3.10 The real advantage of using the Lamé formulation is evident when expressing stress in terms of strain (again, this is all for isotropic materials):

$$\sigma_{ij} = 2\mu\varepsilon_{ij} + \lambda\delta_{ij}\varepsilon_{kk} \qquad i, j, k = 1\text{–}3$$

This equation, when expanded out, is seen to be much simpler mathematically than the engineering constant formulation. The expanded version of the Lamé formulation is as follows:

$$\begin{Bmatrix} \sigma_{11} \\ \sigma_{22} \\ \sigma_{33} \\ \sigma_{12} \\ \sigma_{23} \\ \sigma_{31} \end{Bmatrix} = \begin{bmatrix} 2\mu + \lambda & \lambda & \lambda & 0 & 0 & 0 \\ \lambda & 2\mu + \lambda & \lambda & 0 & 0 & 0 \\ \lambda & \lambda & 2\mu + \lambda & 0 & 0 & 0 \\ 0 & 0 & 0 & 2\mu & 0 & 0 \\ 0 & 0 & 0 & 0 & 2\mu & 0 \\ 0 & 0 & 0 & 0 & 0 & 2\mu \end{bmatrix} \times \begin{Bmatrix} \varepsilon_{11} \\ \varepsilon_{22} \\ \varepsilon_{33} \\ \varepsilon_{12} \\ \varepsilon_{23} \\ \varepsilon_{31} \end{Bmatrix}$$

Show that $\sigma_{11} = E\varepsilon_{11}$ for a uniaxial stress test in the 1 direction. Show also that, for a "confined compression" test (uniaxial *strain* test), the ratio of applied strain ε_{11} to the developed stress σ_{11} is given by

$$\frac{\sigma_{11}}{\varepsilon_{11}} = 2\mu + \gamma = \frac{E(1 - \nu)}{(1 + \nu)(1 - 2\nu)}$$

3.11 Table P 3.11 shows on-axis (in the coordinate system of the principal material axes) elastic properties for human femoral cortical bone. On the basis of these data,

TABLE P 3.11

Anisotropic Elastic Properties of Human Femoral Cortical Bone	
Elastic Constant	
E_1 (GPa)	12.0
E_2 (GPa)	13.4
E_3 (GPa)	20.0
G_{12} (GPa)	4.53
G_{23} (GPa)	6.23
G_{31} (GPa)	5.61
ν_{12}	0.376
ν_{23}	0.235
ν_{31}	0.371

Source: Ashman et al. (1984) *J Biomechanics* 17:349–361.

(a) Calculate values for all stresses that develop when a uniaxial compressive strain of 0.2 percent is applied in the 3-direction (a "confined compression" test); and

(b) Repeat (a), but assuming transverse isotropy, and isotropy. Calculate transversely isotropic values by averaging the properties in the two less stiff directions. For the isotropic values, use the elastic modulus in the stiffest direction and a Poisson's ratio of 0.3 (a common strategy in many structural analyses of cortical bone). Use this result to comment on the importance of the extent (orthotropic vs. transversely isotropic vs. isotropic) of anisotropy of cortical bone in structural applications.

3.12 Figure P 3.12 shows a bone sample subjected to tensile loading at an angle θ with respect to its principal material axis X_3. Assume the material to be

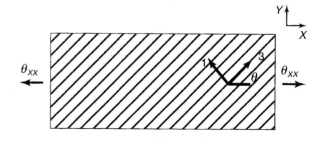

FIGURE P 3.12

orthotropic, with the X_2 axis perpendicular to the load axis. (Data from Turner et al., *J Biomech.* 110:213–214; 1988.)

(a) For plane stress conditions, derive an expression for the apparent modulus in the X direction E_X as a function of the on-axis material properties of an orthotropic material in a single plane and the angle θ, where the 3 axis (principal material axis) is at an angle θ (positive is counterclockwise) to the X axis.

(b) On the basis of the formula you found in (a), plot a single graph of the percentage error in modulus, defined as

$$\% \text{ Error in } E = 100(E_X - E_3)/E_3,$$

as a function of θ (0–10° range only) for the cortical bone properties in P Table 3.11. Do this graph for errors arising from misalignment separately in the 3–1 and 3–2 planes, and explain why the errors are greater for one of the planes.

(c) Repeat (b) for the following trabecular bone on-axis orthotropic properties from the human proximal tibia:

$$E_1 = 237 \text{ MPa}; \quad E_2 = 309 \text{ MPa}; \quad E_3 = 823 \text{ MPa};$$
$$G_{12} = 73 \text{ MPa}; \quad G_{23} = 134 \text{ MPa}; \quad G_{31} = 112 \text{ MPa};$$
$$\nu_{12} = 0.169; \quad \nu_{23} = 0.063; \quad \nu_{31} = 0.423$$

(Data from Turner et.al., *J.Biomech.* 110:213–214; 1988.)

(d) Compare the errors for cortical vs. trabecular bone, and explain the trends. Generalizing your discussion, what are the implications for controlling misalignment errors in mechanical testing of bone?

Tissue Mechanics II: Soft Tissue

In this chapter, we will discuss the major soft tissues encountered in the musculoskeletal system: tendon, ligament, articular cartilage, intervertebral disc, and muscle. As has been stated previously, soft tissues provide connections between bones (ligament and intervertebral disc), excellent joint lubrication (articular cartilage), and actuators for the skeletal system (muscle). These structures work together to control the relative motion of the articulating surfaces.

Soft tissues are also structural elements that must withstand large loads while providing kinematic constraint. In the previous chapter, we saw that bone generally fails at strains of about 5 percent or less and can be considered a linearly elastic material up to the yield point. Soft tissues, by contrast, typically fail at much higher strains and, prior to failure, usually behave nonlinearly. In addition, their load-deformation behavior is time dependent. Consequently, viscoelasticity can be important for soft tissues (as well as bone and many other engineering materials). Therefore, this chapter is also a natural place to discuss viscoelastic material models and the analysis of viscoelastic behavior.

4.1 | Tendon and Ligament

Composition and Microstructure

Tendons and ligaments have similar compositions and microstructures, although subtle differences do exist related to their different functions. Tendons connect muscles to bones, and are therefore loaded in series with the muscles, which can apply large forces to the bone during habitual activities. Ligaments connect bones to bones. As described earlier in our discussion of joint stability, ligament forces are generally small unless the joint is close to its full range of motion. Thus, functional forces are generally higher for tendons than ligaments. As we will see, the two types of tissues are well suited for these different functions.

Both tendon and ligament contain about 60 percent water. By dry weight, tendon contains about 75–85 percent of mostly type-I collagen, about 1–3 percent elastin, and 1–2 percent proteoglycans. Elastin—the most elastic protein known—gives tendon (and particularly ligament, where its concentration can be much higher) substantial elastic properties. The collagen fibrils in tendon are generally aligned with the direction of the tendon, which is along the line of action of the muscle force. Ligament differs from tendon in that it contains slightly less collagen ($\approx 70-80$ percent dry weight), much more elastin ($\approx 1-15$ percent dry weight), and a little more proteoglycan (1–3 percent); it also has a more complex orientation of its fibrils than tendon.

There are a number of hierarchical structures within both tendon and ligament (Figure 4.1). At the lowest scale is the collagen triple helix molecule (1.5 nm diameter); next is the microfibril (3.5 nm diameter), which contains five collagen molecules; then the subfibril (10–20 nm diameter); and finally the fibril (50–500 nm diameter). In tendon, these collagen fibrils are connected to each other by the proteoglycans and noncollagenous proteins and arranged in parallel into discrete packets called fascicles. The collagen fibrils within the fascicle are aligned parallel to each other, but are slightly crimped when unloaded (they straighten out when loaded). The tendon cells, called fibroblasts, are situated between the fibrils.

The different fascicles within the whole tendon are connected to each other and held together by a relatively thick layer of loose connective tissue called the endotenon. The fascicles can slide over each other to some extent, and a variety of nerves, blood vessels, and lymphatics are contained within the endotenon. In regions where tendons slide over bones like pulleys, the tendons have a slightly cartilaginous morphology at the bone contact region to better withstand the compressive contact stresses and the need to reduce friction. Avascular tendons are surrounded by a synovial sheath, which promotes low friction sliding with respect to surrounding tissues,

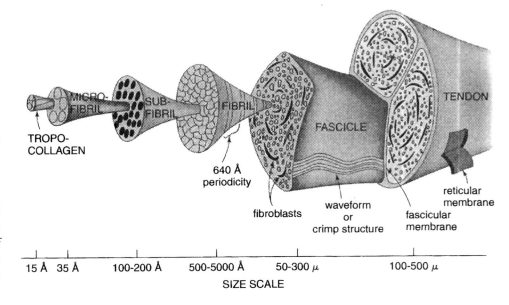

FIGURE 4.1 Arrangement of collagen molecules into tendon, showing the various hierarchical structures and their associated physical scales. (Adapted from Vincent JFV and Curry JD (editors), *The Mechanical Properties of Biologic Materials*. Cambridge University Press, Cambridge, 1980, pp 397–435.)

but restricts blood supply. A thin layer of connective tissue between the tendon and the sheath, the epitenon, secretes lubricating synovial fluid. Vascular tendons do not have a synovial sheath, but are surrounded instead by a thin layer of connective tissue called the paratenon, which facilitates direct blood supply to the interior of the tendon.

In ligament, the collagen fibrils (150–250 nm diameter) are arranged first into crimped fibers ($\approx$1–20 mm diameter) and then into subfascicular units (100–250 μm diameter). Three to twenty of these subfascicular units, each of which is surrounded by a thin endotenon layer, bind together to form fascicles (250 μm to several millimeters in diameter). Each fascicle is surrounded by an epitenon. Fascicles do not have to be aligned with the overall orientation of the ligament, and this occasional lack of alignment is one of the main distinguishing features between tendons and ligaments.

In the anterior cruciate ligament of the knee, for example, the fascicles are spirally wound about each other, whereas in the collateral ligaments they lie parallel to the length of the ligament. The fascicles, or collagen bundles, can slide over each other quite easily. From a biomechanical perspective, the relative independence of the fascicles in both tendon and ligament is important, because it allows these organs to respond in different ways to changing loading conditions. For example, certain fascicles of the anterior cruciate ligament take most of the load for twisting of the knee, whereas other fascicles are dominant for translation. Thus, it is important to realize that tendons and ligaments often have heterogeneous substructures and that their mechanical characteristics therefore can depend on the orientation of the applied loads with respect to the organ.

Mechanical Behavior

The mechanical behaviors of tendon and ligament are qualitatively similar, although tendon is stronger and stiffer because its collagen orientation is generally more aligned. Tendon and ligament have the same general nonlinear stress–strain curve displayed by many biological soft tissues (Figure 4.2—compare with Figure 4.9 for cartilage loaded slowly in tension), with three general regions: the initial nonlinear toe region, where large strains produce only small stresses; the quasi-linear region, where the stress–strain curve is approximately linearly elastic and relatively large stresses develop; and the failure region, where the tangent modulus decreases as collagen fibers become damaged and fracture. The initial nonlinear toe region is generally longer for ligament, since its collagen fibers tend to be less aligned than for tendon.

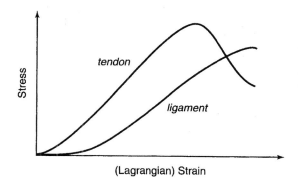

FIGURE 4.2 Typical stress–strain curves for tendon and ligament tissue.

In experimental testing on tendon and ligament tissue, Lagrangian strain or "stretch" is usually used as the measure of strain because of the large values of strain encountered. This is defined as the ratio of the total deformed length to the initial length. It has been found empirically that the nonlinear relationship between tensile stress ($\sigma = F/A_{initial}$) and stretch ($\lambda = L/L_{initial}$) can be described by the following general two-parameter exponential equation up to the start of yielding:

$$\sigma = a(e^{b\lambda} - 1)$$

Here, F, A, and L indicate the force, cross-sectional area, and length, respectively, of the specimen; the subscript "initial" indicates values at the start of testing in the un-loaded state; and the constant parameters a and b are found experimentally by curve fitting. By differentiation of stress with respect to strain, the stress–strain relationship can be converted to a tangent modulus–stress relationship

$$\frac{d\sigma}{d\lambda} = b\sigma + c$$

where c is a constant of integration ($c = ab$) and represents the tangent modulus as $\sigma \to 0$. Thus, tangent modulus increases linearly with increasing stress.

EXAMPLE 4.1 A Micromechanical Model of Collageneous Tissues

Question Various types of fiber-recruitment micromechanical models have been proposed to explain nonlinear stress–strain constitutive behaviors. Consider a model in which the progressive fiber recruitment is modeled as a collection of identical linear springs of stiffness k connected in parallel, but with each linear spring only being recruited at progressively higher strains (Figure 4.3). The final linear region occurs when all fibers have been recruited, say, at a deformation

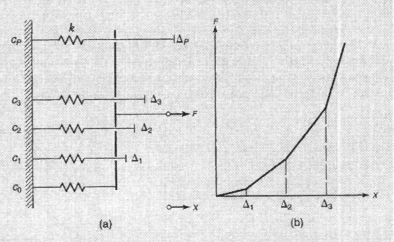

(a)   (b)

FIGURE 4.3 Simple micromechanical parallel-spring model of nonlinear elasticity (a) and the resulting stress–strain curve (b). From Frisen et al. (1969) *J Biomechanics* 2:13.

$x = x_c$, and have a tangent stiffness K_c. Up to this point, there is an equal chance of recruiting any fiber—that is, fiber recruitment length is a random variable. Under these assumptions, at any deformation $0 \le x \le x_c$, the total force sustained by the structure is given by the integral of the extension of its spring times its stiffness, summed over all springs that so far are recruited. What is the expression for the force–deformation relation in terms of x_c and K_c?

Solution   For a discrete number of springs N, the total force at any extension x is

$$F(x) = \sum_{i=1}^{i=N} k(x - \Delta_i), \quad \text{valid in the range } 0 \le x \le x_c$$

in which Δ_i is the clearance length for the ith spring. If N is small, we would need to sum this numerically and would get the stepped response just shown. Real tissues don't show such a stepped response, so we seek a solution for large N. For this case, we can write out an expression for the differential increase in F that would occur with an increment in x, noting that the total stiffness K is now a function of x in the range $0 \le x \le x_c$:

$$dF(x) = K(x)\, dx$$

$$F(x) = \int_0^x K(x)\, dx$$

Since the clearance length is a random variable, there is an equal chance of all clearance lengths occurring. This implies that, as a sample of width W is extended, the fractional width of the test sample that has reached the clearance is equal to the ratio of current deformation to the deformation at which all material has reached the clearance:

$$\frac{w(x)}{W} = \frac{x}{x_c}$$

The term $w(x)$ is the effective width of the specimen. For an axially loaded column, the total stiffness at a deformation $0 \le x \le x_c$ depends on the effective width via the relationship

$$K(x) = \frac{w(x)tE}{L} = \frac{xWtE}{x_c L}$$

in which t is the specimen thickness, E is the Young's modulus (of material that has reached the spring clearance), and L is the specimen length. Thus,

$$F(x) = \int_0^x \frac{xWtE}{x_c L}\, dx = \frac{WtE}{x_c L} \int_0^x x\, dx = \frac{WtE}{2x_c L} x^2 = \frac{1}{2}\frac{K_c}{x_c} x^2$$

and we would expect to see a squared relation between force and deformation for such a material. Note also that $F|_{x=x_c} = \frac{1}{2}K_c x_c$ and that the tangent stiffness is given as

$$K_T(x) = \frac{d}{dx}\left[\frac{1}{2}\frac{K_c}{x_c}x^2\right] = K_c\frac{x}{x_c}$$

Contrast this with a linearly elastic material in which $F = Kx$ and K_T is a constant.

The significance of this nonlinear stress–strain relationship is that the concept of Young's modulus, derived from the stiffness of a linearly elastic Hookean spring, strictly speaking, does not apply, because the tangent modulus of the stress-strain curve depends on the value of strain until all the collagen fibers have been recruited. Even so, the biomechanics literature often cites values of modulus for soft tissues such as tendon and ligament, and care must be exercised when interpreting such values. Also, in comparing values across studies, one must be sure that the tangent moduli being compared were determined at the same strain level.

For porcine anterior cruciate ligament (ACL) tested at a strain rate of 2.5 percent per second, the exponential two-parameter equation has the following values:

$$\sigma = 210(e^{0.63\lambda} - 1)$$

$$\frac{d\sigma}{d\lambda} = 0.63\sigma + 132$$

Thus, the tangent modulus for ligament tissue at zero stress is 132 MPa, while the tangent modulus at the midrange of elastic behavior, which represents strenuous activity ($\sigma \approx 40$ MPa), is 157 MPa. Note that, even at the same strain rate, the effective modulus of the ligament changes with load, which can change with activity level.

Material and Structural Properties

In general, there appears to be a strong dependence of material properties on anatomic site (ligament type) and age for human ligament. Modulus values are in the range 30–500 MPa, depending on the strain rate—we'll see more about this when we discuss viscoelasticity—and the type of ligament, species, age, and disease state. Ultimate tensile stress and strain values are in the range 4–45 MPa and 10–120 percent, respectively. Age is particularly important. For example, the ultimate stress of the young ($\approx$20 yrs) and older ($\approx$50–80 yrs) anterior cruciate ligament is, on average, about 38 and 13 MPa, respectively. The general ranges of tissue material properties for tendon are about 60–2300 MPa for modulus, 25–120 MPa for ultimate stress, and 10–60 percent for ultimate strain. Note again that these properties represent the material behavior of the tissue that makes up whole tendons and ligaments.

When studying ligament–bone or tendon–bone systems, we are generally interested in the strength of the ligament or tendon as an organ—the ultimate load the structure can withstand. Therefore, the structural properties must be used, not the

TABLE 4.1

Typical Whole Ligament Structural Properties (mean ± SD)				
Site	Age Range (years)	Loading Rate (mm/min)	Stiffness (N/mm)	Strength (N)
ACL (knee)	22–35	200	242 ± 28	2160 ± 157
	40–50		220 ± 24	1503 ± 83
	60–97		180 ± 25	658 ± 129
PCL (knee)	55–90	100	145 ± 66	855 ± 225
aPC (knee)	53–98	1000	347 ± 140	1620 ± 500
pPC (knee)	53–98	1000	77 ± 32	258 ± 83
AFTL (ankle)	27–83	125		206 ± 128
cALL (cervical spine)	58–95	20	47.8 ± 8	97 ± 17
lALL (lumbar spine)		6	82 ± 37	742 ± 384
	30–82	60–240	85 ± 33	843 ± 356
		10^4–13800	200 ± 100	1261 ± 369

ACL = Anterior Cruciate Ligament (Knee); **PCL** = Posterior Cruciate Ligament (Knee); **aPC** = anterior Posterior Cruciate (bundle of PCL); **pPC** = posterior Posterior Cruciate (bundle of PCL); AFTL = Anterior FibuloTalar Ligament (Ankle); **cALL** = cervical Anterior Longitudinal Ligament (Spine); **lALL** = lumbar Anterior Longitudinal Ligament (Spine).

stress–strain behavior. Not surprisingly, the stiffness and strength of tendons and ligaments depend very much upon their size and geometry and vary substantially across anatomic sites and species. Some of the most important ligaments, from a biomechanical perspective, are located in the knee, ankle, and elbow joints, and between the vertebral bodies of the spine (Table 4.1). The knee is constrained by the anterior and posterior cruciate ligaments, and the lateral and medial collateral ligaments. The anterior and posterior fibulotalar ligaments, the fibulocalcaneal ligament, and the tibiocalcaneal ligament stabilize the ankle joint. The important ligaments of the elbow include the anterior and posterior bundles of the medial collateral ligament and the radial collateral ligament. The posterior and anterior longitudinal ligaments are the primary connecters of the spinal vertebrae. The range of strengths for these ligaments is large, with mean values from below 100 N for the cervical longitudinal ligament to over 2000 N for the anterior cruciate ligament of the knee. In general, the ligaments of the knee are among the strongest in the body, the ligaments of the ankle and elbow are relatively weaker, and the spinal ligaments vary considerably.

As mentioned previously, some ligaments are composed of smaller substructures, each with their own particular force–deformation characteristics. For example, the ACL can be separated into anteromedial, posterolateral, and intermediate bundles, each of which has distinct properties (Table 4.1 and Figure 4.4). Likewise, the PCL is composed of distinct anterior and posterior bundles, with strengths of about 1600 and 260 N, respectively. Because the force–deformation characteristics and the initial nonlinear toe region vary within subregions of the whole ligament, different bundles take up different loads during *in vivo* functional loading, both singly and in combination. It is important to realize this in surgical reconstruction or replacement of damaged ligaments (or tendons) because failure to reproduce the correct force–deformation characteristics of the composite organ might result in large forces or joint laxity that could jeopardize the longevity of the surgical correction.

FIGURE 4.4 Example of the different force–deformation structural characteristics of the different fiber bundles within the human anterior cruciate ligament. Curves have been shifted along the horizontal axis for clarity. (From Woo and Young in *Basic Orthopaedic Biomech-anics*, ed. Mow and Hayes, pp. 199–243. Raven Press, New York, 1991.)

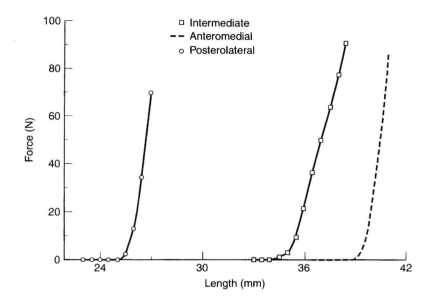

In Vitro and *In Vivo* Behavior

Both tendons and ligaments have an initial nonlinear toe region in the force–deformation curves determined from *in vitro* experiments. *In vivo* behavior is certainly different for tendons and may be different for ligaments as well. Tendons are loaded in series with the muscles. Therefore, it is unlikely that the slack region exists *in vivo*, because the muscle forces will preload the tendon.

The role of the experimentally observed initial nonlinear slack region in the force-deformation curve for ligament in joint stability is less clear. If the slack region observed experimentally exists *in vivo*, the ligaments would allow substantial joint laxity, and the joint would be stabilized primarily by muscle action across the joint. If the ligaments are also preloaded to some extent, then the effective slack region may be relatively small, which would reduce joint laxity and allow the ligaments to play a more direct role in joint stabilization (carry load) for a greater part of the range of motion.

The extent to which the slack region exists for ligaments *in vivo* is at best difficult to determine. It is possible that this region is overestimated in biomechanical tests on excised ligaments. Thus, care must be taken when interpreting this nonlinearity in the context of *in vivo* applications due to possible preloading that is generally not accounted for in typical *in vitro* laboratory experiments.

Although tendons and ligaments consist of soft tissues with large water content (60–80 percent by weight), they do not display substantial time-dependent behaviors (Figure 4.5). Strain rate dependence is relatively weak over physiological loading rates (Table 4.1); an increase in loading rate by four orders of magnitude increases stiffness and strength by a factor of about two. Thus, for physiological strain rates, these tissues, like bone, can be considered relatively insensitive to strain rate. As with bone, we can deal with these relatively minor viscoelastic effects in a quasi-static fashion by performing a time-independent analysis, using elastic modulus and strength properties appropriate to the rate of loading for the given application.

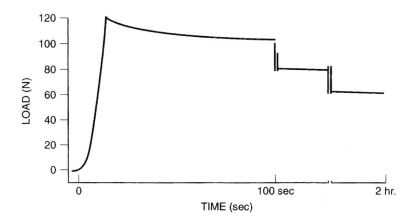

FIGURE 4.5 Example of load-time response to stretching of the anteromedial bundle of a porcine ACL to 5 percent strain by a ramp load at a strain rate of 2.5 percent per second. The specimen was then held at 5 percent strain for two hours and displayed classical stress relaxation behavior. (From Woo and Young in *Basic Orthopaedic Biomechanics*, ed. Mow and Hayes, pp. 199–243. Raven Press, New York, 1991.)

Most experiments on tendons and ligaments are performed by using bone–tendon–bone or bone–ligament–bone constructs, because removal of the soft tissue structure from the bone may damage it and because it is difficult to clamp the ends of an excised tendon or ligament in the jaws of a testing machine. In tests that measure strength, care must be taken to ensure that failure of the soft tissue organ occurs away from the bone junction; otherwise the output of the test may be a measure of the strength of the soft tissue–bone junction, rather than the soft tissue itself.

It was initially argued that strain rate could be used to determine the fracture site, and that tests performed at low strain rates would result in failure at the ligament–bone junction (an avulsion failure), whereas tests at high strain rates would produce failure in the ligament (a midsubstance failure). Consequently, the use of high strain rates was advocated for such tests to produce failure of the ligament itself. It was presumed that, when tested at higher strain rates, the bone would increase in strength more than the ligament, and therefore failure would occur in the ligament, producing a midsubstance failure. This argument is weak because, as we have already seen, bone is not very strain-rate sensitive.

In turns out that age of the animal (level of maturity) may be more important than strain rate, because avulsion failures typically occur if the epiphyseal plate (near the bone–ligament junction) is not closed. (This cartilage-type plate fuses into bone as part of the skeletal maturation process.) The mechanical properties of the ligament and the bone–ligament junction (including the growth plate) increase with age at different rates, the latter being weaker in younger animals, but eventually surpassing the former as the animal ages (Figure 4.6).

Aging, Disease, and Adaptation

Aging and disease also affect the mechanical behavior of tendons and ligaments. The strength of these organs decreases substantially with age. For example, the mean strength of anterior cruciate ligament decreases over threefold, from about 2200 N at age 20–35 to about 650 N at age 60–100 (Table 4.1). Stiffness is also reduced, but not as much. Again, this age-related heterogeneity should be accounted for whenever possible by matching the mechanical properties used in the analysis to the population of interest.

FIGURE 4.6 Schematic diagram showing hypothesized relationship between failure mode vs. age. The bone–ligament–bone complex matures more slowly than the substance, and therefore fails first in younger animals. (From Woo and Young in *Basic Orthopaedic Biomechanics*, ed. Mow and Hayes, pp. 199–243. Raven Press, New York, 1991.)

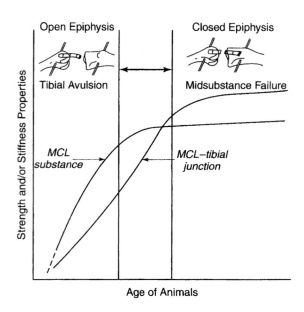

Compared with tendons, ligaments are of more concern clinically, since their failure represents a common and often permanent injury. A common sports injury, for example, is the torn anterior cruciate ligament (ACL), which typically occurs when the knee joint is rotated too much, from skiing, football, basketball, or some other strenuous activity. The lateral collateral ligament at the knee can also be injured when large medially directed forces are placed at the foot, such as during sharp side-steps. These injuries can be particularly serious, since ligaments do not heal well, and therefore surgical repair is often required. No good synthetic replacements for ligaments have yet became available, and grafts obtained post-mortem from donors must be typed against the patient and their biomechanical quality is difficult to ensure.

One common surgical treatment for the ACL is to use a graft constructed from the patient's patellar ligament to replace the damaged ACL. The main surgical challenge is to attach the ligament to the bone. Since this is a difficult task for ACL replacement, part of the bone at each end of the patellar ligament (at the insertion into the patella and proximal tibia) is also removed with the ligament, and the whole construct is then attached to the bone within the knee joint, avoiding any need for reattachment of ligament to bone. The biomechanical principles of the knee joint dictate that the correct tension be obtained in the replacement ligament–bone complex to mimic the natural kinematic function of the joint. Since the graft does not generally have the same structural characteristics of the original ligament, it is a challenging biomechanical problem to obtain a satisfactory approximation of the original kinematics of the knee.

Finally, it should be noted that ligaments and tendons, like most load-bearing biological tissues, remodel in response to changes in the loading environment. Animal studies have shown that, with immobility, ligaments lose mechanical integrity relatively quickly, and upon return to mobility, restoration of properties proceeds at a slower rate, particularly at the insertion site (Figure 4.7). Up to 50 percent of strength can be lost by immobility over a few weeks. The recovery of the strength of

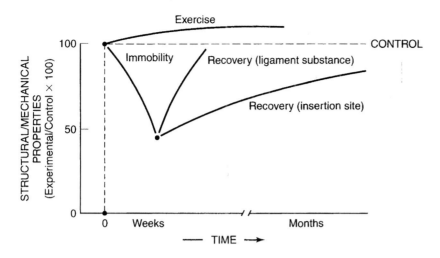

FIGURE 4.7 Schematic representation of the time course and magnitude of effects of immobilization and recovery on biomechanical behavior of ligament. From Woo and Gomez (1987) *J Bone Jt Surg* 69A:1200–1211.

the ligament–bone junction is slower than the recovery of the ligament itself and can take many months for full recovery. As a result of these differential rates of recovery, the ligament–bone junction is the weak link in the remobilized system.

4.2 | Articular Cartilage

Composition and Microstructure

Articular cartilage is a type of hyaline cartilage, as opposed to the other two types of cartilage: fibrocartilage and elastic cartilage. It contains specialized cells called chondrocytes that help maintain its biochemical stasis and structural integrity, but it does not contain any nerves or blood supply. From a biomechanical perspective, articular cartilage can be considered a triphasic material composed of a porous matrix, water, and ions (Figure 4.8a). The porous matrix phase consists of type II collagen (10–20 percent wet weight) and proteoglycans (4–7 percent wet weight). Proteoglycans are complex macromolecules that consist of a central long protein core, which has linkages of long polysaccharide (sugar) chains (Figure 4.8b, top). Most of these proteoglycans in cartilage are the large aggregating types, called aggrecans, that consist of the long protein core to which are attached up to 100 chondroitin sulfate and 50 keratan sulfate glycosaminoglycan chains. Many aggrecan molecules then bind together on a long chain of hyaluronate, thereby forming an aggregate macromolecule that is effectively immobilized in the collagen network due to its bulk (Figure 4.8b, bottom). The second phase, water, accounts for about 70–90 percent of the wet weight and is a crucial contributor to the overall mechanical behavior. The third phase of articular cartilage is a collection of charged molecules and ions. One important feature of the proteoglycans is that their glycosaminoglycan chains contain many carboxyl (COOH) and sulfate (SO_4) groups, which in solution form COO^- and SO_3^- negatively charged ions. These negative ions require positive counter-ions such as Ca^{2+} and Na^+ to maintain electroneutrality. This ionic phase of cartilage also affects its mechanical behavior.

FIGURE 4.8 (a) Three phases of cartilage: porous matrix (made up of the proteoglycan aggrecans and collagen fibers), water, and charged ions associated with the proteoglycans. (b) The molecular structure of the proteoglycan monomer (top) and aggregate (bottom). [Part (b) from Mow et al. in *Basic Orthopaedic Biomechanics*, ed. Mow and Hayes, pp. 143–198. Raven Press, New York, 1991.]

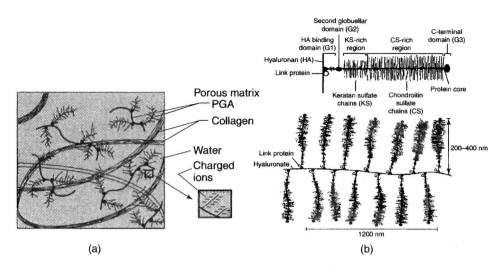

(a)   (b)

Typical thickness values for layers of cartilage vary from 2–4 mm in most human joints. Within any layer, there are four main zones. Close to the surface of the joint is the superficial tangential zone, where the collagen fibers tend to run tangent to the articular surface. Collagen content is also highest, and proteoglycan content is lowest, in this region. It occupies about 10–20 percent of the thickness of the cartilage layer. Immediately below this region is the middle zone, which accounts for about 40–60 percent of the total layer thickness. This region tends to be isotropic. Below this is the deep zone, about 30 percent of the layer thickness, which contains the highest concentration of proteoglycan and the lowest water content. The collagen fibers tend to be thickest in this region. Finally, there is the layer next to the underlying subchondral bone called the zone of calcified cartilage. As the name suggests, it contains a combination of cartilage and mineral. On histological sections, the zone of calcified cartilage can be seen to be separated from the deep zone by a thin line called the tidemark.

Mechanical Behavior and Material Properties

Cartilage material behavior is anisotropic. This aspect of its behavior is difficult to model mathematically and is therefore generally ignored in most structural analyses, but it is important to be aware of anisotropy when interpreting results from experiments on cartilage material behavior. Cartilage also displays heterogeneity in collagen, proteoglycan, and water content, and the material properties vary accordingly.

The material behavior of cartilage can be regarded as that of a poroelastic solid. Its behavior arises from two sources: (1) intrinsic, flow-independent behavior of the collagen–proteoglycan matrix; and (2) flow of the interstitial fluid through the matrix and the resistance of the matrix to this flow. While fluid flow dominates the dynamic, *in vivo* behavior of cartilage, the intrinsic properties determine in large part many of the parameters that restrict such flow. Therefore, intrinsic behavior is an important aspect of cartilage behavior, even though it does not represent typical *in vivo* behavior. The ionic phase also acts to produce swelling in the tissue, which also contributes to the resistance of fluid flow through the matrix. As will be discussed shortly, this swelling depends on the intrinsic properties of the solid matrix. Thus, all three phases are intimately related in how they influence the material behavior.

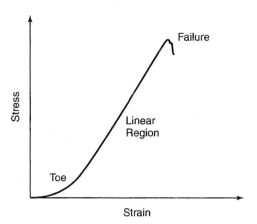

The equilibrium tensile behavior of cartilage can be determined from the steady-state response of tensile creep loading when no fluid flow is occurring. For normal cartilage, the equilibrium stress–strain behavior is linear up to strains of approximately 15 percent, with a modulus value in the range of about 4–10 MPa, depending on the precise location of the specimen within the joint. Degeneration, like that which occurs with osteoarthritis, can reduce values to as low as 1 MPa. The equilibrium tensile modulus can also depend on the orientation of the specimen, since articular cartilage is anisotropic in the surface tangential zone. Values are highest when tested parallel to the split line in the articular surface.

Tensile modulus can also be measured from the more traditional uniaxial tensile test, which is performed at a constant rate of strain, but values are typically higher than equilibrium values due to the dynamic nature of this test. The resulting stress–strain curve exhibits behavior that is characteristic of many biological soft tissues (Figure 4.9). A value of this dynamic Young's modulus can be obtained from the linear region of this stress–strain curve. Typical values range from 40–400 MPa, depending on the depth and orientation of the specimen and strain rate. It should be noted that this type of tensile test does cause flow of fluid from the cartilage specimen. Therefore, the tensile modulus measured in these experiments is not a true intrinsic property, although if the test is performed very slowly, the equilibrium modulus is better approximated. For faster testing, tensile modulus increases with increasing strain rate.

The intrinsic compressive properties of cartilage are usually obtained by the confined compression creep test (Figure 4.10). Here, a cartilage-bone plug is placed tightly in a cylindrical rigid chamber, where deformation can occur only in the direction of loading. This is a uniaxial strain test. During loading, fluid can escape only from the top of the specimen through a porous platen, which also loads the specimen with a constant stress. (The pores in the platen are carefully designed to allow fluid to escape from the cartilage and yet still apply a uniform displacement to the top surface of the specimen without allowing the specimen to enter the pores.) As fluid is forced out of the specimen, creep occurs, and eventually a steady state is reached when all fluid flow stops. Analysis of the steady-state stress–strain response provides the equilibrium compressive modulus. If the test is repeated at successively higher levels of applied stress, the overall stress–strain envelope is approximately linear for strains

FIGURE 4.10 Setup for the confined compression test of articular cartilage. (From Mow et al. in *Basic Orthopaedic Biomechanics*, ed. Mow and Hayes, pp. 143–198. Raven Press, New York, 1991.)

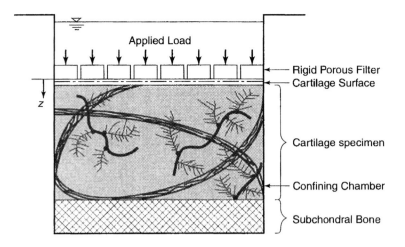

below about 20 percent. Equilibrium compressive behavior is usually expressed in terms of the *aggregate modulus* H_A (terminology borrowed from poroelasticity theory and the soil/rock mechanics literature) and equals the ratio of the equilibrium stress to the equilibrium strain. Typical H_A values are in the range 0.3–1.3 MPa, depending on location within the joint.

Intrinsic properties are strongly affected by tissue composition and disease. The tensile equilibrium modulus is not affected by water or proteoglycan content, but increases with increasing collagen content. The analogy here is that of a rope, in which the equilibrium tensile behavior is determined mainly by the collagen network. Shear behavior also involves stretching of the collagen (Figure 4.11), which is conceptually consistent with the fact that a pure shear stress is equivalent to a combination of tension and compression applied at ±45° to the plane of shear. Thus, shear testing can also be used to learn about intrinsic behavior and the effects of composition and disease on collagen behavior. Such tests confirm that increasing collagen content increases the shear modulus (Figure 4.12). Dynamic viscoelastic shear testing (see Example 4.5), because it induces no change in volume and therefore no fluid flow, can also be used to determine the intrinsic viscoelastic properties of the proteoglycan–collagen matrix. Results from these studies indicate that the solid matrix is only slightly viscoelastic, but more viscoelastic than pure collagen. The implication is that the substantial viscoelastic behavior of cartilage is due mainly to fluid flow within the matrix.

Increasing collagen content has no effect on the compressive equilibrium aggregate modulus, because resistance to compression is provided mainly by the repulsive negative charges of the trapped proteoglycan molecules—the collagen, like rope, cannot sustain compression. The collagen does, however, play a role in compressive intrinsic behavior by constraining the separation and free expansion of the proteoglycan molecules. Recall that they are negatively charged, and this tends to make them swell. The collagen constrains this swelling and, in doing so, develops internal tensile stresses. Cartilage has a volume of only about 20 percent of the free-swelling volume of its proteoglycans. Not surprisingly, then, equilibrium compressive aggregate modulus of cartilage increases with increasing proteoglycan content (Figure 4.13). It also decreases with increasing water content (Figure 4.14), presumably because if there is

Pure Shear

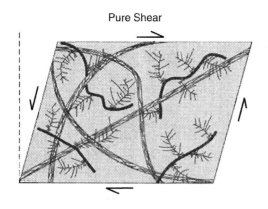

FIGURE 4.11 Proposed mechanism for cartilage resistance to shear loading, where collagen fibers are stretched. From Mow et al. (1984) *J Biomechanics* 102:73–84.

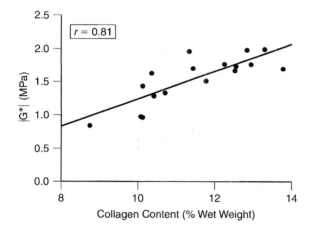

FIGURE 4.12 Positive correlation between the magnitude of the dynamic shear modulus (as measured in dynamic viscoelastic tests) and collagen content for bovine cartilage, confirming the mechanism proposed in Figure 4.11. (From Mow et al. in *Basic Orthopaedic Biomechanics*, ed. Mow and Hayes, pp. 143–198. Raven Press, New York, 1991.)

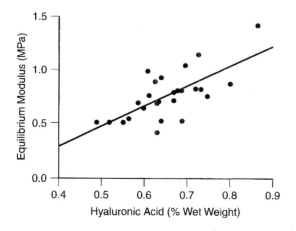

FIGURE 4.13 Dependence of equilibrium compressive aggregate modulus for human patellar cartilage on hyaluronic acid content (a surrogate measure of proteoglycan content). (From Armstrong and Mow in *Clinical Trends in Orthopaedics*, ed. Wilson and Straub, pp. 189–197. Thieme-Stratton, New York, 1982.)

more water, there must be less proteoglycan per unit volume, and therefore less repulsive electrostatic internal stresses to resist external loading. Degenerative changes during osteoarthritis include a decrease in proteoglycan content and an increase in water content, both of which degrade intrinsic compressive properties.

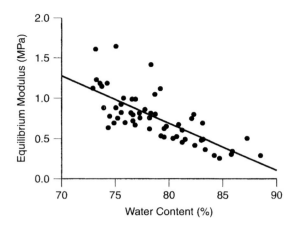

FIGURE 4.14 Dependence of equilibrium compressive aggregate modulus for human patellar cartilage on water content. From Armstrong and Mow (1982) *J Bone Jt Surg* 64A:88–94.

Dynamic Loading

The increased stiffness of cartilage under dynamic loading compared with its intrinsic static behavior—that is, its viscoelastic behavior—is due primarily to the flow of fluid through the proteoglycan–collagen matrix and the resistance to such flow offered by the porous elastic matrix. Because of this interaction of fluid flow and matrix elasticity, collagen is often modeled as a biphasic material, consisting of the water and solid (proteoglycan/collagen matrix) phases.

The relationship between the pressure gradient and fluid flow rate through a permeable material can be described by Darcy's law. For a specimen with a pressure gradient across its ends, but which is not otherwise compressed, this law can be written as

$$Q = \frac{\kappa A \Delta P}{t}$$

where Q is the volumetric flow per unit time, κ is the hydraulic permeability coefficient, A is the cross-sectional area of the specimen, t is the thickness, and ΔP is the pressure differential between the top and bottom of the specimen. The hydraulic permeability coefficient κ is a material property, which determines the relationship between local pressure and local flow rate. Values of κ for healthy cartilage are very low, in the range 10^{-15}–10^{-16} m^4/Ns. The implications of such low values are that very large viscous frictional drag forces are developed between the fluid and matrix, such that large pressure gradients are required to force fluid through the specimen. For example, a typical cartilage thickness for the human proximal tibia is about 3 mm. Thus, with $\kappa = 1 \times 10^{-15}$ m^4/Ns, a one-dimensional flow speed (Q/A) of 10 μm/s for such a specimen requires a pressure differential of 30 MPa.

If the tissue is compressed and then the pressure gradient applied, permeability decreases due to both closing of the pores (compaction) and an increase in the fixed charge density (which slows the flow of water through the matrix). Thus, the permeability of articular cartilage decreases with increasing applied strain (Figure 4.15a), the so-called strain-dependent permeability effect. Permeability also decreases with increasing pressure gradient. One implication of this strain and pressure dependence of the permeability is that, while Darcy's law can be used to measure permeability of

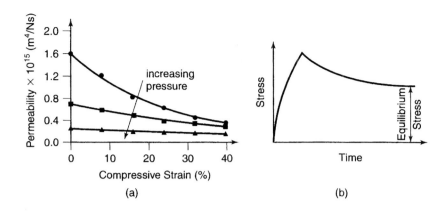

FIGURE 4.15 (a) Dependence of permeability of articular cartilage on compressive clamping strain and applied pressure gradient. Modified from Mow et al. (1980) *J Biomech Eng* 102:73–84. (b) Typical response for a stress relaxation test of articular cartilage, where a uniform displacement is applied and the stress relaxes over time to its steady-state equilibrium value.

cartilage, the hydraulic permeability coefficient κ should not be treated as a constant in structural applications.

More importantly, as cartilage is compressed and fluid is forced out, its permeability decreases, which has the effect of preventing further loss of fluid (Figure 4.15b). Thus, the cartilage decreases its own permeability as it is loaded more, increasing its dynamic stiffness and thereby stopping itself from bottoming out. So, when you stand still for a long while, cartilage can continue to sustain your body weight without your losing too much body height.

Compression of the specimen also compacts the matrix, thereby increasing fluid pressure. The extent to which fluid pressure increases by this mechanism depends in part on the permeability. In this way, external dynamic loads are supported by a complex interaction of stress in the matrix and pressure in the fluid—biphasic poroelastic behavior. The decrease in proteoglycan content and increase in water content that accompany osteoarthritis also increase permeability. These biochemical changes not only degrade the intrinsic properties of the matrix, but also the fluid pressurization mechanism of load support, leading to a cascade of events that compromise the load-carrying capacity of the cartilage.

The third phase of cartilage is its ionic content. When this ionic phase is considered together with the solid and fluid phases, the tissue is referred to as a triphasic material, which may provide direct support of external loads through development of fluid pressure by swelling. Swelling arises from two related mechanisms. First, because of the mutually repulsive electrostatic negative charges of the proteoglycans and their close confinement due to their entrapment by the surrounding collagen, a fluid swelling pressure is generated within the tissue, called the chemical expansion stress. Second, positive ions are attracted into the cartilage in order to attain electroneutrality, because of the high density of negative charges of the proteoglycans within the cartilage. This results in an increase in ion concentration within the tissue, compared with its external fluid environment, and that in turn attracts fluid into the tissue in an attempt to reduce the concentration gradient. This produces another aspect of swelling pressure within the tissue called the Donnan osmotic pressure. The degree to which the Donnan osmotic pressure develops depends on the fixed charge density of the cartilage relative to the ionic concentration of the external fluid. The fixed charge density for healthy cartilage is in the range 0.1–0.5 mEq/ml H_2O at physiologic pH; with osteoarthritis, it decreases as a result of the decrease in proteoglycan content. It's difficult to separate out the effects of the chemical expansion stress and Donnan osmotic pressure, but this can be done by altering the concentration of the bathing solution, since this will alter only the osmotic effect.

The total swelling pressure within cartilage is the sum of the chemical expansion stress and the Donnan osmotic pressure and is equilibrated against the elastic constraint of the stretched collagen fibers and any externally applied stress. Typically, total swelling pressure for cartilage under no external load is in the range 0.1–0.25 MPa, of which about 50 percent is due to the osmotic component. Since the swelling pressures are resisted in part by the tensile stress generated in the collagen elastic matrix, if the intrinsic tensile stiffness of the collagen decreases—as it does with osteoarthritis—the swelling volume will increase and swelling pressure will decrease, thus reducing the contribution of this mechanism to load bearing.

The contribution of swelling pressure to resistance of dynamic loads is not well understood, but is probably much less than the biphasic mechanisms associated with frictional drag of the fluid through the matrix. For this reason, in most biomechanical analyses of whole bone structures, the triphasic nature of cartilage is not included explicitly. Instead, the simpler (but still complex) biphasic model is used. Indeed, depending on the objectives of the analysis, it is often reasonable to model cartilage as a linearly elastic material with a modulus equal to a typical dynamic tangent modulus for a specified loading rate (typically 10–20 MPa). Such modulus values can be calculated from biphasic or triphasic constitutive models of cartilage; the quantitative study of these theories is beyond the scope of this text.

EXAMPLE 4.2 Dynamic Stiffness of Cartilage

Question   As we have seen, the aggregate compressive modulus of collagen is only on the order of 1 MPa. During gait, there is about 3–4 times body-weight acting on the knee, associated with contact stresses σ on the cartilage of up to 8 MPa. If the thickness t of the cartilage at the knee is 5 mm, what is the predicted deformation of the cartilage?

Solution   If we assume that we have elastic behavior and small strains, then $\sigma = E\varepsilon$. (This, of course, is not a valid assumption, since cartilage is not a purely elastic material and strains can be very large; but it is reasonable for obtaining a gross estimate of strains and deformations in cartilage when loaded.) Since, for these conditions, strain ε is the ratio of deformation δ to original thickness t, it follows then that $\delta = t\sigma/E$.

For the preceding numbers, this indicates that the deformation in the cartilage at the knee during gait is expected to be on the order of 40 mm! Even if our calculation is off by one order of magnitude due to our simplifying assumptions, it would still indicate a very large deformation—if the hip, knee, and ankle all deformed by about 4 mm, we would sink by about one half inch for each step we took, which is not reasonable. This calculation indicates that cartilage must be a lot stiffer than its equilibrium aggregate modulus for *in vivo* dynamic loading.

If we do the reverse problem and ask what cartilage modulus is required to give a deformation at the knee of, say, 0.4 mm, we find a value of 100 MPa. This simple calculation therefore suggests that cartilage should be about 10–100 times stiffer when loaded dynamically than when loaded statically. Direct measurements of the dynamic compressive modulus of cartilage provide support of this argument—values are typically on the order of 10 MPa. An elastic modulus value of 10–20 MPa is often used in elastic structural analysis problems to account for the increased stiffness of cartilage under dynamic loading conditions.

4.3   Intervertebral Disc

Composition and Microstructure

There are 23 intervertebral discs in the spinal column that connect adjacent vertebral bodies. The discs allow a limited amount of relative motion between the bones, while transmitting most of the compressive load in the spine. An intervertebral joint is classified as an amphiarthrodial symphysis type joint, as opposed to the diarthrodial synovial joints of the hip, knee, elbow, shoulder, and facet joints. Disc height varies from 4–5 mm at C2–C3 in the cervical spine to about 11–12 mm for L5–S1 at the base of the lumbar spine.

The disc itself is a heterogeneous organ, consisting of three elements: the nucleus pulposis, annulus fibrosis, and cartilaginous endplates (Figure 4.16). The nucleus pulposis, located in the middle of the disc and occupying up to about 50 percent of the volume, is a fluid-like viscous gel. It is composed mostly of water (70–90 percent content, highest at birth, steadily decreasing with age), proteoglycans, and a randomly oriented network of type II collagen. As with articular cartilage, the proteoglycans contain many negatively charged ions that attract water by a Donnan osmotic effect, causing the nucleus to swell. Unlike cartilage, however, the main resistance to this swelling is provided not by interspersed collagen, but instead by the surrounding annulus fibrosis. The annulus is intimately connected to the nucleus, and is composed primarily of 20–25 alternating thin sheets (lamellae) of type I collagen, similar to what occurs in lamellar bone, but without any mineral. Moving radially outward from the nucleus, the type I collagen content increases, reaching a maximum of about 70 percent at the outside surface, and the water content decreases. The lamellae within the annulus are stacked alternatively, with collagen fiber orientations of approximately ±30–35° to the endplate. The annulus is connected directly into the vertebral body similar to the ligament–bone interface. A thin layer ($\approx$0.6 mm thick) of hyaline

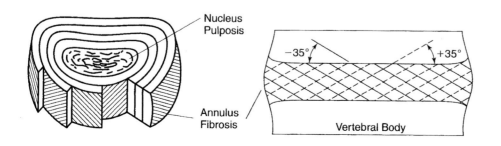

FIGURE   4.16   Schematic diagram of the structure of the intervertebral disc, showing the lamellar arrangement of the annulus fibrosis and the ±30–35° arrangement of the individual lamellae. (Adapted from White and Panjabi, *Clinical Biomechanics of the Spine,* 2d ed. JB Lippincott, Philadelphia, 1990.)

cartilage, similar to articular cartilage, serves as the interface between the bone of the vertebral body and each of the annulus fibrosis and nucleus pulposis of the disc. This is called the cartilaginous endplate. It is water permeable, allowing water to be transported in and out of the nucleus to the underlying trabecular bone within the vertebral body when the disc is loaded.

With aging, the distinction between the nucleus and annulus fades, with the former becoming more solid like. As will be described, this has profound effects on the biomechanics of this complex structure. Like articular cartilage, there is no blood supply to the intervertebral disc. (It is the largest organ without a blood supply.) Cell nutrition therefore occurs by fluid transport, which is determined by the biomechanical properties of the disc. Consequently, if the biomechanical properties are altered, say, by injury or degenerative changes, cell nutrition may be adversely affected, which in turn may lead to biochemical degradation by altered cellular activity. Like cartilage, there is no nerve supply, so the body has no direct sensory mechanism to detect damage within the disc.

Material and Structural Characteristics

Biomechanically, the intervertebral disc displays poroelastic characteristics typical of cartilage and nonlinear elastic characteristics like those of tendon and ligament. A healthy disc supports its mainly compressive loads, similar to the way inflated tires support the weight of automobiles (Figure 4.17a). The nucleus pulposis acts as a pressurized fluid and is contained by development of tension in the annulus fibrosis. The annulus develops tension in both the axial and circumferential directions, thereby subjecting the periphery of the underlying vertebral body endplates to tension in the inferior–superior (axial) direction. Meanwhile, the hydrostatic pressure developed in the nucleus pulposis applies an approximately uniform compressive stress (pressure) to the central portion of the endplates of the vertebral body. The total vertical compressive force on the vertebral body is equal to the integral of these axial compressive and tensile stresses acting on the endplates.

The mechanism of pressure generation and therefore load bearing of a healthy disc is as follows. The negative charges of the proteoglycans cause water to be transported osmotically into the nucleus pulposis from the vertebral body. The resistance to swelling offered by the surrounding annulus fibrosis generates an osmotic pressure in the nucleus. This results in a pressure vessel type behavior, whereby tensile

FIGURE 4.17 Load-bearing mechanisms for a healthy disc loaded by (a) a uniaxial compressive force and (b) anterior bending. (Adapted from White and Panjabi, *Clinical Biomechanics of the Spine*, 2d ed. JB Lippincott, Philadelphia, 1990.)

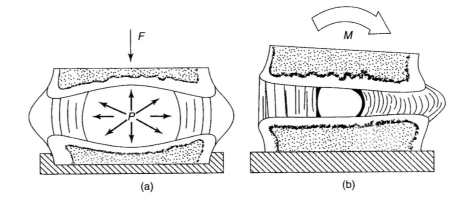

(a)   (b)

hoop and axial stresses are developed within the annulus (the vessel). If a large compressive external load is placed on the disc by the vertebral bodies, there will be a slight reduction in height, the annulus will bulge slightly but remain in tension, and some water will be forced back out of the nucleus into the vertebral body. When the load is removed, the water returns to the nucleus, height is regained, and the annulus straightens out. In this way, normal compressive loading causes cyclic transport of water, and therefore nutrients, in and out of the nucleus.

EXAMPLE 4.3 Mechanism of Axial Load Bearing in the Disc

Question Consider a vertebral disc subjected to an axial compressive load F. How is the load shared between the nucleus and the annulus?

Solution We use thick-pressure-vessel theory to model the annulus. Internal pressure p (in the nucleus) causes tensile axial σ_a stresses in the vessel (the annulus), which are constant across the thickness of the vessel, and which serve to equilibrate the internal pressure. This internal pressure is generated by osmotic water intake associated with the negatively charged proteoglycans in the nucleus. Compressive radial stresses σ_r and tensile hoop σ_h (circumferential) stresses also develop, which change in a nonlinear fashion through the thickness of the vessel. We therefore have a triaxial state of stress in the vessel. Theory of elasticity can be used to show that these stresses are given by

$$\sigma_a = C_1, \sigma_r = C_1 - \frac{C_2}{r^2}, \sigma_h = C_1 + \frac{C_2}{r^2}$$

$$C_1 = \frac{pr_i^2}{r_o^2 - r_i^2}, C_2 = \frac{pr_i^2 r_o^2}{r_o^2 - r_i^2}$$

in which r_i and r_o are the internal and external radii of the vessel and r is the radial coordinate for stress calculation. When an external axial force F is then added to the top of the vessel (the endplate), we must make assumptions as to how that load is shared between the nucleus and annulus. At one extreme, we can assume that the entire external axial load is taken by the vessel wall—that is, not transferred at all to the nucleus. In this case, the theory would dictate that the axial stress in the vessel walls σ_a must now equilibrate both the internal pressure and the external load:

$$\sigma_a = p\pi r_i^2 - \frac{F}{\pi(r_o^2 - r_i^2)}$$

This scenario would suggest that axial loading of the spine has no effect on disc pressure and would ultimately cause the annulus to fail by buckling, as its stress state would go from tension to compression as F increases.

At another extreme, we can assume that the vessel wall takes none of the axial load, and so the total internal pressure p_{total} must now balance the added external compressive force:

$$p_{total} = p + \Delta p = p + \frac{F}{\pi(r_o^2 - r_i^2)}$$

In this case, the tensile axial stress in the vessel wall remains unchanged, but the tensile hoop and compressive radial stresses are now increased due to the increase of pressure. This scenario would suggest that the pressure in the nucleus increases linearly with applied axial load, with concomitant increases in tensile hoop and radial compressive stresses in the annulus. Annulus failure would ultimately occur by tearing due to excessively high tensile stresses.

The truth is likely in between these extreme cases, since the load transfer of the external axial load to nuclear pressure depends on the poroelastic behavior of the disc, as well as the elastic properties of the endplate—a very complex structural problem. Further, it is thought that with disc degeneration, less of the external axial load is taken by the nucleus as it loses its ability to pressurize in a fluid-like manner.

Anterior bending of the healthy spine, common during daily activities such as lifting heavy objects and leaning forward, shortens the anterior aspect of the annulus fibrosis and lengthens the posterior aspect (Figure 4.17b). This decreases the axial tension in the annulus anteriorly and increases it posteriorly. Development of sufficient hydrostatic pressure in the nucleus, however, maintains net tension in the annulus anteriorly such that collapse of the annulus does not occur. (The healthy annulus, composed primarily of aligned collagen fibers similar to tendon, would collapse if it alone were subjected to compression.) In this way, the axial stresses on the underlying endplates of the vertebral body during bending change only slightly at the periphery and, for the most part, remain the same as for compressive loading. This ensures that the vertebral body of the healthy spine is subjected to similar stress distributions, whether loaded in compression or bending. Essentially, this biological design ensures that the vertebral body acts as a fulcrum, and all external bending moments are resisted by the action of the musculature about this fulcrum. It should be noted that stresses in the disc for combined axial compression and anterior bending add—but not linearly, since the disc is not a linearly elastic material and the pressure development does not scale linearly with the applied force F; stress analysis of the disc is a complex problem and is usually done with nonlinear computational models.

Due to the substantial changes that occur in the composition and microstructure of the disc with aging, the biomechanics of the aged disc are much different than those for a young healthy disc. Most importantly, the nucleus dehydrates with aging, and instead of behaving in a fluid-like manner, it acts more like a highly viscous gel, which is unable to develop large hydrostatic pressures. This reduced ability of the nucleus to develop hydrostatic pressure when loaded alters the overall mechanics of the disc, with serious implications (Figure 4.18). Compressive loads of the spine now result in direct axial compression of the annulus, since the pressurized tire analogy no longer holds. For bending, the situation is worse, as the annulus is subjected to even higher axial compressive stresses anteriorly. In an adaptive response to these new functional stresses, the annulus thickens over time, encroaching on the nucleus, and in some cases becomes mineralized. The stresses on the endplates of the vertebral body are changed, too, now being subjected to nonuniform compression, particularly for anterior bending. It is likely that these age-related changes in loading of the vertebral body by the disc are directly related to the large

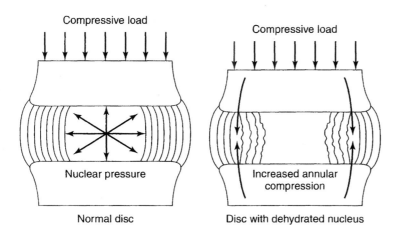

FIGURE 4.18 Comparison of the load-bearing mechanisms for a healthy (left) and degenerated (right) disc for uniaxial compression. (From Colliou, O.K., "Role of Mechanical Loading in Intervertebral Disc Degeneration," PhD diss., University of California–San Francisco, 1998.)

number of spinal anterior wedge fractures (in the vertebral body) that occur with aging. Thus, structural analyses of the vertebral body, particularly in the context of aging and osteoporosis, must ultimately account for how changes in the disc change the stress boundary conditions on the vertebral body. This is an example of the interaction between hard and soft tissue mechanics. It is important to consider the system, not just the components of the system in isolation.

The strength properties of the intervertebral disc are usually of interest because of clinical problems such as disc prolapse (damage of the annulus so that the nucleus can escape) and instability. If the internal pressure is too large on the annulus, or if pathological compressive stresses are too large, failure of the annulus can occur. To analyze such behavior, we must consider the material properties of the tissue, which, as with ligaments, are usually obtained by tension testing with the adjacent bone attached (Figure 4.19). Tensile modulus of the annulus tissue can vary from as low as 0.15 MPa for transverse loading (perpendicular to the lamellae) to over 400 MPa for longitudinal loading (parallel to the fibers); corresponding tensile strengths vary from 0.2 MPa to over 100 MPa. Because of the specific orientation pattern of the fibers within the lamellae of the annulus, maximum strength and stiffness occur for a fiber orientation that is oblique to the longitudinal axis of the spine. This configuration is optimized

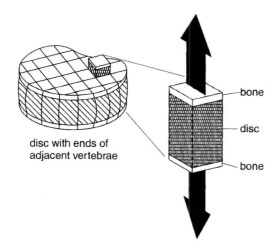

FIGURE 4.19 Specimen preparation used for tensile testing of disc tissue properties. (Adapted from White and Panjabi, *Clinical Biomechanics of the Spine*, 2d ed. JB Lippincott, Philadelphia, 1990.)

FIGURE 4.20 Standard linear solid viscoelastic spring–dashpot model for intervertebral bone–disc complex.

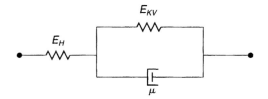

for resisting the fiber biaxial hoop and axial stresses that occur due to the pressure-vessel type behavior of the disc (see homework problem). Within the whole disc, there is a characteristic heterogeneity of tensile properties of the annulus, with specimens being strongest when taken from the anterior and posterior regions. These regions correspond to those where axial stresses are expected to be highest *in vivo* from common activities such as anterior (forward) bending. The central region is weakest.

For the whole disc, compressive stiffness is in the range 2500–3500 N/mm, depending on the level tested and state of disc, with a compressive strength of about 5000 N. Bending stiffness is in the range 600–8500 Nm/rad, depending on the plane of bending. Stiffness is highest for flexion–extension.

Because of its substantial water content, the disc is highly viscoelastic. To a first approximation it may be represented by a standard spring–dashpot model (Figure 4.20). This viscoelastic behavior is important for prolonged static loading, such as sitting for a long period, particularly with poor posture for which static loads of over one times body weight are easily developed within the disc. Typically, when a compressive axial load is applied to the disc and held constant, there is an instantaneous elastic response, followed by a creep response in which deformation slowly increases to an equilibrium value (Figure 4.21). It takes a healthy disc a few hours to reach its equilibrium configuration for normal habitual loads. If that load is then removed after reaching the equilibrium value, there is another instantaneous elastic response, followed again by a nonlinear creep response. However, the final equilibrium configuration does not return to the zero position—there remains a residual deformation. This loss of disc height is due to fluid loss. As a result, over a typical day, the combined shortening of all the discs is about 15–20 mm. Fortunately, this height is recovered during sleep, as the fluid reenters the disc while stresses are low due to the reclining posture and relaxed musculature.

FIGURE 4.21 Typical creep curve for an intervertebral body–disc complex, showing the nonzero deformation that develops after complete unloading. This latter feature is not typical of classical viscoelastic materials, but instead is due to water loss from the disc during loading. During sleep, this height loss is regained as the disc is rehydrated. [From Fig. 16, page 112, Goel and W einstein, *Biomechanics of the Spine: Clinical and Surgical Perspective.* CRC Press, Boca Raton, FL, 1990; originally Burns et al. (1984) *J Biomechanics* 17:117.]

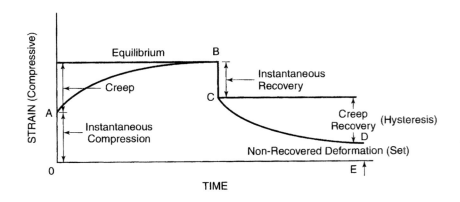

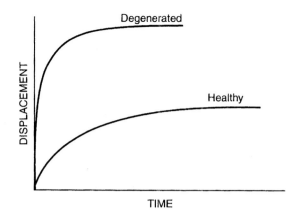

The creep response under a static load depends strongly on the state of disc degeneration (Figure 4.22). In general, the nondegenerated disc creeps more slowly than the degenerated one, reaches its final equilibrium configuration after a longer time, and deforms less. Thus, viscoelastic and stiffness properties are decreased with disc degeneration.

EXAMPLE 4.4 Loss of Disc Height Due to Compression

Question   Assume that, during any activity, most disc height is lost due to the combined shortening of the thoracic and lumbar bone–disc complexes. The intervertebral bone–disc complex can be characterized as a viscoelastic standard linear solid type of spring–dashpot model (Figure 4.20), in which the material constants have been quantified as $E_H = E_1 = 5.1$ MPa; $E_{KV} = E_2 = 7.6$ MPa; and $\mu = 19.6$ GPa-s. Assume that a stress of 0.55 MPa is developed during standing and is the same in all discs, regardless of their level or size. Assume also that the vertebra is relatively rigid, compared with the disc, and that the height of the disc H_i (in mm) varies in a linear fashion from T1/2 through L4/5, as follows:

$$H_i = 1/3(i - 1) + 3.6$$

In this case, the subscript i refers to the disc level: $i = 1-12$ corresponding to discs T1/2 – T12/L1, and $i = 13-16$ corresponding to discs L1/2 – L4/5.

   (a) What is the time it takes for the discs to reach steady state under constant stress loading conditions?

   (b) What is the total loss of body height for standing for this amount of time? (Think of the guards standing to attention outside some government buildings.)

Solution   As we will derive later in Section 4.5, the strain response to an applied uniform stress σ for the standard linear solid is as follows:

$$\varepsilon(t) = \sigma\left\{\frac{1}{E_1} + \frac{1}{E_2}(1 - e^{-t/\tau_1})\right\} \text{ where } \tau_1 = \frac{\mu}{E_2} = \frac{19.6 \times 10^3}{7.6} = 2580 \text{ s}$$

Thus, the relaxation time τ_1 is 43 minutes, indicating that about 63 percent of the steady-state deformation will have been reached by this time. If we approximate that steady state is reached when the exponential term has decreased to 2 percent, then this will take 3.9 times the relaxation time, or a little under 3 hours.

Inserting all parameter values into the strain equation, we obtain the total strain at this time:

$$\varepsilon(t)\big|_{t=3.9\tau_1} = 0.55\left\{\frac{1}{5.1} + \frac{1}{7.6}(1 - e^{-3.9})\right\} = 0.18$$

This strain value is constant for each disc, and thus the deformation of each vertebral–disc complex is obtained by calculating the sum of the products of the strain × height for each of the 16 complexes, since we assumed that the deformations in the vertebrae are negligible. Doing this summation over all 16 thoracolumbar complexes yields a total deformation of 17.6 mm. Thus, we would expect this loss of height after about three hours of standing. Care to do the experiment to test this prediction?

Damage and Failure

One clinically important spinal injury to the intervertebral disc is a tear or rupture in the annulus, termed a disc prolapse or, more colloquially, a slipped disc (Figure 4.23). In some cases, disc prolapse allows the annulus itself or the nucleus pulposis (by leakage) to come into contact with the spinal cord or other nerves exiting the spinal cord. This causes severe pain and in some cases loss of neuromuscular function in the lower extremity. The mechanism for this injury varies. One cause, arising from trauma, is the development of large circumferential hoop stresses in the annulus due to the high external loads. Another is collapse of the annulus, which can occur with disc degeneration, as the nucleus no longer develops sufficient hydrostatic pressure to keep the annulus inflated when loaded in compression. Since there is no blood supply to the disc, tears or damage within the annulus cannot be

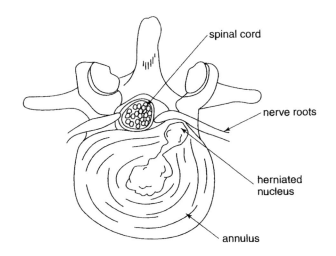

FIGURE 4.23 Herniated, or slipped, disc. Neuromuscular function can be compromised if there is significant impingement of the herniated disc against the nerve roots that exit laterally from the spinal cord.

repaired biologically, and therefore may accumulate over time. Thus, a third mechanism for disc prolapse is a failure mechanism that is similar to what occurs in trauma, but that occurs under apparently normal loads due to the compromised nature of the disc from previous, nonpainful microprolapses. A variety of approaches are concurrently being investigated to inhibit degeneration, repair injured discs, or replace the entire disc.

Another important clinical problem arising from disc degeneration or damage is instability. This term refers to when the disc deforms too much under functional loads, due most often to the loss of its ability to maintain sufficient hydrostatic pressure within the nucleus pulposis. When this occurs, disc height is lost, the surrounding ligaments become slack, and the entire motion segment (bone–disc–bone unit) loses the ability to remain upright under applied loads. The resulting gross movement of the motion segment can lead to physical impingement of the bone and disc elements against surrounding nerves or even the spinal cord, leading to pain and possible impairment of neuromuscular function.

4.4 | Muscle

Composition and Microstructure

Muscle is the largest tissue mass in the body, making up 40–50 percent of body weight. There are over 700 muscles, which have a variety of mechanical characteristics specific to their function. The muscle tissue of the musculoskeletal system is classified as striated voluntary muscle, since it has a grain to it (striations) and can be controlled by voluntary contraction (as opposed to involuntary muscle, such as cardiac muscle). As an organ (Figure 4.24), a single muscle consists of a collection of muscle cells, soft connective tissue, and an organized network of nerves and blood vessels. Muscles as organs vary greatly in their size, shape, ability to produce force, and fiber architecture (Figure 4.24, right).

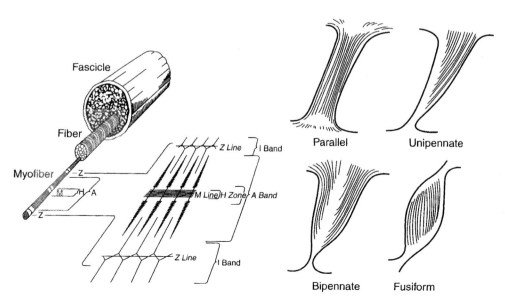

FIGURE 4.24 Schematic of the molecular structure of muscle (left) and the different gross architectures at the organ level, showing various arrangements of muscle fibers and fascicles (right). From *Orthopaedic Basic Science*, 2nd Edition, Buckwater et al, Editors, AAOS, 2000.

Parallel muscles, such as the biceps brachii and sartorius, have the muscle fibers aligned parallel to the overall axis of the muscle (the line of action between the tendons), whereas pennate muscles, such as the extensor digitorum longus, have their fibers oblique to the axis. Each of these structures is associated with specific functions. The pennate muscles are generally more powerful than their weight-matched parallel counterparts, since they allow recruitment of more fibers. Parallel muscles, however, allow for greater contraction, since their fibers are generally longer than those in pennate muscles.

The basic and most important structural element of muscle tissue is the muscle fiber, or muscle cell (Figure 4.24, left), which is about 10–100 microns in diameter, but generally extends along the entire muscle. Within the muscle cell are a large number of parallel smaller myofibrils (or myofibers), about 1–2 microns in diameter, which do not extend along the length of the cell. Within the myofibers there are two types of even smaller fibers, called thin (6 nm diameter) and thick (16 nm diameter) myofilaments. Thin and thick filaments are composed mostly of long aggregate chains of the proteins actin and myosin, respectively. Specifically, thin filaments are long rod-like chains of the protein actin, with a small amount of the other proteins troponin and tropomyosin. The latter proteins sit on the actin, covering sites that can form bonds with the myosin. Thick filaments are also rod-shaped proteins, but contain a round head at the end and project away from the main body of the rod. This projection is called a cross-bridge and can rotate about a pivot point when the molecule adenosine triphosphate (ATP) attaches to the myosin. The thin and thick filaments are arranged in parallel and slightly offset from each other in discrete units called sarcomeres. Each sarcomere is about 2.6 microns long. When a muscle is relaxed, the thick and thin filaments overlap slightly, giving muscle its striated appearance; when it is contracted, they overlap more as the sarcomeres shorten.

According to the widely accepted sliding filament theory for muscle contraction, chemical energy stored from the breakdown of ATP when it attaches to the myosin is stored as mechanical potential energy by way of a change in the shape of the myosin molecule. The cross-bridge rotates about its pivot point analogous to a wound-up torsional spring. This energy is released when the energized cross-bridge attaches to the actin thin filament at a specific binding site. The myosin molecule then reverts back to its original shape. Since the actin and myosin are still connected to each other at the cross-bridge, the actin is forced to slide along the myosin molecule as it rotates about its fixed pivot back to its low energy conformation (shape). The result of this is a shortening of the length of the sarcomere, although the lengths of the actin and myosin filaments remain constant. Continued supply of a new ATP molecule then breaks the bond between the actin and myosin, but energizes the myosin, and another cross-bridge cycle occurs. Thus, muscle contraction is the result of continuous cross-bridge cycling, which occurs at multiple sites along the thick–thin filament interface.

The strength of a muscle contraction depends on how many cross-bridges occur within a muscle fiber, and their rate. When the appropriate nerve cell (motor neuron) stimulates a muscle fiber, the concentration of calcium increases inside the muscle cell. This causes the binding sites on the actin to open, allowing bonds with the myosin to occur in the presence of ATP. Specifically, a calcium ion binds to the troponin protein on the thin filament, causing conformational changes in the tropomyosin protein, thereby exposing the myosin-specific binding site on the actin.

Thus, regulation of muscle contraction is controlled by the stimulation from nerve cells, but is mediated by intracellular calcium. When the body cannot absorb adequate calcium from food through the intestine to maintain adequate muscle function, it will take what it needs from other sources, such as the bone. For this reason, it is important to maintain adequate dietary calcium. This is particularly a problem in the elderly, who have a lower rate of absorption of calcium through the gut and therefore need a greater dietary calcium intake than younger people do.

Mechanical Behavior and Active Force Generation

Since muscle is mechanically active and can produce a force without deformation, it is unique among biological tissues. Motor neurons innervate a muscle by sending a short electrical potential to the muscle cells. A single motor neuron nerve cell innervates a number of muscle fiber cells, from about 10 to 2000, depending on the type of muscle.

In mammals, a single muscle fiber receives a stimulus from only one motor neuron. Therefore, a single motor neuron and the muscle fibers to which it is attached are referred to as a motor unit. Muscle fibers also obey the all-or-none principle: if stimulated above some threshold value, all muscle fibers in a motor unit will contract to the fullest extent; if stimulated below the threshold value, there will be no contraction; there is no middle ground. This does not imply that the strength of the contraction will always be constant for stimulation of a given motor unit; that depends on other factors such as oxygen supply to the muscle and ATP levels, both of which can be depleted during strenuous or cyclic activities. Therefore, the nervous system controls the magnitude of force produced by muscles by varying the number of motor neurons that are active and their frequency of activation, but this is mediated by a number of biochemical factors that can change with aging, disease, and activity.

At the organ level, when a muscle receives an electrical stimulus from a motor neuron, the response is discrete and highly repeatable (Figure 4.25). For the first 3–5 milliseconds after receiving the stimulus, there is no production of force, but the stiffness of the muscle increases. Then, after a latency period of about 15 milliseconds during which time the muscle still produces no force, the muscle produces a transient force, which rises to a peak and quickly falls off. This transient force acts for little more than one second and is known as the twitch response. The magnitude

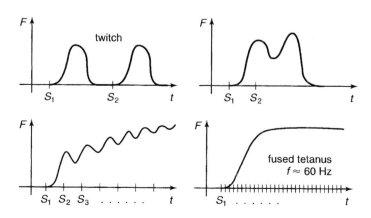

FIGURE 4.25 Response of muscle to an applied electrical stimulus. As the time between stimuli decreases, the identical twitch responses of each stimulus superimpose until, at high enough frequency, there is fused tetanus. (vertical scale not uniform across panels.)

of the force produced during a twitch depends on the type of muscle and the number of fibers stimulated. If the magnitude of the electrical stimulus is too small, there will be no production of force, but once it is above a threshold level, the magnitude of the force is independent of the magnitude of the stimulus.

If a series of electrical stimuli are delivered to the muscle, the force–time twitch responses add, which is evidence of some elasticity within the muscle constituent materials. If the frequency of stimuli is low, the overall response is termed unfused tetanus, in which there is a substantial ripple in the force–time response. If the frequency is increased to some threshold (about 30 Hz in frogs at 0 °C—a common experimental model used in muscle mechanics—or 60 Hz in humans at body temperature), fused tetanus occurs, in which the force–time response reaches a plateau with only a tiny ripple. Further increases in the frequency of the stimulus have no effect. The twitch–tetanus ratio—the ratio of maximum force in a single twitch compared with that in a fused tetanus—varies across muscle types from about 1:1.5 to 1:10.

Force–Length Behavior

Muscle force consists of both passive and active components. The passive component is simply the viscoelastic mechanical response to deformation. Inactivated muscle displays characteristics similar to passive tissues, such as tendon and ligament, that produce force only when deformed. If a piece of unstimulated muscle is clamped and extended, the force–deformation curve is qualitatively similar to that of collagenous soft tissue, with a notable initial toe region and nonlinearity (Figure 4.26 solid points; compare with Figure 4.2).

When the muscle is fully stimulated to tetanus, it produces additional force. Interestingly, it turns out that at full stimulation (all the fibers stimulated at tetanus) the magnitude of this force depends on the length of the muscle at which the electrical stimulation is applied. Experimentally, the procedure is as follows. A living muscle is excised and placed between two fixed grips that are set a certain length apart from each other. The muscle is held by its tendons at each end (Figure 4.26, left). It is then stimulated to full tetanus in isometric (constant length) contraction, and a load cell connected in series with the grips measures the total force exerted on the grips by the muscle. Thus, one data point is collected, namely, the current length of the muscle (distance between the grips less the length of the tendons) and the measured tensile force. Then the stimulus is removed, the length between the grips is changed, the muscle is stimulated to tetanus again, the force is again measured, and the second length–force data point is acquired. The process is repeated a number of times to generate a complete tension–length curve for the muscle. Typically, this

FIGURE 4.26 Left: Schematic of the experimental setup for conducting the tension–length experiment on live (excised) muscle. Right: Resulting tension–length curves (X points—active; • points—passive).

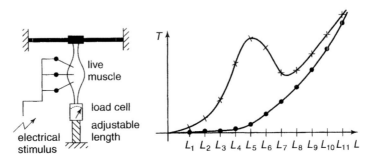

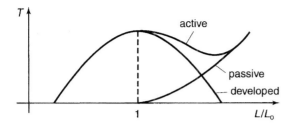

FIGURE **4.27** Tension–length curve for muscle, showing the active, passive, and developed tension responses. The length variable is nor malized by the resting length L_o.

curve has a local maximum followed by a dip and a rise (Figure 4.26, right). The precise shape of this active response curve response depends on the architecture of the muscle (parallel versus pennate, etc.) and the orientation of its fibers.

If one subtracts the passive response from the active response, one can extract the force produced exclusively by the contractile machinery of the muscle, the developed tension (Figure 4.27). This tension–length response is typically quadratic shaped, in which the maximum tension developed occurs at the resting length of the muscle, the length of the muscle in an anatomically relaxed configuration. If the muscle length is too small, it cannot produce force when stimulated, and if the muscle is extended too much, it cannot produce force from electrical stimulation (although it is clearly stretched elastically, thereby producing a large passive force).

One clinical implication of the nonlinear shape of the active tension–length curve is that there is typically a particular length—the resting length—at which a muscle can produce a local maximum force when stimulated. If the muscle resting length is changed surgically, then the muscle strength will be reduced. One example of this is in lateralization of the greater trochanter, in which the greater trochanter (and gluteal hip abductors) during total hip replacement is sometimes displaced slightly laterally and distally in an attempt to reduce the required muscle forces for joint stabilization, and concomitant with that, a reduction of the hip-joint contact force. But the price required is lengthening of the abductors, which will reduce the maximum possible force they can generate. Thus, the overall efficacy of this procedure is not clear, and we see a classic example of competing objectives in the overall outcome.

It should be noted that the tension–length characteristics described so far are for fully stimulated muscles. For most activities, we do not fully stimulate our muscles, because not all motor neurons are firing, and thus not all motor units and fibers within the muscle are active. As a result, the tension–length curve for muscle does not dictate what the tensile force in the muscle will be at any given length. Instead, it describes the maximum possible tensile force that the muscle can produce when all motor units within the muscle are active.

Force–Velocity Behavior

The amount of force that an active muscle can produce also depends upon how fast the muscle is contracting. Common experience tells us this: You can do an elbow flexion dumbbell exercise faster when the weight in your hand is lighter. It turns out that, for shortening of muscle (the usual type of physiological activity), the maximum force produced occurs when the muscle is at rest—isometric contraction. At any given muscle length, this force would be the value measured in tension–length experiments in which the muscle is held fixed between two grips and then fully stimulated. As the velocity of shortening increases, the force–velocity profile exhibits the

FIGURE   4.28 Force–velocity and power–velocity relations for muscle. The maximum velocity v_{max} is used to normalize the velocity values. Maximum power is produced at about one-third of the maximum shortening velocity.

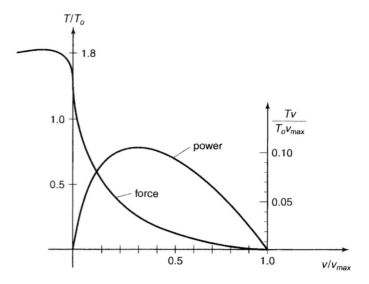

shape of a hyperbola, in which the force quickly falls off as the shortening velocity increases (Figure 4.28). For muscle lengthening (while the muscle is still contracting), the maximum possible force is much higher than for shortening. It has a plateau value of about 1.8 times the isometric contraction value, which is independent of the velocity of lengthening. So, if one wants to apply as large a force as possible to one's muscles during an exercise routine, the muscles should be lengthening. If one wants to avoid lengthening exercises (difficult to do safely), then isometric contractions will maximize forces applied to the muscle.

One important aspect of the dynamic nature of muscle force production is in the associated power–velocity characteristics. Power is the product of force and velocity. The power–velocity curve for shortening has a parabolic shape (Figure 4.28), and the local maximum typically occurs at a shortening velocity of about one-third the maximum possible velocity. A practical application of this is in the design of gear systems in bicycles. Maximum human power can be output if the leg muscles contract at about one third of their maximum shortening velocity. The gears then allow you to control the rate of rotation of the legs, thereby controlling muscle contraction velocity and optimizing power output. Advanced exercise machines are designed to control for the force–length and power–velocity characteristics of muscle in an attempt to maximize performance parameters such as muscle force and power over as wide a range of motion as possible.

Muscle Force Modeling

As discussed earlier in our treatment of the force distribution problem in joint mechanics, the maximum possible stress in most muscles is about 0.2 MPa, regardless of the size or shape of the muscle. This allows us to scale the relative force-producing capacity of different sized muscles, since this uniform stress principle dictates that maximum muscle force scales with physiological cross-sectional area of the muscle. This scaling law refers only to the maximum force capacity of the muscle, when all motor units are active. Unless we know the percentage of the motor units within a muscle that have been stimulated—a very

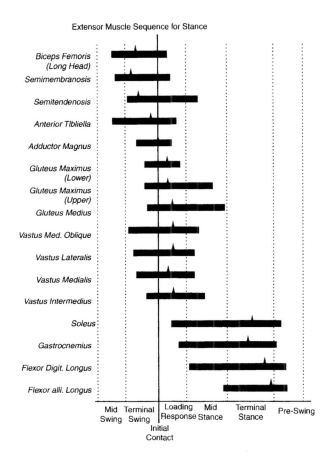

FIGURE 4.29 On–off diagram of EMG muscle activity for the extensor muscle sequence for the stance phase of gait. From Perry J., *Gait Analysis-Normal and Pathological Function*, Thorofare, NJ: Slack 1992.

difficult task—it is not possible to determine the tensile force in an active muscle from its size or length. Even so, one common strategy is to assume that the scaling law also applies at any level of stimulation. This, of course, assumes that muscles uniformly scale the percentage of muscle fibers being stimulated, which is somewhat tenuous. Results from such analyses should be interpreted with these limitations in mind.

The best available tool to directly measure muscle stimulation is electromyography (EMG), whereby the muscle's electrical activity is detected by surface electrodes or, preferably, by thin needle electrode probes placed within the muscle. The main drawback of this technology is that it is difficult to calibrate the transducer to actual force measurement, since the probes can detect electrical activity only in their immediate vicinity. If probes are placed such that they miss some motor units, or the position of the probe with respect to the motor units changes (as it does during length changes of the muscle), the activity of these motor units will go undetected. For this reason, EMG is used most reliably to determine simply if a muscle is active or not (Figure 4.29). EMG is widely used in studies of human activity and is used to validate muscle loading about joints predicted by theoretical models. For example, a subject can be asked to perform different tasks without removing the EMG probes to confirm which muscles become active for the various tasks.

4.5 | Viscoelasticity

Most biological materials, many polymers, and almost all metals at high temperature have material properties that depend on the temporal loading history, including the time rate of applied loads. When such materials are loaded to stress or strain levels that do not cause any type of irreversible failure, the resulting time-dependent behavior is referred to as viscoelasticity. The first part of this term refers to the viscous nature of the material, in which the applied stress is proportional to the time rate of change of the strain, a simple example being a Newtonian fluid. The second part of the term refers to its elastic behavior, in which the stress is proportional to the instantaneous magnitude of the strain, as with a Hookean spring. Thus, viscoelastic materials display characteristics of both viscous fluids and elastic solids, cartilage being a classic example.

Viscoelastic behavior has a number of different manifestations. The most common is a sensitivity of material properties to the rate of applied loading (Figure 4.30, left). Typically, strength and stiffness both increase with increasing rate of loading. A second manifestation is the phenomenon of hysteresis (Figure 4.30, right), in which the trajectory of the stress–strain curve for unloading is lower than it is for loading, even though the start and end points of the loading and unloading stress–strain curves are identical. In this case, the stress–strain curves for loading and unloading form a closed loop, and the area contained within the loop represents mechanical energy that is dissipated between loading and unloading.

A third manifestation of viscoelastic behavior is the phenomenon of creep and its inverse, stress–relaxation (Figure 4.31). Creep refers to the situation in which a material

FIGURE 4.30 A classical effect of viscoelasticity is an increase in both stiffness and strength with increasing strain rate $\dot{\varepsilon}$ (left). A second manifestation is the phenomenon of hysteresis, in which the loading and unloading stress–strain curves do not coincide away from the end points (right). The shaded area denotes the energy loss in one complete loading–unloading cycle.

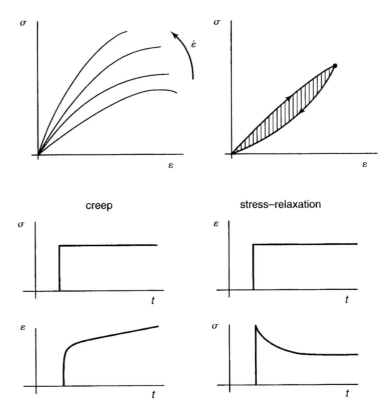

FIGURE 4.31 Creep (left) and stress–relaxation (right). In a creep test, a constant stress σ is applied; in a stress–relaxation test, a constant strain ε is applied.

continues to deform under a constant stress; stress–relaxation refers to the opposite situation, in which the stress decreases over time when a material is held at a fixed strain.

Bone, tendon, ligament, cartilage, and the intervertebral disc all display characteristics of viscoelasticity to various extents. From an analysis perspective, it is important to be able to discern when it is necessary to explicitly include viscoelastic behavior and when it is more reasonable to perform simpler linear elastic analyses, but somehow account in an implicit manner for changes in material properties that might arise from strain rate or other viscoelastic effects. This situation is analogous to study of dynamic effects in analysis of forces and motion of the skeleton. In some cases it is crucial to include inertial effects explicitly and use the equations of motion, whereas in other cases a quasi-static analysis with appropriate boundary conditions is sufficient. Whether to use one approach or another is problem dependent, and the same is true in analysis of viscoelastic effects. The remainder of this section will address the theory of linear viscoelasticity, followed by a series of examples that illustrate some practical applications. We address the theory from a one-dimensional perspective, since this captures the dominant concepts and yet avoids being encumbered by the complex mathematics associated with a fully three-dimensional treatment.

Linear Viscoelastic Models

The constitutive equations for linear viscoelastic materials are mathematically quite complicated, even in one-dimensional systems. Thus, in order to gain an intuitive understanding of viscoelasticity, engineers have devised a phenomenological approach for formulating the time-dependent constitutive equations in which the behaviors of Hookean elastic spring and Newtonian viscous dashpot elements are combined in various configurations (Figure 4.32). The constitutive equations for a linear spring and linear dashpot are

$$\text{elastic spring:} \quad \sigma = E\varepsilon$$
$$\text{viscous dashpot:} \quad \sigma = \mu\dot{\varepsilon}$$

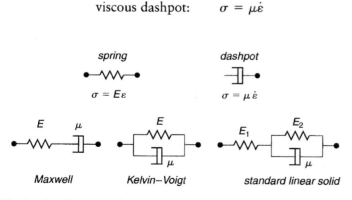

FIGURE 4.32 In the phenomenological approach to viscoelasticity, the overall constitutive equations are based on the behavior of a combination of spring and dashpot elements. Top: In linear viscoelasticity, we use a linear spring and a linear dashpot, in which the constants of proportionality between stress and strain or strain rate (E and μ, respectively) are truly constant. Bottom: Shown here are three common phenomenological models used in viscoelasticity: the Maxwell, Kelvin–Voigt, and standard linear solid. One can develop stress–strain relations by using any combination of the spring and dashpot elements.

where E is the Young's modulus of elasticity (units Nm^{-2} or Pa) and μ is the coefficient of viscosity (units Nm^{-2} s), both of which are constant during the deformation. $\dot{\varepsilon} = d\varepsilon/dt$ is the strain rate. In one of the simplest combinations of the spring and dashpot elements, the two elements are arranged in series, resulting in what is known as the Maxwell model. Its stress–strain relation is as follows:

$$\mu\dot{\sigma} + E\sigma = E\mu\dot{\varepsilon}$$

When they are arranged instead in parallel, we obtain the Kelvin–Voigt model, with its characteristic constitutive equation:

$$\sigma = E\varepsilon + \mu\dot{\varepsilon}$$

These two equations represent examples of one-dimensional constitutive equations for a viscoelastic material.

Unfortunately, these two types of models are inadequate for describing the behavior of most real materials. A simple model that has been applied successfully to many biological materials is the standard linear solid, a parallel combination of a spring and dashpot, all connected in series to a second spring (Figure 4.32). Its stress–strain constitutive relation is

$$\dot{\sigma} + \frac{1}{\mu}[E_1 + E_2]\sigma = E_1\dot{\varepsilon} + \frac{E_1E_2}{\mu}\varepsilon$$

One could derive stress–strain relations from models that contain the standard linear solid connected in series to a second dashpot, or indeed any parallel and series combination of any number of spring and dashpot elements—the more elements there are, the more degrees of freedom there are, and the more complex are the resulting constitutive equations. The challenge in practical situations is to use the simplest model that adequately captures the experimentally observed behavior of the material.

Stress–Strain Behavior for Simple Loading

It is instructive to study in more detail the behavior of these three models, since doing so helps to develop an intuitive understanding of the behavior of viscoelastic materials. Consider first the case of the Maxwell model subjected to a constant stress. For simplicity, we will assume that the magnitude of the applied stress is one unit, $\sigma(t) = 1$. Since the rate of change of stress with time in this application is zero, $\dot{\sigma} = 0$, the governing differential equation reduces to the following:

$$\dot{\varepsilon} = \frac{1}{\mu}$$

In general, when a stress is applied to a dashpot, it takes a finite amount of time for the dashpot to move. Thus, this element is infinitely stiff at the instant of any load application. As a result, when a stress is initially applied to the Maxwell model, all deformation will instantaneously occur in the elastic spring. The initial condition for this situation is that the initial strain at time zero is the ratio of the applied stress to the elastic modulus of the spring:

$$\varepsilon(0) = \frac{\sigma(0)}{E} = \frac{1}{E}$$

The solution to this problem is therefore given as

$$\varepsilon(t) - \varepsilon(0) = \int_0^t \frac{1}{\mu} dt = \frac{t}{\mu}$$

$$\varepsilon(t) = \frac{1}{E} + \frac{1}{\mu} t$$

So, $\varepsilon(t)$ is the elongation produced in a creep test in which there is the sudden application at time $t = 0$ of a constant stress of magnitude unity. We designate this particular solution as the function $c(t)$, known as the "creep" function and given by

$$c(t)_M = \frac{1}{E} + \frac{1}{\mu} t$$

where the subscript M signifies that this function is for the Maxwell model. For the Kelvin–Voigt model, the corresponding creep function is

$$c(t)_{KV} = \frac{1}{E}(1 - e^{-t/\tau_R})$$

in which we define the quantity $\tau_R = \mu/E$ as the "relaxation time" or "retardation time." This parameter designates the time at which the creep strain has increased to 63.2 percent of its equilibrium steady-state value.

We can also obtain equations for the response to the equivalent stress–relaxation test. In this case, a constant strain of magnitude unity is applied to each model, resulting in stress histories that we now term "stress–relaxation" functions $s(t)$, given by

$$s(t)_M = Ee^{-t/\tau_R}$$
$$s(t)_{KV} = \mu\delta(t) + E$$

where $\delta(t)$ is the Dirac–delta singularity function, a mathematical operator defined as

$$\int_{-\Delta}^{\Delta} f(t)\delta(t) \, dt = f(0), 0 < \Delta \ll 1$$

$$\text{and } \delta(t) = 0 \quad \text{for} \quad \begin{matrix} t > 0 \\ t < 0 \end{matrix}$$

These stress–relaxation functions describe the stress–time response in a stress–relaxation test in which there is the sudden application at time $t = 0$ of a constant strain of magnitude unity. One can derive stress–relaxation and creep functions for any combination of spring and dashpot elements. These functions for the standard linear solid are

$$c(t)_{SLS} = \frac{1}{E_1} + \frac{1}{E_2}(1 - e^{-t/\tau_1})$$

$$s(t)_{SLS} = \frac{E_1 E_2}{E_1 + E_2}\left\{1 + \frac{E_1}{E_2} e^{-t/\tau_2}\right\}$$

where

$$\tau_1 = \frac{\mu}{E_2} \text{ and } \tau_2 = \frac{\mu}{E_1 + E_2}$$

are the relevant relaxation times.

It is instructive to qualitatively compare the creep and stress–relaxation functions for the Maxwell, Kelvin–Voigt, and standard linear solid models (Figure 4.33). It is seen that for the Maxwell model, the sudden application of a stress produces an instantaneous deflection in the spring, followed by a linear deformation of the dashpot. By contrast, application of a constant strain produces an instantaneous stress in the spring followed by a reduction in stress. In the Kelvin–Voigt model, the application of a constant stress produces no initial deformation, because the dashpot cannot respond instantaneously to the application of stress. Since it is connected in parallel with the spring, the deformation of the spring is therefore constrained. When the system does deform, deformation increases exponentially due to the influence of the dashpot. The stress relaxation of the Kelvin model displays a mathematical discontinuity at the application of the initial strain, reflecting again the inability of the dashpot to respond instantaneously to a step input in stress or strain. The response of the standard linear solid shows characteristics of both responses. Initially, the response is determined by the spring that it is attached in series to the Kelvin–Voigt element. Under steady-state conditions, the dashpot has ceased to deform and the system behaves like two springs in series. Note that when the loads are removed, the response is simply the equal, but opposite, of the original loading response. This is an example of linear superposition, which is a characteristic of linear viscoelasticity. This concept will be discussed later in more detail.

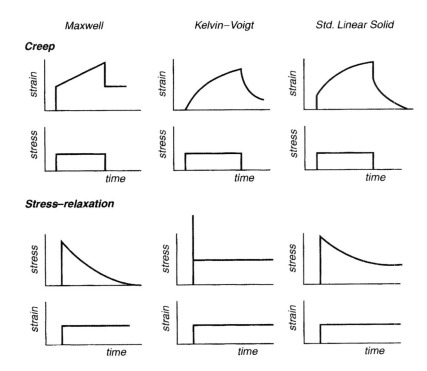

FIGURE 4.33 The creep and stress–relaxation functions for the Maxwell, Kelvin–Voigt, and standard linear solid models, in response to the stress and strain time histories, as shown.

Another interesting manifestation of viscoelasticity is that even though a viscoelastic material contains linear springs and a linear dashpot, when a constant rate of deformation is applied to the material, a nonlinear stress–strain response is observed (Figure 4.34). The standard linear solid model demonstrates this effect nicely. When the strain rate is constant ($\dot{\varepsilon} = R$), the initial conditions dictate that both the stress and strain are initially zero: $\sigma(0) = \varepsilon(0) = 0$. For these conditions, the governing differential equation is

$$\dot{\sigma} + a\sigma = E_1 R + bRt$$

where the constants are

$$a = \frac{1}{\tau_2} = \frac{E_1 + E_2}{\mu} \text{ and } b = \frac{E_1 E_2}{\mu}$$

The resulting stress-vs.-time solution (derive as an exercise) is

$$\sigma(t) = R\left[\frac{aE_1 - b}{a^2}\right](1 - e^{-t/\tau_2}) + \frac{b}{a}Rt$$

Noting that $\varepsilon = Rt$, a graph of stress versus strain (Figure 4.34) illustrates the main characteristics of this solution. Initially, the tangent modulus (the instantaneous slope of the stress–strain curve) is equal to E_1. This is followed by a nonlinear portion of the stress–strain curve that has a decreasing tangent modulus. At steady state ($\varepsilon = Rt \rightarrow \infty$), the stress–strain curve becomes a straight line, characteristic of a system that acts as two elastic springs in series, having slope $E_1 E_2/(E_1 + E_2)$.

Stress–Strain Behavior for General Loading

So far, we have mostly discussed the response to a single input stress or strain. More practically relevant is the response of the viscoelastic material to an arbitrary history of either stress or strain. For an elastic material, once either the stress or strain at any instant is specified, the corresponding stress or strain at that instant can be calculated from the elastic constitutive properties. Time is not relevant for elastic materials. However, for a viscoelastic material, because its material properties depend on

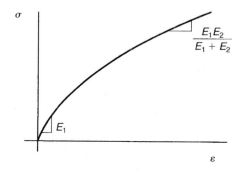

FIGURE 4.34 Illustration of the nonlinearity of the monotonic stress–strain response for a constant strain-rate loading experiment of a standard linear solid material. At steady-state (large values of strain), the response is approximately linear.

FIGURE 4.35 Example of discrete (left) and continuous (right) load histories. Linear superposition theory dictates that the overall response to an arbitrary load history is the sum of the individual responses to each increment in load.

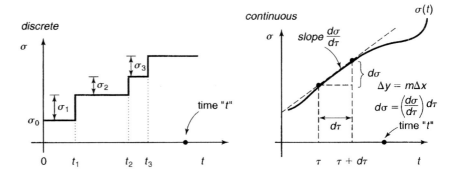

time, the past history of mechanical loading can also influence the instantaneous response to any new load application. Thus, the stress–strain curve can be nonlinear for a linear viscoelastic material, as seen by the preceding example of the standard linear solid subjected to a constant strain rate. The defining characteristic of a *linear* viscoelastic material is that linear superposition can be used to determine the response to a combination of loading cases. A nonlinearly viscoelastic material contains nonlinear springs and/or dashpot elements, and thus the linear superposition of loading cases does not apply.

Armed with the principle of linear superposition, the response of a linear viscoelastic material to an arbitrary load history can be found with knowledge of only the creep and stress–relaxation functions. Consider the case in which a constant stress σ_0 is applied to a linear viscoelastic material at time t_0. The strain response to this stress is given by $\varepsilon(t) = c(t)\sigma_0$, where $c(t)$ is the creep function previously described. Now consider the situation when the stress is increased by an amount σ_1 at t_1, σ_2 at t_2, and, finally, σ_3 at t_3 (Figure 4.35, left). Then the resulting strain $\varepsilon(t)$ will simply be the linear combination of the strain histories produced by applying each of the incremental stresses acting at the time that those stresses were applied; that is,

$$\varepsilon(t) = \sigma_0 c(t - 0) + \sigma_1 c(t - t_1) + \sigma_2 c(t - t_2) + \sigma_3 c(t - t_3)$$

$$\text{i.e., } \varepsilon(t) = \sum_{i=0}^{3} \sigma_i c(t - t_i)$$

where σ_i is the *incremental* stress.

Consider now the case where, instead of having discrete increments in stress, the stress history over time $\sigma(t)$ is mathematically continuous and smooth (Figure 4.35, right). In this case, the increment in stress, $d\sigma$, that occurs over a time increment, $d\tau$, is $d\sigma = (d\sigma/d\tau)d\tau$. Expressing the equivalent of the foregoing summation in integral form in which the incremental stress σ_i is set equal to $d\sigma$, we arrive at an expression that gives a value of the total strain at any time t as an integral function of the entire preceding stress history:

$$\varepsilon(t) = \int_{-\infty}^{t} \frac{d\sigma(\tau)}{d\tau} c(t - \tau)\, d\tau$$

This integral is called a "hereditary" integral. This equation states that the strain $\varepsilon(t)$ at any time, t, depends on the entire load history $\sigma(t)$ up to that time—the material has memory. For example, one can have the same stress acting on two specimens of the same viscoelastic material at a particular instant, but if the *previous* stress histories differ, the resulting strains in the two specimens can differ. Note that if the stress is zero at the start of an experiment (i.e., if there are no residual stresses in the material), then the aforementioned time integral extends only from time $t = 0$, and the hereditary integral is

$$\varepsilon(t) = \int_0^t \frac{d\sigma(\tau)}{d\tau} c(t - \tau)\, d\tau$$

EXAMPLE 4.5 Stress–Strain Behavior Under Sinusoidal Loading

Question   Consider a viscoelastic material with no residual stress that can be characterized by the three-parameter standard linear solid model. What is the strain response to the imposed sinusoidal stress history $\sigma(t) = \sigma_0 \sin \omega t$?

Solution   The strain response is given by the heriditary integral

$$\varepsilon(t) = \int_0^t \frac{d\sigma(\tau)}{d\tau} c(t - \tau)\, d\tau$$

where $\sigma(\tau) = \sigma_0 \sin \omega \tau$, and thus

$$\frac{d\sigma(\tau)}{d\tau} = \sigma_0 \omega \cos \omega \tau$$

From our earlier discussion of the creep function for the standard linear solid, we see that

$$c(t - \tau) = c(t - \tau)^{SLS} = \frac{1}{E_1} + \frac{1}{E_2}(1 - e^{-(t-\tau)/\tau_1})$$

Inserting these expressions into the heriditary integral, we obtain

$$\varepsilon(t) = \int_0^t \sigma_0 \omega \cos \omega \tau \left\{ \frac{1}{E_1} + \frac{1}{E_2}(1 - e^{-(t-\tau)/\tau_1}) \right\} d\tau$$

Performing the easier integrals first, we obtain the intermediate result

$$\varepsilon(t) = \sigma_0 \sin \omega t \left\{ \frac{1}{E_1} + \frac{1}{E_2} \right\} - \frac{\sigma_0 \omega}{E_2} \int_0^t \cos \omega \tau \{ e^{-(t-\tau)/\tau_1} \}\, d\tau$$

and by completing the integration by parts, we obtain the following solution:

$$\varepsilon(t) = \sigma_0 \sin \omega t \left(\frac{1}{E_1} + \frac{1}{E_2} \right) - \frac{\sigma_0 \omega \tau_1}{E_2(1 + \omega^2 \tau_1^2)} \{ \cos \omega t - e^{-t/\tau_1} + \omega \tau_1 \sin \omega t \}$$

For steady state—that is, when $t \gg \tau_1$—the exponential term vanishes. Thus, for steady state, standard algebra further simplifies this expression to

$$\varepsilon(t) = \varepsilon_0 \sin(\omega t - \delta)$$

where

$$\varepsilon_0 = \sqrt{\left\{ \frac{\sigma_0 \omega \tau_1}{E_2(1 + \omega^2 \tau_1^2)} \right\}^2 + \left\{ \sigma_0 \left(\frac{1}{E_1} + \frac{1}{E_2} \right) - \left(\frac{\sigma_0 \omega^2 \tau_1^2}{E_2(1 + \omega^2 \tau_1^2)} \right) \right\}^2}$$

and

$$\delta = \tan^{-1} \left\{ \frac{\left(\dfrac{\sigma_0 \omega \tau_1}{E_2(1 + \omega^2 \tau_1^2)} \right)}{\sigma_0 \left(\dfrac{1}{E_1} + \dfrac{1}{E_2} \right) - \left(\dfrac{\sigma_0 \omega^2 \tau_1^2}{E_2(1 + \omega^2 \tau_1^2)} \right)} \right\}$$

As can be seen from this expression, the strain response is out of phase with the input stress by the phase angle δ, but has the same frequency. Note that E_0 and δ are both functions of the material parameters and the frequency of loading.

We are now ready to address the response of a viscoelastic material to some typical types of loads that might be encountered in biomechanical applications. Consider the case when cyclic sinusoidal stresses are applied to a viscoelastic material,

$$\sigma(t) = \sigma_0 \sin \omega t$$

Consistent with the results of the last example, it is typically found in experiments on real tissues that the resulting strains will also vary sinusoidally (Figure 4.36) and will have the same frequency as the applied stresses, but will be out of phase with the stresses. The strain response to a sinusoidal applied stress is given by

$$\varepsilon(t) = \varepsilon_0 \sin(\omega t - \delta)$$

Special terms have been developed to describe this sort of behavior. In particular, the *storage modulus* E_S and the *loss modulus* E_L are defined as

$$E_S = \frac{\sigma_0 \cos \delta}{\varepsilon_0} \quad \text{and} \quad E_L = \frac{\sigma_0 \sin \delta}{\varepsilon_0}$$

in which the *loss tangent* is defined as the tangent of the phase angle, $\tan \delta$, by which the resulting strain is out of phase with the applied stress. In general, a large

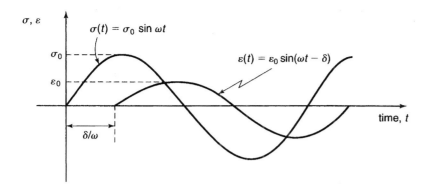

FIGURE 4.36 Typical phase lag response seen in a viscoelastic material in response to a sinusoidal loading regimen. In this case, the strain response is out of phase with the input stress history, but has the same frequency.

value of loss tangent will be associated with larger increases in stiffness properties as the loading rate is increased, and shorter times to equilibrium in creep and stress relaxation loading conditions.

4.6 | Summary

The main soft tissues of the musculoskeletal system are the tendons and ligaments, articular cartilage, intervertebral discs, and muscles. Tendons connect muscles to bones; ligaments connect bones to other bones; articular cartilage lines the ends of long bones and provides a very low-friction articulation between the bones; intervertebral discs allow limited relative motion between vertebral bodies; and muscles serve as the actuators that convert biochemical energy into the forces that provide motion and stability. Like bone, all these tissues are anisotropic and display substantial heterogeneity across individuals, anatomic site, over time, and with disease.

Tendons and ligaments are composed primarily of water (60–80 percent by wet weight) and an aligned array of type I collagen fibers and have similar material behavior in a number of ways. They are nonlinearly elastic, for which the stress–strain curve is well described by a two-parameter exponential model. Tendon tissue tends to be stiffer and stronger than ligament because of the greater alignment of its collagen fibers. At the organ level, there is tremendous variety in strength, since the size of whole tendons and ligaments varies so much with anatomic site. Aging is accompanied by large reductions in strength, and disuse can also produce atrophy, leading to loss of mechanical performance.

Cartilage is composed primarily of water (70–90 percent by wet weight) and a porous matrix phase consisting of type II collagen (10–20 percent wet weight) and proteoglycans (4–7 percent wet weight). Its dynamic mechanical behavior depends mostly on the interaction of the fluid and matrix components, which is influenced by the ionic charges associated with the proteoglycans. These charges cause the proteoglycans to swell, which is resisted by the collagen network, creating internal pressure. The fixed negative charges also draw water into the tissue by osmosis. The resulting low permeability makes it difficult for water to escape when loaded. As a result, this tissue is highly viscoelastic and can withstand much higher stresses when loaded dynamically than statically. An avascular organ without a nerve supply, cartilage is prone to damage and has very limited ability to self-heal.

The intervertebral disc is a complex organ composed of the nucleus pulposis, annulus fibrosis, and cartilaginous endplates. The nucleus pulposis, located in the middle of the disc and occupying up to about 50 percent of the volume, is a fluid-like viscous gel and is composed mostly of water (70–90 percent; decreases with age) and proteoglycans. Similar to cartilage, its negative fixed charge pressurizes it via an osmotic mechanism, but the fluid pressure for the disc is resisted by development of tension in the surrounding annulus fibrosis, a set of about 20 thin layers of oriented lamellae of type I collagen. Another avascular organ without a nerve supply, the disc undergoes substantial degeneration with aging, primarily characterized by dehydration and depressurization of the nucleus, fundamentally altering the load transfer characteristics of the disc.

The muscle tissue of the musculoskeletal system is classified as striated voluntary muscle, since it has a grain to it (striations) and can be controlled by voluntary contraction. Muscles as organs can be thought of biomechanically as actuators, because they can produce force independent of tissue deformation. At the molecular level, it is the "cross-bridging" of the proteins actin and myosin that generates such force. Muscle has a characteristic tension–length relation, which dictates the maximum force sustainable by a muscle at a given length. Muscle force capacity is greater for lengthening than shortening and decreases with increasing muscle velocity. Even so, maximum power output during shortening is achieved at about one-third of the maximum muscle velocity. Despite the huge range in muscle output force and power capacity, reflecting differences in muscle geometry and orientation, the maximum stress sustainable by muscle tissue is relatively constant.

Viscoelasticity is manifested in a number of ways, including strain-rate sensitivity, creep and stress relaxation, hysteresis, and certain types of nonlinearities in the stress–strain curve for monotonic loading. Linear viscoelasticity refers to the combination of linear elastic and linear viscous behaviors, for which the responses for different loading conditions can be superimposed. For sinusoidal loading, the stress and strain histories are out of phase. The storage and loss moduli are parameters derived from sinusoidal loading responses that describe the relative elastic versus viscous characteristics of the overall responses. These moduli are a function of the loading frequency. In some cases, a material can behave in a primarily elastic fashion at certain frequencies and a more viscous fashion at different frequencies. This frequency dependence is a characteristic of most viscoelastic materials.

4.7   EXERCISES

4.1 Discuss the viscoelastic properties of ligaments. Address the following: (i) preconditioning; (ii) creep; (iii) stress relaxation; (iv) strain-rate effects on stress–strain behavior; and (v) strain-rate effects on *in vivo* damage mechanisms (i.e., when connected to bone). Suggest a spring-dashpot model that can explain some of these characteristics.

4.2 (a) For the confined compression test on a piece of cartilage, assume that Darcy's law holds; that is,

$$Q = \frac{\kappa A \Delta P}{t}$$

where Q is the volumetric flow per unit time, κ is the hydraulic permeability coefficient (m^4/Ns), A is the cross-sectional area of the specimen, t is the thickness, and ΔP is the pressure differential between the top and bottom of the specimen. Assume also that the cartilage deforms under load such that its axial displacement rate is dominated by the volume loss of fluid, and further that it is given by the ratio Q/A. For a specimen thickness of 2.5 mm, and assuming a constant permeability of 10^{-15} m^4/Ns, show that the total change in height over a 250 second period is 1 mm—corresponding to a strain of 40 percent—when the specimen is loaded by a constant stress of 10 MPa.

(b) Assume instead that the permeability decreases in a linear fashion with increasing strain according to the equation $\kappa = \{1.6 - 3.25\varepsilon\} \times 10^{-15}$, in which ε is expressed as percent strain. What is the change in height for this situation? On the basis of these results, discuss the biological significance of strain-dependent permeability for articular cartilage.

4.3 The annulus fibrosis of the healthy intervertebral disc has its fibers oriented at approximately $\pm 35°$ to the vertebral endplate. When the disc is carrying load, the nucleus pulposis acts as a pressurized fluid that is contained by the annulus fibrosis, much as an inflated tire supports the weight of an automobile. Some insight into the structure of the annulus fibrosis with its characteristic fiber orientation can be gained by this analogy.

(a) Idealizing the intervertebral disc as a thin-walled pressure vessel, derive expressions for the hoop and axial stresses in the pressure vessel (radius R, thickness t, and internal pressure P).

(b) Show that the angle γ of the fibers in the walls of this pressure vessel—if it were reinforced by unidirectional fibers—should be oriented at 35° with respect to the endplate in order to resist best the hoop and axial stresses.

(c) Discuss the implications of these findings, if any, for the structure–function relationships of the intervertebral disc.

4.4 The risk of disc herniation is increased if fissures are present within the annulus. These fissures may be caused by age, disease, or an overload to the spinal column. We seek here to determine the effects of different types of fissures on the likelihood of disc herniation.

(a) Assume that the disc is a thick-walled pressure vessel with inner radius, $r_i = 5$ mm, and outer radius, $r_o = 20$ mm. Assume that a strenuous loading condition develops a nucleus pressure of 2.3 MPa and that the external axial compressive load is supported entirely by the nucleus. A fissure of length 5 mm develops in the annulus, which effectively reduces its load-carrying cross-sectional area (i.e., its radius is changed by the fissure length). Determine the percent increase in maximum tensile and/or compressive stress if (1) the fissure develops from the interior annulus to the outer annulus and (2) the fissure develops from the outer annulus to the inner annulus.

(b) According to these results, what is the worst type of fissure to have and why? How does this compare against clinical experience?

(c) On the basis of your knowledge of the morphology of the annulus, discuss physical failure mechanisms suggested by your results. Discuss also possible treatments.

4.5 Vertebral fractures may occur as the spine undergoes sudden axial loading. Under high strain rates, the discs can stiffen substantially, causing excessive loading of the adjacent vertebrae.

Here, we seek to evaluate vertebral fracture risk for a high rate of loading. Assume that the disc and vertebra undergo a total axial deformation of $\varepsilon_t = 10\%$ at a strain rate of $d\varepsilon_t/dt = 30\%$/sec. The strain rate in the vertebra is $d\varepsilon_b/dt = 0.5\%$/sec. Furthermore, assume that the disc behaves as a standard linear solid (E_1, E_2, μ) and that the vertebra behaves as a simple spring (E_b).

(a) Derive an expression for the axial stress in the bone as a function of ε_t, $d\varepsilon_t/dt$, $d\varepsilon_b/dt$, E_1, E_2, μ, and E_b.

(b) Figure P 4.5 shows the stress–strain response of the disc under quasi-static and high strain-rate loading. Use these data to determine the elastic constants E_1 and E_2. (Use experimental data only.)

(c) Under the given loading conditions, will the bone fail? Assume that $\mu = 100$ MPa/sec, and use reasonable values for the elastic modulus and strength of the vertebral trabecular bone.

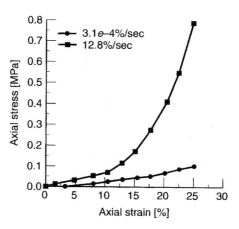

FIGURE P 4.5 (Data courtesy of Dr. Jeffrey Lotz, UCSF.)

4.6 The force–velocity characteristics of muscle for shortening can be described quite well by the hyperbolic function

$$v^* = (1 - T^*)(1 + T^*/k)$$

where v^* is the ratio of the shortening velocity to the maximum velocity, and T^* is the ratio of the tension to the resting length tension; k typically varies in the range 0.15–0.25 for most muscles. Derive the equation of the power–velocity behavior, and from that plot a graph to show how the maximum power output of the muscle depends on k.

4.7 (a) Read the classic research paper "An analysis of the mechanical components in frog's striated muscle," by B.R. Jewell and D.R. Wilkie (1958, *J Physiology* 143:515–540). With the aid of your own schematic of their experimental setup, describe the "quick-release" experiment that is now commonly used in studies on muscle mechanics.

(b) Plot graphs of tension vs. time and displacement vs. time that would be typical for this experiment.

(c) Describe a spring–dashpot–actuator model that can be used to describe this behavior. Label the series elastic, parallel elastic, and contractile (actuator) components of this model.

(d) What does the series elastic component represent physically?

(e) Describe how the data from the graphs in (b) can be processed to give a tension–length curve for the series elastic component and a force–velocity curve for the contractile component of your model.

4.8 One of the simplest possible models of muscle is the spring–dashpot–mass-actuator model shown in Figure P 4.8, characterized by the constants k, c, m, and F, respectively. The actuator represents the active contractile tensile component of the muscle and is assumed to be a constant force $F(t) = F$, $t \geq 0$, while the spring and damping parameters also do not change with time. For critical damping (i.e., when $c = \sqrt{4mk}$), show that the elastic force $K(t) = kx(t)$, where $x(t)$ is the motion of the mass, is given by

$$K(t) = K_{max}\{1 - (1 + \omega t)e^{-\omega t}\}$$

where ω is the natural frequency of the system ($\omega = c/2m$) and K_{max} is the maximum elastic force generated. As it turns out, muscle does in fact appear

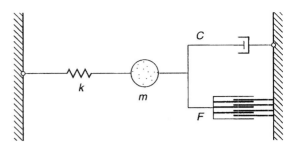

FIGURE P 4.8 Simple four-parameter model of muscle. (Adapted from Figure 4.4.10, page 412, in *Biomechanics of the Musculo-skeletal System*, ed. B.M. Nigg and W. Herzog. Wiley & Sons, Chichester, UK, 1994.)

to be critically damped (typical values for ω are 10–20 sec^{-1} for the biceps brachialis, for example), suggesting that muscles are tuned.

4.9 Derive expressions for the frequency responses of loss modulus and storage modulus for the Maxwell, Kelvin–Voigt, and standard linear solid models. Your responses should look like Figure P 4.9.

4.10 Compare quantitatively the strain rate responses of cortical bone vs. articular cartilage vs. ligament. Compare also the creep responses for these three tissues. Identify and use spring–dashpot type models for these tissues as part of your comparison.

4.11 (a) Derive expressions for, and compare, the steady-state strain responses to an applied stress $\sigma(t) = \sigma_0 \sin \omega t$ for the three spring–dashpot models shown in Figure P 4.10.

(b) Does the standard linear solid model behave more as a solid or a fluid? Explain.

(c) The standard linear solid model is composed of a spring connected in series to a Kelvin–Voigt model. Show that this is mathematically equivalent to a model in which a spring is connected in parallel to a Maxwell model.

4.12 (a) To develop a physical understanding of the frequency response of various linear viscoelastic models, consider first the stress response of purely elastic and viscous materials to a time-dependent strain of the form

$$\varepsilon(t) = \varepsilon_0 e^{i\omega t},$$

where ε_0 is the initial strain and ω is the angular frequency. Determine expressions for the storage (E_S) and loss (E_L) moduli for, first, a purely elastic material

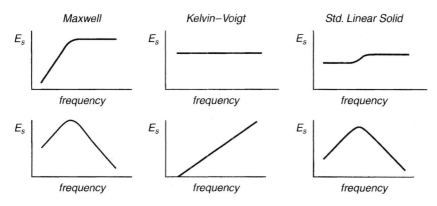

FIGURE P 4.9   Examples of typical frequency responses for various spring–dashpot models. E_s–loss modulus; E_s–storage modulus.

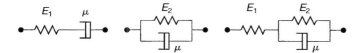

FIGURE P 4.11   Maxwell, Kelvin–Voigt, and standard linear solid spring–dashpot models.

of Young's modulus, E; and second, a purely viscous material of viscosity μ. For each material, what is the dependence of E_S and E_L on frequency, and how does this change if the Young's modulus and coefficient of viscosity are increased?

(b) The frequency response of the standard linear solid model of Figure P 4.11, having $E_1 = 20$ MPa, $E_2 = 30$ MPa, and $\mu = 0.1$ N/mm^2*s, as a function of the given sinusoidal loading, is shown in Figure P 4.12.

Notice that the storage modulus (E_S) makes a transition from a constant value of 12 MPa at low frequencies to a value of 20 MPa at high frequencies and that the loss modulus is only nonzero during the transition phase. By analyzing the behavior of the spring–dashpot model at steady state for various frequencies, provide a mechanistic explanation of this behavior. On the basis of this behavior, for what loading conditions would you say that this viscoelastic material can be well approximated as an elastic material?

Plot the storage and loss moduli as a function of frequency for the cases in which each parameter in the model (E_1, E_2, μ) is independently increased or decreased by one order of magnitude. Provide a mechanistic explanation for the trends.

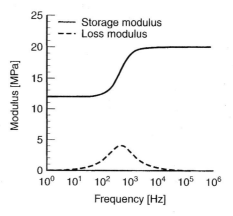

FIGURE P 4.12   The frequency response of the standard linear solid model (on a semi-log plot) to a sinusoidal loading, showing the storage and loss moduli.

CHAPTER 5

Structural Analysis of Musculoskeletal Systems: Beam Theory

Whenever stresses are calculated in a structure like a bone or a bone-implant system, a model lies behind the equations that we use. The model is an idealization of the structural behavior and leads to equations that describe the behavior. The same underlying idealization can lead to different equations. For example, the equations for beam theory are different for symmetrical and unsymmetrical cross sections.

Some models result in relatively simple equations like those from strength of materials for beam theory; the most complex models, like those for finite element analysis, can only be solved numerically by using a computer. In between these extremes lie methods based on advanced strength of materials or theory of elasticity. Each model and the equations associated with it can provide useful information if used within their limitations. The skill to be developed is to be able to choose the simplest model to do the job.

The value of simpler models is that the resulting closed-form equations provide visual relationships among key factors affecting structural performance. Furthermore, since the results from simpler models are embedded in more complex models, knowledge of their results provides data that can be used to check the output from more general theories. For example, simple beam theory can be used to check finite element analysis results in regions of the finite element model where beam theory applies. This is good practice; there is really no other analytical way to verify that the more complex model is producing results that make sense.

The structural behavior of a number of skeletal structures, including bone-implant systems, may be described by beam theory. In some cases, these structures may be modeled as one-material beams. In others, we will have to consider them to be composite structures that consist of more than one material. A bone strut, the neck of the femoral component for a total hip replacement, the elastic behavior of bone specimens, and the overall behavior of a long bone are examples of structures that can be modeled as one-material beams.

A fractured long bone may be treated with a plate attached with screws (Figure 5.1) or with a rod down its center. In both cases, after healing has occurred,

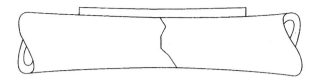

FIGURE 5.1 Long bone with a fracture fixation plate. The bone and plate, which is fixed to the bone with screws, form a composite beam.

the bone and the device form a composite beam, which may be modeled as a two-material beam. Bone specimens from the longitudinal axis of a bone may also be modeled as a two-material beam when tested in bending to failure. These specimens bend inelastically. As yielding begins, part of the cross section will behave elastically and part inelastically. The specimen can be modeled as a two-material beam, where one of the materials represents the elastic portion of the cross section and the other the yielded portion of the cross section.

When stems are used to fix components of total joint replacements to bone, a three-material beam results. For example, the femoral component of a total hip replacement (Figure 5.2) may be fixed to the femur with polymethyl methacrylate bone cement. The fixation stem, the cement, and the bone form a three-material composite beam. For cementless fixation, the interface between the stem and the bone may be a fibrous tissue layer, or in the absence of fibrous tissue, the interface may be modeled as a thin layer of the bone itself.

Beam theory, if used within its limitations, provides an excellent model for understanding the overall behavior of these bone-implant systems. In the sections that follow, we first develop the equations for symmetric one-material and multimaterial beams. The results are then generalized for unsymmetric bending.

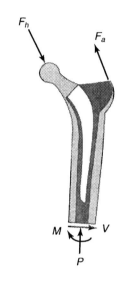

FIGURE 5.2 Proximal femur with prosthesis. This bone–stem–cement system may be analyzed as a composite beam.

5.1 | Basic Concepts

Our goal in beam theory is to determine the stresses in the structure as a function of the geometry, loads, and material properties of the structure. The derivation of beam theory equations is based on three elements: a strain–displacement relationship, equilibrium relationships, and material behavior.

All beam theory (one-material, multimaterial, inelastic material) is based on the assumption that plane sections before loading remain plane after loading. This establishes the displacement field and the strain–displacement relationship. For axial loading, this results in the strain being constant over the cross section; for bending, the strain varies linearly from the neutral axis.

5.2 | Symmetric Beams

One-Material Beams: Axial Loading

Two fundamental assumptions of beam theory are that plane sections before loading remain plane after loading and that the only stress is the longitudinal stress, σ_x, in the x direction. All other stress components are assumed to be zero.

FIGURE 5.3 Deformation of an axially loaded beam.

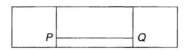

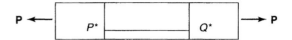

Since plane sections remain plane, the strain may be defined as follows (see Figure 5.3):

$$\varepsilon_x = \lim_{PQ \to 0} \frac{P^*Q^* - PQ}{PQ}$$

Since P^*Q^* is constant with respect to y, the strain is constant over the entire cross section.

For elastic behavior, from Hooke's law, we have

$$\sigma_x = E\varepsilon_x$$

where E is the elastic modulus of the material. Because ε_x is a constant, the stress may be written

$$\sigma_x = CE$$

From equilibrium (Figure 5.4),

$$P = \int_A \sigma_x \, dA$$

Substituting for σ_x produces

$$P = \int_A CE \, dA$$

Since C and E are not functions of position in the cross section, this integral simply becomes

$$P = CEA$$

from which C can be determined and substituted into the equation for stress

$$\sigma_x = CE$$

FIGURE 5.4 The axially loaded beam must be in equilibrium. The force due to the distributed stress must equal the applied load.

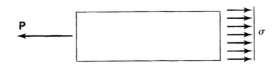

which gives us the familiar equation

$$\sigma_x = \frac{P}{A}$$

Notice that the elastic modulus, E, drops out; the stress in a one-material beam is independent of material.

One-Material Beams: Bending

For symmetric beams, we assume that the bending moment is applied about an axis perpendicular to the plane of symmetry, so that there is no out-of-plane bending. For bending, it is also assumed that plane sections before loading remain plane after loading. This leads to the deformation shown in Figure 5.5. The deformations vary linearly across any cross section, and we choose as the reference axis the axis that neither shortens nor lengthens (the neutral axis). We consider a short section at a distance t from the neutral axis.

The longitudinal strain is again given by

$$\varepsilon_x = \lim_{PQ \to 0} \frac{P^*Q^* - PQ}{PQ}$$

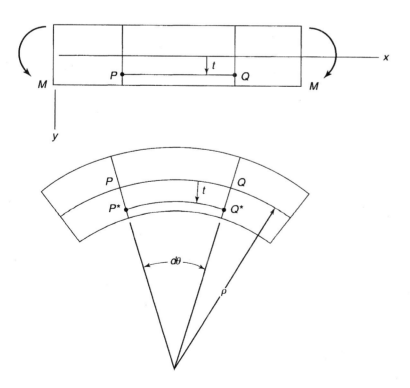

FIGURE 5.5 Deformation of a beam in pure bending.

Substituting for P^*Q^* and PQ yields

$$\varepsilon_x = \lim_{PQ \to 0} \frac{(\rho - t)\, d\theta - \rho d\theta}{\rho d\theta}$$

In the limit, this reduces to the strain–deformation relationship for bending, namely,

$$\varepsilon_x = -\frac{t}{\rho},$$

where ρ is the radius of curvature of the neutral axis. Again, for elastic behavior, Hooke's law applies, so

$$\sigma_x = E\varepsilon_x$$

From equilibrium considerations (Figure 5.6), the resultant moment at a cross section (Figure 5.7) is given by

$$M_z = -\int_A \sigma_x t\, dA$$

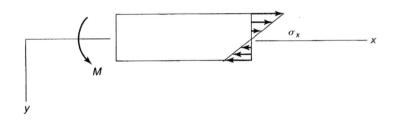

FIGURE 5.6 Equilibrium of a beam in pure bending. The moment of the distributed stresses must equal the applied moment; the axial load due to the stress distribution must be zero.

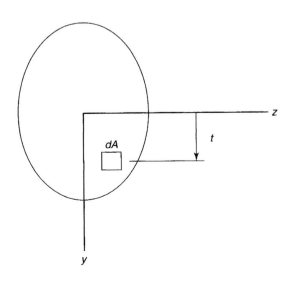

FIGURE 5.7 Cross section of a beam in bending.

The strain–deformation relationship and Hooke's law can be used to write the stress, σ_x, in terms of t and ρ, which gives us the following equation for the resultant moment:

$$M_z = \frac{E}{\rho} \int_A t^2 \, dA$$

E and ρ can be taken outside the integral, because they are not functions of position in the cross section. The integral on the right-hand side of this expression is just the definition of the second moment of area with respect to the neutral axis. Solving for $1/\rho$ and substituting this result into Hooke's law produces the well-known equation for bending of a one-material beam:

$$\sigma_x = -\frac{Mt}{I}$$

The location of the neutral axis is determined from the axial force at a section, which is given by

$$P = \int_A \sigma_x \, dA = 0$$

The integral is zero, because there is no axial force in the beam for pure bending. When the Hooke's law and the strain–deformation relationship are substituted into this equation, we find that

$$-\frac{E}{\rho} \int_A t \, dA = 0$$

The integral in this expression is the first moment of area with respect to the neutral axis and must be zero for a nontrivial solution. This can occur only if the first moment is computed with respect to the centroidal axis. Therefore, we deduce that the centroidal axis is the neutral axis of bending for a one-material beam.

Three-Material Beams: Axial Loading

In this section and those following, equations will be derived for beams made of more than one material, which are symmetric about the x,y plane. We will first develop the equations for three-material beams and then generalize the results for symmetric beams made of n materials.

The bone-implant system shown in Figure 5.2 is an example of a three-material beam that occurs frequently in orthopaedic biomechanics. It consists of three components: bone, a fixation stem, and an interface layer, which could be bone cement, cancellous bone, or fibrous tissue. A schematic of the cross section of a symmetric, three-material beam is shown in Figure 5.8.

The composite beam is assumed to deform as a one-material beam. That is, cross sections that were plane before loading remain plane after loading. Consequently, the strain relationships obtained for the one-material beam also apply for the composite beam. Therefore, for axial loading,

$$\varepsilon_x = C$$

FIGURE 5.8 Cross section of a three-material beam consisting of bone, cement, and prosthesis.

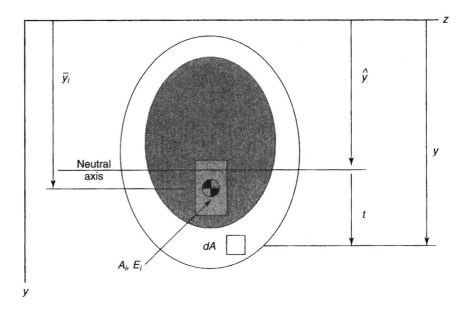

and for bending,

$$\varepsilon_x = -\frac{t}{\rho}$$

Linearly elastic behavior is assumed for each material; consequently, Hooke's law applies for each component of the composite beam, and we have

$$\sigma_i = E_i \varepsilon_i$$

(The stress and strain in this expression are in the x direction.)

Consider first a beam loaded by an axial load alone that is applied along the neutral axis of the beam so that no bending is introduced. From equilibrium conditions, the resultant load is given by

$$P = \int_{A_B} \sigma_x \, dA + \int_{A_C} \sigma_x \, dA + \int_{A_P} \sigma_x \, dA$$

where the subscripts B, C, and P indicate the bone, cement, and prosthesis, res-pectively.

Using Hooke's law and the strain–deformation relationship, and then integrating, we may write this equation as

$$P = C(E_B A_B + E_C A_C + E_P A_P)$$

where P is the total load acting on the cross section. Solving for the constant C and substituting into the stress-strain relationship, we obtain

$$\sigma_j = \frac{E_j P}{E_B A_B + E_C A_C + E_P A_P}$$

where σ_j is the normal stress in the x direction in the jth material. For an n-material beam,

$$\sigma_j = \frac{E_j}{\sum_{i=1}^{n} E_i A_i} P$$

where P is the total load applied to the beam.

Three-Material Beams: Bending

For a composite beam in *pure bending*, the equilibrium relationships are as follows. Referring to Figure 5.8, the resultant moment at a section is

$$M_z = -\int_{A_B} \sigma_x t \, dA - \int_{A_C} \sigma_x t \, dA - \int_{A_P} \sigma_x t \, dA$$

The resultant axial force at a cross section is zero for pure bending and is given by

$$P = \int_{A_B} \sigma_x \, dA + \int_{A_C} \sigma_x \, dA + \int_{A_P} \sigma_x \, dA = 0$$

After substituting the stress–strain and stress–deformation relationships into the moment equation and integrating, it becomes

$$M_z = \frac{1}{\rho} (E_B I_B + E_C I_C + E_P I_P).$$

Solving for $1/\rho$ and substituting into the material relationship, we obtain the equation for the bending stress in the jth material:

$$\sigma_j = \frac{-E_j M t}{E_B I_B + E_C I_C + E_P I_P}$$

Here, t is the distance from the neutral axis and E_j is the corresponding modulus. The minus sign comes from the convention for moment and curvature shown in Figure 5.6. It is very important to note that the second moments of area, I_B, I_C, and I_P, are computed with respect to the *neutral axis*. In general, the neutral axis of a composite beam is not located at the geometric centroid of the beam. The location is affected by the positions and material properties of the various components of the beam.

As is the case for one-material beams, the location of the neutral axis for a composite beam is determined from the equilibrium condition for the axial force. Substituting the stress–strain and strain–deformation relationships into the axial force equation, we can show that the location of the neutral axis for a three-material beam is given by

$$\hat{y} = \frac{\bar{y}_B E_B A_B + \bar{y}_C E_C A_C + \bar{y}_P E_P A_P}{E_B A_B + E_C A_C + E_P A_P}$$

where $\bar{y}$ is the location of the centroidal axis of the ith material.

The equations for stress and the location of the neutral axis may be generalized for symmetric beams made of n materials. The bending stress is given by

$$\sigma_j = \frac{-E_j M t}{\sum_{i=1}^{n} E_i I_i}$$

and the location of the neutral axis is given by

$$\hat{y} = \frac{\sum_{i=1}^{n} \bar{y}_i E_i A_i}{\sum_{i=1}^{n} E_i A_i}$$

EXAMPLE 5.1 Two-Material Beam Under Load

Question Consider a two-material beam consisting of bone and stainless steel that is subjected to axial loading.

Given that

$$E_1 = 17 \text{ GPa} \quad \text{and} \quad E_2 = 200 \text{ GPa}$$
$$A_1 = 560 \text{ mm}^2 \quad \text{and} \quad A_2 = 50 \text{ mm}^2$$
$$P = 1000 \text{ N}$$

what is the portion of the load carried by component 1 (bone)?

Solution The stress in component 1 is

$$\sigma_1 = \frac{17}{17(560) + 200(50)} 1000 = .87 \text{ MPa}$$

Note that the stress in component 1 of the composite can also be written as

$$\sigma_1 = \frac{P_1}{A_1}$$

from which we see that

$$\frac{P_1}{A_1} = \frac{E_1 P}{\sum_{i=1}^{2} E_i A_i},$$

and then obtain

$$\frac{P_1}{P} = \frac{E_1 A_1}{\sum_{i=1}^{2} E_i A_i} = \frac{17(560)}{1.952 \times 10^4} = .49$$

5.3 | Unsymmetrical Beams

We now turn to a more general formulation of the equations describing the structural behavior of composite beams. In general, the composite beams encountered in bone-implant systems are not symmetric. The cross sections of bones are not symmetric, and even though an implant may be symmetric about its own axis, it may not be placed symmetrically with respect to the cross section of the bone at the time of surgery. Therefore, even though composite beam theory for symmetric cross sections (described in the previous section) is extremely useful, there may be structural questions that can be answered only with the more general theory. A cross section of an unsymmetric composite beam is shown in Figure 5.9.

The cross section is placed arbitrarily with respect to the yz coordinate system. The origin of the ts system is defined to be located at the modulus-weighted centroid of the cross section, denoted by the coordinates $\hat{y}$ and $\hat{z}$.

The cross section can be defined by several regions, each with its own area A_i and elastic modulus E_i. In a bone-implant system, one of these regions might be bone, another the implant, and another an interface layer between the bone and the implant. In a whole bone system, the different regions might represent cortical and trabecular bone regions, or trabecular regions having different values of Young's modulus.

It is assumed that the composite structure behaves as a beam, such that plane sections before bending remain plane after bending. We will show that the neutral axis coincides with the modulus-weighted centroid.

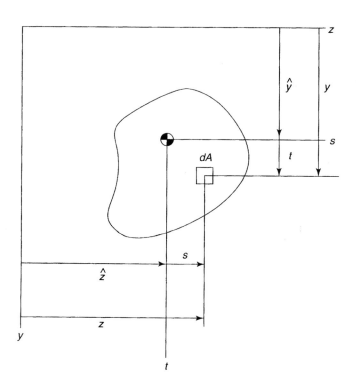

FIGURE 5.9 Cross section of an unsymmetric composite beam, denoting the modulus-weighted centroid at coordinates $\hat{y}$ and $\hat{z}$.

The strain at any point t, s in the cross section is given by

$$\varepsilon(t, s) = C_1 + C_2 t + C_3 s$$

The stress in the x direction, σ_x at point t, s, is given by

$$\sigma(t, s) = E(t, s)(C_1 + C_2 t + C_3 s)$$

where E is the Young's modulus, which can vary with position. The stress distribution on any section must be equivalent to the resultant forces acting on the beam. For axial loading,

$$P = C_1 \int_A E dA + C_2 \int_A Et dA + C_3 \int_A Es dA$$

For bending moments M_z and M_y, the following equations must hold (here, we're taking moment with respect to the modulus-weighted centroid):

$$M_y = C_1 \int_A Es dA + C_2 \int_A Ets dA + C_3 \int_A Es^2$$

$$-M_z = C_1 \int_A Et dA + C_2 \int_A Et^2 dA + C_3 \int_A Ets dA$$

Note that the negative sign in the latter equation is consistent with the right-hand rule convention. From Figure 5.9, it can be seen that $t = y - \hat{y}$ and $s = z - \hat{z}$. Therefore, the above equations become

$$P = C_1 \int_A E dA + C_2 \int_A E(y - \hat{y}) dA$$
$$+ C_3 \int_A E(z - \hat{z}) dA$$
$$M_y = C_1 \int_A E(z - \hat{z}) \, dA + C_2 \int_A E(y - \hat{y})(z - \hat{z}) dA$$
$$+ C_3 \int_A E(z - \hat{z})^2 dA$$
$$-M_z = C_1 \int_A E(y - \hat{y}) \, dA + C_2 \int_A E(y - \hat{y})^2 dA$$
$$+ C_3 \int_A E(y - \hat{y})(z - \hat{z}) dA$$

The second and third of these equations are associated with bending. The first equation is associated with axial loading. Since, for pure bending, $P = 0$ for all values of y and z, we must have

$$C_1 = 0$$

$$\int_A E(y - \hat{y}) dA = 0$$

$$\int_A E(z - \hat{z}) dA = 0$$

Because $C_1 = 0$, the neutral axis coincides with the modulus-weighted centroid. As with the symmetrical beam, these equations therefore define the location $(\hat{y}, \hat{z})$ of the modulus-weighted centroid and give information about the location of the neutral axis.

For a beam made of n materials,

$$\int_A E(y - \hat{y})dA = \sum_{i=1}^{n} \int_{A_i} E_i(y - \hat{y})dA = 0$$

Recognizing that, by definition, $\bar{y}_i = (1/A_i)\int_{A_i} y dA$, we can solve this equation to obtain the following expression for $\hat{y}$, the location of the modulus-weighted centroid in the y direction:

$$\hat{y} = \frac{\sum_{i=1}^{n} \bar{y}_i E_i A_i}{\sum_{i=1}^{n} E_i A_i}$$

Similarly, the location of the modulus-weighted centroid in the z direction can be found from

$$\hat{z} = \frac{\sum_{i=1}^{n} \bar{z}_i E_i A_i}{\sum_{i=1}^{n} E_i A_i}$$

We now look at the bending moment equations. Consider the equation for M_y. As we have discussed, the first term in this equation is zero. The second term can be expanded as follows:

$$\int_A E(z - \hat{z})^2 \, dA = \sum_{i=1}^{n} E_i \int_{A_i} (z^2 - 2z\hat{z} + \hat{z}^2)dA$$

The right-hand side integrand can be written as

$$= \sum_{i=1}^{n} E_i(I_{yy_i} - 2\hat{z}\bar{z}_i A_i + \hat{z}^2 A_i)$$

where $I_{yy_i} = \int_{A_i} z^2 \, dA$ is the second moment of area about the y axis. Using the parallel axis theorem, we can write $I_{yy_i} = \bar{I}_{yy_i} + \bar{z}_i^2 A_i$, where $\bar{I}_{yy_i}$ is the second moment of area about an axis that is parallel to the y axis, but through the centroid of A_i. After some algebraic manipulation, we arrive at the following expression:

$$\int_A E(z - \hat{z})^2 \, dA = \sum_{i=1}^{n} E_i \left[\bar{I}_{yy_i} + (\bar{z}_i - \hat{z})^2 A_i \right] = I_{yy}^*$$

Similarly, the term $\int_A E(y - \hat{y})^2 \, dA$ may be written

$$\int_A E(y - \hat{y})^2 \, dA = \sum_{i=1}^{n} E_i \left[\bar{I}_{zz_i} + (\bar{y}_i - \hat{y})^2 A_i \right] = I_{zz}^*$$

The third term to be evaluated in the M_y equation is $\int_A E(y - \hat{y})(z - \hat{z})dA$. Using the parallel axis theorem for products of area $[I_{yz_i} = \bar{I}_{yz_i} + \bar{y}_i \bar{z}_i A_i]$ and expanding the preceding equation, we obtain

$$\int_A E(y - \hat{y})(z - \hat{z}) \, dA = \sum_{i=1}^{n} E_i \left[\bar{I}_{yz_i} + (\bar{y}_i - \hat{y})(\bar{z}_i - \hat{z})A_i \right] = I_{yz}^*$$

These expressions can now be substituted into the previous equations for M_x and M_y to yield the following two simultaneous equations in C_2 and C_3:

$$M_y = C_2 I_{yz}^* + C_3 I_{yy}^*$$

$$-M_z = C_2 I_{zz}^* + C_3 I_{yz}^*$$

Solving for C_2 and C_3 and substituting them into the equation for the normal (bending) stress, we obtain

$$\sigma_{x_i} = E_i \frac{(M_y I_{zz}^* + M_z I_{yz}^*)s - (M_y I_{yz}^* + M_z I_{yy}^*)t}{I_{yy}^* I_{zz}^* - I_{yz}^{*\,2}}$$

Note that, for a single material beam where the product of inertia $I_{yz} = 0$, the equation simplifies to

$$\sigma_x = \frac{M_y s}{I_{yy}} - \frac{M_z t}{I_{zz}}$$

which is the sum of the familiar bending expressions for the two axes. Now consider the cross section shown in Figure 5.10, where the moment M is applied to the cross section at angle θ and the neutral axis of the cross section is at angle α with respect to the z axis. It can be shown that α is given by

$$\tan \alpha = \frac{M_y I_{zz} + M_z I_{yz}}{M_z I_{zz} + M_y I_{yz}}$$

Note that the angle α depends upon both the angle at which the moment is applied and the cross-sectional geometry of the beam and that, in general, the neutral axis does not coincide with the bending axis, which is given by

$$\tan \theta = \frac{M_y}{M_z}$$

FIGURE 5.10   Cross section of a bone, showing the y–z reference coordinate system, and vector representation of the applied moment M, at an angle θ to the z axis, and the neutral axis at an angle α to the z axis. Note that the sign convention for moments follows the right-hand-screw rule.

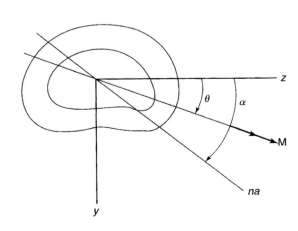

We saw that the equation for unsymmetrical bending is simplified when $I_{yz} = 0$, which is the case when coordinate axes are the principal axes of the cross section. If the coordinate axes are not the principal axes, the principal axes can always be found from the following transformation relationships:

$$I_1 = \frac{I_{zz} + I_{yy}}{2} + \frac{I_{zz} - I_{yy}}{2}\sec(2\phi)$$

$$I_2 = \frac{I_{zz} + I_{yy}}{2} - \frac{I_{zz} - I_{yy}}{2}\sec(2\phi)$$

$$\phi = \frac{1}{2}\tan^{-1}\left(\frac{2I_{yz}}{I_{zz} - I_{yy}}\right)$$

Then the stresses in the principal coordinate system become

$$\sigma_x = \frac{M_{y'}s'}{I_1} - \frac{M_{z'}t'}{I_2}$$

where s' and t' are measured from the neutral axis in the z' and y' directions respectively, and

$$\alpha' = \tan^{-1}\frac{M_{y'}I_1}{M_{z'}I_2}$$

EXAMPLE 5.2 Bending Stresses on a Tibial Cross Section

Question Assume that the cross-sectional properties of a human tibia are

$$I_z = 15{,}820 \text{ mm}^4, \quad I_y = 10{,}820 \text{ mm}^4, \quad \phi = 35°,$$

where ϕ is the angle from the medial-lateral z axis (Figure 5.11).

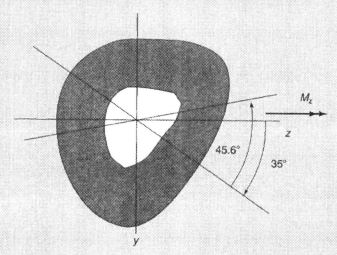

FIGURE 5.11 Tibial cross section with a moment applied about the transverse z axis. The principal axis z' is 35 degrees from the z axis.

We will assume that a moment is applied about the lateral (z) axis. What is the maximum bending stress? How does it compare to result obtained symmetric beam theory?

Solution   The moment components about the principal axes are

$$M_{z'} = M_z \cos 35° \qquad M_{y'} = M_z \sin 35°$$

Consider the point P on the periosteal surface along the y axis ($z = 0$). The bending stress is:

$$\sigma = \frac{M_{z'}y'}{I_{z'}} - \frac{M_{y'}z'}{I_{y'}} = \frac{(M_z \cos 35°)(y \cos 35°)}{15{,}820} - \frac{(M_z \sin 35°)(-y \sin 35°)}{10{,}820}$$

$$= 7.28(10^{-5})M_z y$$

where the units for M_z and y are N-mm and mm, respectively.

If we were doing a one-dimensional analysis, we would use the standard expression

$$\sigma = \frac{M_z y}{I_{zz}}$$

Then, by the transformation equations,

$$I_{zz} = \frac{15{,}820 + 10{,}820}{2} + \frac{15{,}820 - 10{,}820}{2} \cos 70° = 14{,}180 \text{ mm}^4$$

The corresponding stress value would be

$$\sigma = \frac{M_z y}{14{,}180} = 7.06(10^{-5})M_z y$$

The error in the calculated stress along the y axis is actually fairly small in this case, ~3 percent. The actual neutral axis orientation is

$$\tan \alpha' = \frac{M_z(\sin 35)(15{,}820)}{M_z(\cos 35)(10{,}820)} \quad \Rightarrow \quad \alpha = 45.6°$$

Hence, the neutral axis is approximately 11.6° off the axis of the moment. In order to locate the point of maximum bending stress, *the point on the perimeter of the cross section that is the farthest from the neutral axis must be located* (see Figure 5.11). It could be either on the tensile or the compressive side of the neutral axis, depending on the exact shape of the cross section. Thus, while the calculated stress along the y axis obtained by the simple symmetric beam formula has a fairly small error, the actual maximum stress could occur elsewhere and be substantially different in value.

5.4 | Case Studies: Whole Bone Mechanics

The analysis of whole bones represents an engineering challenge because bone geometries and the spatial distribution of material properties within bones are complex. Most engineered structures are made of uniform materials, possess planes of symmetry, have mathematically well-defined shapes, and are usually mass produced. If this were not the case, it would be too expensive and time consuming to design, construct, and repair most engineered objects.

Bones are not engineered structures, and their geometries and material property distributions typically reflect the result of complex adaptations to multiple mechanical and biochemical environmental stimuli, as well as genetic programming and possible evolutionary forces. As a result, bone is a geometrically irregular structure with substantial biological heterogeneity across the population. (Compare the young versus old vertebral bodies in Figure 5.12, for example.)

Thus, a whole bone is a difficult structure to analyze, and it is a challenge to generalize from analysis of a single bone to the entire population—issues that rarely arise in conventional engineering analysis. As with all mathematical modeling of the musculoskeletal system, a critical part of the process is to choose the most appropriate model for the problem at hand by balancing the need for fidelity with the available resources.

Since the central portion of long bones, such as the mid-diaphysis of the femur, can be modeled quite well as a beam, we will use beam theory for these types of applications. However, since bones are not symmetric, we may need to incorporate beam theory for nonsymmetric cross sections. Furthermore, since bones are never homogeneous in material properties, we will also need to account for the composite nature of the system. Our approach will be to analyze several common whole bone problems as examples to illustrate the various theories and address some important modeling issues.

In some cases, closed-form analytical solutions are inadequate, because the objective of the analysis may call for a more detailed modeling of the actual physical structure, such as inclusion of the anisotropic material properties of the bone tissue or the fine geometric detail of trabecular bone that is typically not captured with analytical solutions. Finite element computer modeling has been used extensively for analysis of whole bone (and bone-implant) systems when simpler models are insufficient.

Whole bone mechanics is a central theme in both clinical and biological problems. One important clinical example is age-related bone fracture, which arises

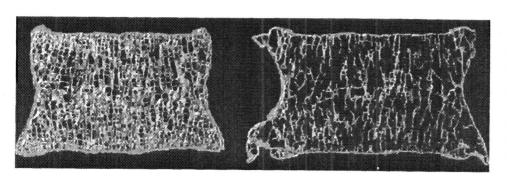

FIGURE 5.12 Midsection coronal slice (0.6 mm thick) of a T-10 vertebral body. The image is at 60 μm resolution, obtained from micro-CT imaging. Left: 54-year-old female; Right: 82-year-old female. Note the substantial increase in porosity with aging.

mostly as a result of the bone-wasting condition of osteoporosis. Although various definitions have been employed over the years, osteoporosis is essentially the reduction in bone mass and deterioration of its microstructure, accompanied by an increased susceptibility to fracture. In the United States alone, there are well over one million osteoporotic fractures each year, occurring most often in the spine, hip, and wrist (in order of prevalence). Women are more affected than men, primarily because of the complex effects of differences in hormonal status between the sexes and in part because women live longer. As engineers, we seek to understand those geometric and material properties that most affect the strength of whole bones such as the proximal femur, vertebral body, and distal radius. This information can be used by radiologists to develop noninvasive imaging techniques for measurement of the critical biomechanical parameters that most affect fracture risk. In this way, diagnostics of fracture risk can be optimized, and patients can be advised on the best course of preventative action or treatment. Similar concepts can be applied to determine a risk of fracture for patients with bone tumors; if the risk is high, prophylactic fracture-fixation surgery will often be performed in order to avoid a future traumatic fracture and the associated uncontrolled pain.

Understanding the mechanics of whole bones is also important biologically, since it provides insight into the structure–function relations of bones in various species and how bones adapt to their environment during growth and maturation within a lifetime. With the advent of drugs that can change normal bone biology and thus alter bone adaptation and growth, it is a necessary part of drug development to measure whole bone strength in animal models as an outcome of the effectiveness of candidate drug treatments. A detailed understanding of the biomechanical behavior of the whole bone is required to properly interpret the results of such experiments and, indeed, to design biological strategies for possible future development of drugs that might be used to tailor the mechanical properties of bone.

CASE STUDY 5.1 | Compression Analysis of the Vertebral Body—Load Sharing Between the Cortical and Trabecular Bone

Spine fractures are the most prevalent type of osteoporotic fractures, with upwards of 700,000 occurring annually in the United States alone. These types of fractures are unique, since they typically are manifested not by a complete separation of bony fragments, but instead by a permanent deformity, the anterior wedge fracture being the most common (Figure 5.13). The etiology of spine fractures may not be clear. For example, wedge fractures might occur from an isolated overload, from cumulative damage, or from longer-term creep or fatigue. Regardless of which mechanism is most important, a key issue is the relative role of the cortical shell versus trabecular centrum in load sharing within the vertebral body. This is important clinically, since it determines which bony compartment of the whole bone, cortical or trabecular, needs to be monitored most closely during screening for osteoporosis or targeted for drug treatment. The morphology of the cortical shell is complex (Figure 5.14), and it is difficult to determine its thickness and material

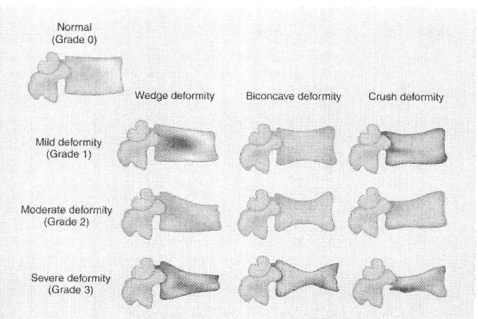

FIGURE 5.13   Basis for radiographic classification of spine fractures. The fracture is classified according to the changes in geometry of the vertebra with respect to normal adjacent vertebrae. Wedge fractures are the most common in the elderly, whereas biconcave and crush fractures, indicative of high-speed injuries, are more common in younger individuals. (from *Osteoporosis*, 2nd Edition, Riggs and Meltor editors, Lippincott–Raven, Philadelphia 1995.)

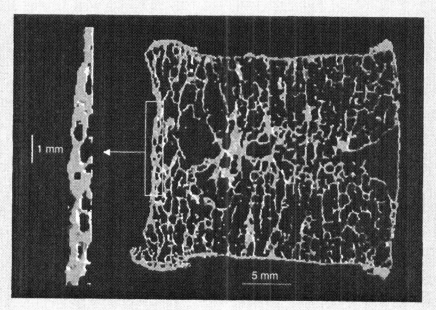

FIGURE 5.14   Sagittal slice (0.3 mm thick) of T-10 vertebral body (76 years old, female) at 60 μm resolution, showing the thin, porous nature of the cortical shell. The magnified portion at left shows that the shell is indeed more of a fused set of trabeculae than a continuous thick cortex.

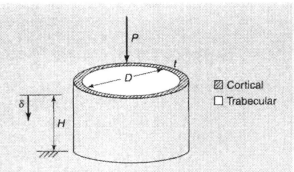

FIGURE 5.15 Simple circular cylindrical model of the vertebral body (without posterior elements). The top of the model is loaded by a central compressive force P via a rigid plate (not shown), ensuring that both the cortical and trabecular compartments displace by equal amounts δ—a uniform displacement boundary condition.

properties and how these parameters change with age. These uncertainties complicate and sometimes even confound biomechanical analysis of the vertebral body.

Since the question here is broad—How much load does the cortical shell carry?—we seek a simple model that can be easily generalized. The model is composed of a composite column, essentially two springs in parallel; the cortical shell is in parallel with the trabecular centrum (Figure 5.15). For mathematical simplicity, the cross section is assumed to be circular, and the sides are assumed to lack any curvature. It is unlikely that a more complex cross-sectional geometry would alter our general conclusions, given the parallel spring nature of the model. Also, curvature effects are expected to be minor, although this may require validation by a more complex analysis. Since the density of the bone is expected to affect how much load each type of bone tissue will take, it should be possible to vary this parameter.

From direct measurements of the cortical shell, its thickness is on the order of one-third to one-half of a millimeter, although this can vary across the vertebra, across individuals, and with aging. The material properties of the shell are also uncertain. Since the shell is so thin, it is not obvious that material properties derived from a uniaxial test on a relatively large and uniform specimen of machined diaphyseal cortical bone will reflect those of such a thin and irregular shell. Given these uncertainties, it should be possible to vary shell thickness and material properties in the model.

We will restrict our attention to the role of the shell for the special case of uniaxial compression. Our model of the vertebral body therefore consists of two concentric circular cylinders, the outer cylinder being the thin cortical shell. For two springs in parallel, loaded on top by a uniform displacement δ, the strain $\varepsilon = \delta/H$ is the same in each compartment. If the overall applied axial compressive force for δ is given by P, then P is shared between the cortical (P_c) and trabecular (P_t) compartments as follows:

$$P_c + P_t = P$$

Assuming linear elastic behavior, we can easily show that the fraction of load taken by the cortical shell P_c/P is

$$\frac{P_c}{P} = \frac{E_c A_c}{E_c A_c + E_t A_t}$$

where A is the cross-sectional area of each compartment, E is Young's modulus, and the subscripts c and t refer to the cortical and trabecular bone, respectively. This is the governing equation for this model for the assumed loading conditions.

Given the uncertainty of some of the parameters in the system, we seek to determine the role of the trabecular bone density ρ, cortical shell thickness t, and cortical shell elastic modulus E_c on the fraction of load carried by the cortical shell. Let's assume that t is uniform around the perimeter, and that the diameter of the trabecular centrum is D. As we saw in a previous chapter, the modulus of vertebral trabecular bone can be related to its density by an equation of the form $E_t = m\rho$. Then, the load sharing by the cortex is given by

$$\frac{P_c}{P} = \frac{1}{1 + \dfrac{E_t A_t}{E_c A_c}} = \frac{1}{1 + \dfrac{m\rho}{E_c\{(1 + 2t/D)^2 - 1\}}}$$

Typically, t is about 0.35 mm, and D has a characteristic dimension on the order of 30 mm. Inserting these values indicates that

$$\frac{P_c}{P} \approx \frac{1}{1 + \dfrac{m\rho}{0.05 E_c}}$$

Before looking at the behavior of this model, let's look at some of its bounds to develop our intuition for what to expect. If E_c is typical of cortical bone, namely, on the order of 17,000 MPa, and the product of $m\rho$ is on the order of 300 MPa, then $m\rho/E_c = 0.018$ and $P_c/P \approx 74$ percent. By contrast, if the effective modulus of the cortical shell is much lower (because it is not a contiguous structure), say, $m\rho/E_c = 0.5$, then $P_c/P \approx 9$ percent. This result therefore suggests that the mechanical behavior of the vertebral body depends very much on the relative stiffness of the cortical to trabecular bone and that the role of the shell may be important.

Now we can use this model to investigate in more detail how the load-carrying capacity of the cortical shell might change with aging. Let's assume that the cortical thickness remains constant with aging, but that the trabecular bone density changes with age. Since so little is known about the material properties of the thin cortical shell, we need to include this parameter as an uncertainty variable in the model. Aging can be captured as a variation in density of the trabecular bone (m is about 2200 MPa/g/cm^3 and is assumed to be constant with aging); variations in cortical modulus are also included as an uncertainty variable. Figure 5.16 shows the predicted load-carrying capacity of the cortical shell versus trabecular bone density for different values of the assumed cortical modulus. It is seen that the relation is nonlinear, and—as expected from our analysis on the bounds of the behavior—the solution

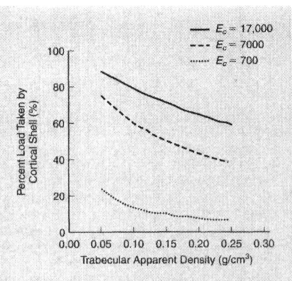

FIGURE 5.16 Dependence of loading of the cortical bone within a vertebral body on the apparent density of the vertebral trabecular bone. Over a lifetime in some individuals, trabecular bone density in the spine might decrease from about 0.25 to 0.05 g/cm^3—a worst-case scenario. The behavior of the model is shown for three different values of effective modulus of the cortical shell E_c (in MPa), since so little is known about the value of this material property. Although the load carried by the shell increases nonlinearly with loss of trabecular bone, it is clear that the assumed value of the effective modulus for the cortical shell dominates the magnitude of the density effect.

depends very much on the assumed value of the cortical modulus. Without information on the latter, it is not possible to quantify the portion of the load carried by the cortical shell. Even so, we can conclude that, regardless of how much load is taken by the cortical shell, its share of the load will increase with loss of trabecular bone and that this effect increases as the trabecular density decreases.

Interpretation of the results is critical. In this analysis, we included a value of cortical bone modulus of only 700 MPa, over 20 times lower that the standard value often used for diaphyseal cortical bone. How can such a low value be justified? Since the cortical shell is so thin, and since it is curved and irregularly shaped and contains many tiny vascular channels, it may not be able to resist mechanical loads very well. Thus, while the material that makes up the cortical shell may be similar to the constituents of diaphyseal cortical bone, and while nano-indentation measurements have shown that the modulus of the cortical shell is not too different from that of diaphyseal cortical bone, the vertebral shell as a structure at the scale of about one millimeter may be much more compliant. Thus, the effective modulus of the shell may be many times lower than the modulus of a larger, more continuous and solid volume of the same material. By considering the structure of the shell, we can make plausible arguments for why the effective cortical modulus of the shell may be very low. Unfortunately, we must look elsewhere for other evidence to support the results of this analysis, since it is currently not clear if the effective modulus of the vertebral cortical shell is closer to 17,000 or 700 MPa.

CASE STUDY 5.2   Composite Beam Analysis of Femoral Neck Fractures

Hip fracture (Figure 5.17) is the most devastating type of osteoporotic fracture. In the elderly, about 90 percent of hip fractures occur as the result of a fall, but only about 2 percent of falls result in a hip fracture. Thus, falling may be a necessary, but not sufficient, condition to break a hip. One possibility is that the type of fall is important, and indeed, epidemiology studies have shown that a fall to the side of the hip is most dangerous. In addition, the strength of the proximal femur will determine whether or not the hip will fracture. This analysis addresses both factors.

Our goal here is to determine the relative role of bone density and whole bone structure on the risk of a fracture, for a fall to the side of the hip. Our focus will be on the mechanics of cervical (neck) hip fractures, but we will also comment on the behavior for habitual loading conditions such as gait. We will develop an analytical expression that relates the relevant structural parameters of the problem to the maximum stress that develops in the femoral neck during a fall. Those stresses will be divided by the strength of the bone tissue at that location in order to calculate a risk of fracture. (Risk > 1 suggests that the bone will fracture.) This is a common approach in biomechanics fracture risk assessment and is the inverse of the safety factor used in traditional engineering design analysis.

With a fall to the side of the hip, a medially directed compressive impact force is applied by the ground to the body. Some portion of this force, F, is eventually applied through the surrounding soft tissue at the hip to the greater trochanter (Figure 5.18). This femoral impact force in turn generates a joint contact force on the femoral head at some angle θ to the femoral neck axis and some distal equilibrating loads.

It is assumed that the external shapes of the trabecular and cortical regions are both circular, as shown, with the trabecular region displaced superiorly by a

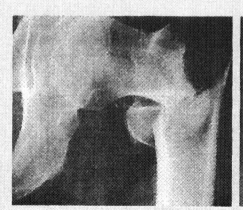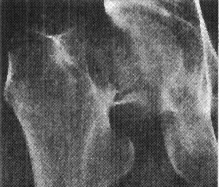

FIGURE 5.17   Example AP X-rays of intertrochanteric (left) and femoral neck (right) fractures of the hip. [From *Fractures in the Elderly*, Koval and Zuckerman (editors), Lippincott and Raven, Philadelphia, 1898.]

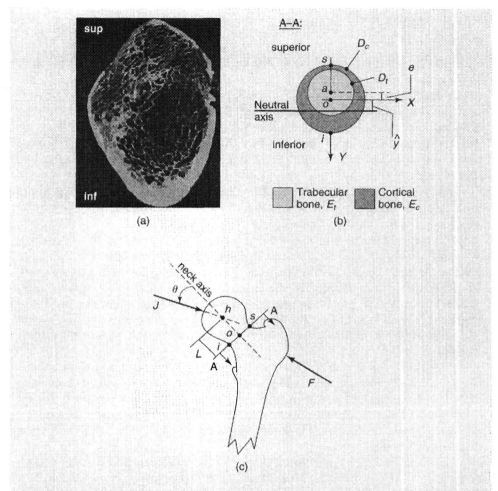

FIGURE 5.18   (a) High-resolution image (20 μm) of femoral neck cross section. (b) Schematic of the narrowest cross section of the femoral neck, A–A at right, assuming circular cross sections for simplicity. (c) Free-body diagram of the femur during a fall (muscle and distal equilibrating loads not shown). (a) and (b) from Fox and Keaveny (2001) *Journal of Theoretical Biology* 212:211–221.

distance e. The center of the cortical external circle is at Point o; the center of the trabecular region is at Point a. The diameters of the cortical and trabecular bone regions are D_c and D_t, respectively, with corresponding moduli of E_c and E_t. The X–Y coordinate system has its origin at Point o, and positive directions are as indicated. The neutral axis of the composite beam is at a distance $\hat{y}$ from the X axis. Symmetry is assumed about the Y axis. Stresses will be calculated at the most inferior point of the cortical surface, Point i, and also at the most superior aspect, Point s. A trochanteric contact force, F, produces a femoral head reaction force, J, producing tensile bending stresses on the inferior aspect (Point i). For habitual loading conditions such as gait, there would be no force F, and the joint contact force, J, would act at a negative angle to what is shown, producing compressive bending stresses at Point i.

The femoral neck is modeled here as a composite beam, composed of cortical and trabecular regions, each having a circular cross-sectional geometry (Figure 5.18). The circular region of trabecular bone is eccentrically placed in a superior position with respect to the midplane of the neck, with eccentricity e. According to composite beam theory, the bending stress in the cortical bone at a distance t from the neutral axis of the beam is given by:

$$\sigma_{\text{bend}} = \pm \frac{ME_c t}{E_c \hat{I}_c + E_t \hat{I}_t}$$

where

M is the bending moment at the cross section resolved to the neutral axis—that is, the axis along which all bending stresses are zero;

E_c is the Young's modulus of the cortical bone;

E_t is the Young's modulus of the trabecular bone;

$\hat{I}_c$ is the areal moment of inertia of the cortical bone with respect to the neutral axis; and

$\hat{I}_t$ is the areal moment of inertia of the trabecular bone with respect to the neutral axis.

Each of these terms will be derived next. To simplify the mathematical expressions, the following nondimensional parameters are introduced:

$$\alpha = \frac{D_t}{D_c} \qquad \beta = \frac{E_t}{E_c} \qquad \delta = \frac{L}{D_c} \qquad \gamma = \frac{\hat{y}}{D_c}$$

In these equations, D_c and D_t are the outside diameters of the cortical and trabecular bone, respectively. The use of nondimensional parameters is common in such analyses, since it enables one to determine the effects of various parameters without having to choose specific values of any of the parameters. Instead, only relative values are used, which makes the model more robust.

The total bending moment acting on the cross section A–A about the neutral axis is the sum of the moments produced by the transverse component of the joint contact force ($J \sin \theta$), which acts through the femoral head center h at a distance L from the cross section of interest, and the now eccentric compressive axial force $J \cos \theta$, which acts at the midpoint of the overall cross section at Point o, which is a distance $\hat{y}$ superior to the neutral axis:

$$M = J(L \sin \theta + \hat{y} \cos \theta) = JD_c(\delta \sin \theta + \gamma \cos \theta)$$

For the loads as shown in Figure 5.18 (which represents one possible type of fall condition, having J act at an angle inferior to the neck axis), the eccentric compressive axial force produces a moment that reinforces the moment produced by the transverse component of the joint contact force. This occurs because, as will be shown, $\hat{y}$ is always inferior to the Point o for superiorly eccentric trabecular bone. Thus, one biomechanical effect of the superior eccentricity of the trabecular bone in the femoral neck is to increase the internal effective bending moment on the cross section, compared with what would occur if there were no trabecular eccentricity ($\hat{y} = 0$, for that case). This occurs even though the external forces have not changed. If J acts at a negative angle superior to the neck axis—as it does for habitual activities such as gait—then the eccentricity tends to reduce the internal effective bending moment. Thus, the cross-sectional shape of the neck tends to minimize bending stresses in the neck for habitual activities. However, the magnitude of the bending stress depends on a number of other factors, and it is not possible from the analysis so far to ascertain whether the eccentricity increases or decreases cortical bending stresses.

The value for $\hat{y}$ is derived from the condition that, for the case of pure bending, there is no resultant axial force acting on the cross section (Section 5.1), which leads to the equation

$$\hat{y} = \frac{E_c A_c \bar{y}_c + E_t A_t \bar{y}_t}{E_c A_c + E_t A_t}$$

where $\bar{y}_c$ and $\bar{y}_t$ are the geometric centroids of the cortical and trabecular bone regions, respectively, and A_c and A_t are the corresponding cross-sectional areas. Realizing that the positions of the centroids with respect to the X axis are given by

$$\bar{y}_c = \frac{e\alpha^2}{1 - \alpha^2} \qquad \bar{y}_t = -e$$

one can show that the position of the neutral axis with respect to the X axis is given by

$$\hat{y} = \frac{e\alpha^2(1 - \beta)}{1 - \alpha^2(1 - \beta)}$$

where e has a positive value when the trabecular region is superiorly placed within the cortical region, as shown in Figure 5.18. A positive value of $\hat{y}$ indicates that the neutral axis is located inferior to the X axis. This equation indicates that $\hat{y}$ will always be positive for $e > 0$, $\beta < 1$, and $\alpha < 1$, as they are for the femoral neck. Thus, a second biomechanical effect of the superior eccentricity of the trabecular bone in the femoral neck is to shift the neutral axis of bending inferior to the center of the neck.

We now calculate stresses at the inferior and superior periosteal surfaces of the cortical bone (Points i and s in Figure 5.18). For Points i and s, t is given by the following equations:

$$\text{At } i, t = \frac{D_c}{2} - \hat{y} = \frac{D_c}{2}(1 - 2\gamma); \qquad \text{at } s, t = \frac{D_c}{2} + \hat{y} = \frac{D_c}{2}(1 + 2\gamma)$$

It can be seen that a third biomechanical effect of the trabecular eccentricity is to decrease the distance from the neutral axis to the inferior periosteal surface of the bone (and a corresponding increase on the superior side).

The areal moments of inertia about the neutral axis for the cortical and trabecular bone regions, $\hat{I}_c$ and $\hat{I}_t$, respectively, are found from the parallel axis theorem:

$$\hat{I}_c = \frac{\pi D_c^4}{64} + \frac{\pi D_c^2}{4}\hat{y}^2 - \hat{I}_t \qquad \hat{I}_t = \frac{\pi D_t^4}{64} + \frac{\pi D_t^2}{4}(\hat{y} - \bar{y}_t)^2$$

After some algebra, it can be shown that the cortical bending stresses σ_{bend}^{inf} at Point i on the inferior periosteal surface and σ_{bend}^{sup} at Point s on the superior periosteal surface are given by

$$\sigma_{bend}^{inf} = \frac{32J(\delta \sin \theta + \gamma \cos \theta)(1 - 2\gamma)}{\pi D_c^2 \left\{ 1 - \alpha^4(1 - \beta) + 16\gamma^2 \left(1 - \frac{\beta^2}{\alpha^4(1 - \beta)} \right) \right\}}$$

and

$$\sigma_{bend}^{sup} = -\frac{32J(\delta \sin \theta + \gamma \cos \theta)(1 + 2\gamma)}{\pi D_c^2 \left\{ 1 - \alpha^4(1 - \beta) + 16\gamma^2 \left(1 - \frac{\beta^2}{\alpha^4(1 - \beta)} \right) \right\}}$$

Remember that

$$\alpha = \frac{D_t}{D_c} \qquad \beta = \frac{E_t}{E_c} \qquad \delta = \frac{L}{D_c} \qquad \gamma = \frac{\hat{y}}{D_c}$$

These equations reveal that, for the bending stresses, there is a complex interaction between the effects of eccentricity and bone density, as reflected in the parameters γ and β, respectively, and interactions also exist between eccentricity and all other geometric parameters in the model.

To complete the stress calculations, we add any axial compressive stresses to these bending stresses. For all points on the cross section, the uniform (negative) compressive stress in the cortical bone due to the action of the axial component of J acting on the composite column is given by

$$\sigma_{axial} = -\frac{J \cos \theta E_c}{E_c A_c + E_t A_t} = -\frac{4J \cos \theta}{\pi D_c^2 \{1 - \alpha^2(1 - \beta)\}}$$

By linear superposition of stresses, the total stress is $\sigma_{total} = \sigma_{axial} \pm \sigma_{bend}$, where the latter term will depend on the location of the point of interest within the cross section.

To perform a failure risk analysis, we need to compare these stresses with the strength of the tissue. Typically, in a clinical setting, we calculate a risk factor, defined as the ratio of functional stress to tissue strength (inverse of engineering factor of safety), such that failure is predicted when the risk factor exceeds unity. Although we should perform a nonlinear analysis to compute stresses once the bone behaves in a nonlinear fashion, if we are comparing stresses against yield strength values, for which there is little inelastic deformation of the bone, the error we introduce by using a linear analysis for risk factor calculation is often small. Because the strength properties of cortical bone tissue are asymmetric, it is necessary to compare tensile stresses with the tensile strength, and compressive stresses with the compressive strength. Since in this analysis all calculated stresses act along the axis of the neck, we would use the longitudinal strength values for the cortical bone.

Figure 5.19 shows some typical results, which indicate that risk factors are generally greater on the superior aspect for a fall, and that increasing eccentricity increases the risk factor. Further, as the trabecular bone density is decreased relative to the cortical density, the effects of eccentricity are accentuated, indicating an interaction between the effects of bone loss and eccentricity.

If we were to investigate effects of aging in the preceding analysis, we could use equations that relate cortical strength to its porosity in the fracture risk calculations, and we would use a similar approach to vary the modulus of the trabecular bone and cortical bone (although the latter appears to vary little, if at all, with age). Indeed, a substantial challenge in failure analyses of whole bone structures is to account for the biological heterogeneity in the bone material properties; another challenge is the need to account for variations—either within an individual over time or across a population—in bone density and how this affects both elastic and failure properties.

Finally, the trends predicted by this model provide insight into bone adaptation. A typical value for the eccentricity e is about 1 mm, whereas a typical value of D_c is about 28 mm, such that we have $\lambda = e/D_c = 0.036$. Thus, for a pure bending load case, we see from the foregoing equations that the ratio of the magnitude of the inferior to superior bending stresses is given by

$$\frac{\sigma_{bend}^{inf}}{\sigma_{bend}^{sup}} = \frac{(1 - 2\gamma)}{(1 + 2\gamma)} = 0.87$$

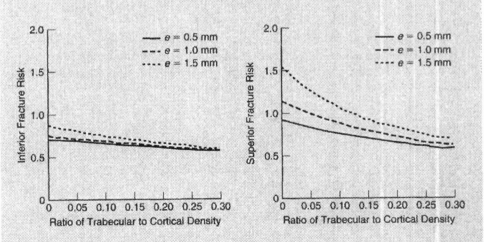

FIGURE 5.19 Risk factors at the inferior (left) and superior (right) aspects of the periosteal femoral neck for a sideways fall. A value greater than 1 indicates that failure is predicted. As trabecular bone density is preferentially lost, the effects of eccentricity are accentuated, indicating an interaction between the effects of bone loss and eccentricity.

This result indicates that the magnitude of the bending stresses in the femoral neck, regardless of the loading conditions, will always be lower on the inferior than superior aspect. For a fall loading condition, compressive bending stresses develop on the superior aspect, whereas tensile bending stresses develop there for gait conditions. Cortical bone tissue is weaker in tension than compression, and this suggests that the eccentricity has a protective effect by reducing tensile risk factors for gait conditions, but this protective effect puts the structure at risk for nonhabitual loading conditions, such as a sideways fall.

CASE STUDY 5.3 | Asymmetric Bending of the Rat Femur

Perhaps the greatest hope for treatment of osteoporosis is through drug therapy, and a number of drugs are now FDA-approved. As part of the assessment process in the ongoing development of candidate drug treatments, the drugs are tested for biomechanical efficacy on animal models. A common model is the rat, since it can be bred in a uniform fashion, has a relatively short lifespan, and after ovariectomy shows characteristics of osteoporotic bone loss. Three-point bending of the rat femur is a common test by which drug treatments can be tested in the early stages of the development process.

One important testing issue is whether or not it is necessary to use asymmetric beam theory to assess the structural characteristics of treated and untreated bones. If symmetric beam theory were good enough, its use would simplify the post-processing of the data from such experiments. We will address this issue in this analysis by comparing results predicted by both asymmetric and simple beam theories for different loading conditions. All this will be done under the assumption that the beam is composed of a single, uniform material—a reasonable assumption, given that the diaphysis is composed of only cortical bone. (However, the cortical bone is not necessarily uniform, particularly in a drug-treated animal in which the newly formed bone may have properties different from the native bone in response to the drug treatment.)

A schematic of a typical experimental setup is shown in Figure 5.20, together with a typical cross section of a rat femur. The x–y–z axes show the laboratory coordinate system; in the y–z plane of the cross section, the coordinate system is centered on the centroid. Recall that for a single-material beam, the neutral axis goes through the centroid, but for an asymmetric beam, its orientation is unknown and must be calculated as part of the analysis.

Let's look first at the case in which a moment M_z (about the AP or z axis) is created by applying a vertical force to the top of the bone, at the midpoint between the supports, three-point bending with $x = 0$ at this plane. (Let the X axis be along the length of the femur.) Application of asymmetric beam theory for a single material beam for this situation results in the following equation for the elastic bending stress σ_x at a point having coordinates $(0, y, z)$:

$$\sigma_x = \frac{M_z(I_{yz}z - I_{yy}y)}{I_{yy}I_{zz} - I_{yz}^2}$$

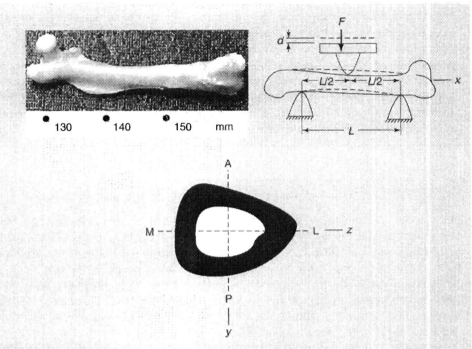

FIGURE 5.20 A rat femur (top left), a schematic of the experimental setup for the rat diaphysis three-point bend test (top right), and a typical cross section of a rat femur at mid-diaphysis (above centre), with aspects labeled (A—anterior, etc.). Schematic taken from Figure 7.9 from *Cowin Bone Biomechanics Handbook*, by Turner.

Here, all areal moments and products of inertia are calculated with respect to the y and z axes, which pass through the centroid.

Next, let's find the orientation θ of the neutral axis for this load condition. By definition, the neutral axis is the line along which all bending stresses are zero for pure bending. Setting $\sigma_x = 0$ in the preceding equation therefore produces the condition $I_{yz}z - I_{yy}y = 0$, from which we can find θ, as shown in Figure 5.21:

$$\theta = \tan^{-1}\left\{\frac{I_{yz}}{I_{yy}}\right\}$$

With this relationship, we now have sufficient information to find the maximum stress in the cross section. For a given bending moment and bone geometry, the only variable is the location of the point at which we evaluate the stress. For an irregular cross section in which there is no analytical relation between the independent coordinates, the maximum stress must be found by trial and error.

For the asymmetrical bending analysis, a maximum compressive stress of 128 MPa occurred on the lateral exterior surface of the diaphysis, while a maximum tensile stress of 130 MPa was generated at the medial exterior surface (Figure 5.21). Symmetrical bending analysis produced similar results for the locations of the maximum compressive and tensile stresses. However, the magnitudes were slightly higher, with a 140 MPa maximum compressive stress and a 143 MPa maximum tensile stress resulting from the applied moments. The neutral axis of

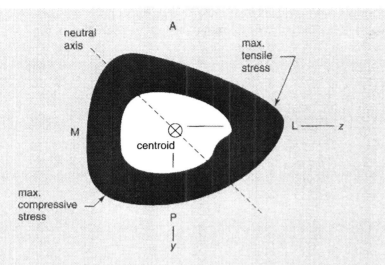

FIGURE 5.21 Cross section of the rat femur, showing the neutral axis, which goes through the centroid and has an orientation with respect to the ML axis. Note that for this example, the bending moment is applied only about the AP axis. Also shown are the locations of maximum tensile and compressive bending stress, respectively.

the cross section for the asymmetrical analysis is oriented at 58° with respect to the z axis, while symmetrical analysis resulted in a neutral axis orientation of 56°.

These results indicate that, for this application, the asymmetrical and symmetrical bending analyses yield similar results in terms of the locations of the maximum compressive and tensile stresses and the orientation of the neutral axis. The similarities between the two analyses may be attributed to the fact that the product of inertia is small ($I_{yz} = -267$ mm^4), compared with the moments of inertia ($I_{zz} = 2696$ mm^4, $I_{yy} = 3317$ mm^4). This is a reflection of the relatively high degree of symmetry of the cross section about the y and z axes. We conclude therefore that application of the mathematically simpler symmetric theory is reasonable for this application and provides measures of maximum stress that err slightly on the high side.

5.5 | Summary

Structural analysis is a key tool for understanding the mechanics of the musculoskeletal system and designing implants and devices for skeletal reconstruction. Many problems involving long bones can be examined by modeling the structure as a beam. Elastic models of beams subjected to axial and bending loads involve a number of simplifying assumptions, particularly that the beams are of sufficient length, are approximately straight, and are approximately prismatic. A major fundamental assumption consistent with these assumptions is that, in bending, plane cross sections remain plane. These assumptions, along with the necessary conditions for equilibrium and the linear stress–strain relations, provide the required model equations for elastic beam analysis.

A number of problems of interest involve the nonhomogeneous nature of cross sections, which is due either to variation in stiffness properties of the bone (especially cortical versus cancellous bone regions) or to multiple materials resulting from adding an implant. These add complications to the details of the model, but present no conceptual difficulties. Composite beams with two and three material cross sections illustrate the concept. This is obviously extendable to as many material regions in a cross section as one might wish.

Unsymmetrical bending analysis shows that bending moments about an arbitrary axis can produce bending about the corresponding axis and the perpendicular axis as well. Typically, long-bone cross sections are not symmetric, so unsymmetrical bending is the normal situation. Assuming that the bone bends symmetrically may lead to errors in both the magnitude and the location of the maximum bending stresses.

Three case studies illustrate the merit of these simple models in parametric studies and for understanding the significance of basic geometric and material properties of skeletal elements. Examples in subsequent chapters will further illustrate the utility of these models in design applications.

5.6 EXERCISES

5.1 Consider a model of a bone with a cemented prosthesis, where the outside radius of the bone is r_o, the radius of the medullary cavity is r_m, and the radius of the prosthesis is r_p. The prosthesis is exactly centered in the cavity. For the case of pure bending, determine how the ratio of the moment carried by the prosthesis to the total moment, M_p/M_{tot}, varies as a function of r_p/r_m. How will this result change if the cortex is thicker (i.e., if r_o/r_m increases)?

5.2 Calculate the flexural stiffness about the neutral axis of this composite beam (Figure P 5.2):

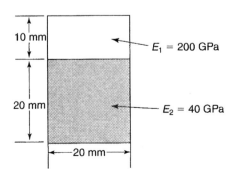

FIGURE P 5.2 Cross section of a composite beam made of two materials (E_1 and E_2).

5.3 Figure P 5.3 shows an anterior–posterior slice of a tibial component of a metal-backed knee prosthesis. This portion of the prosthesis can be modeled as a

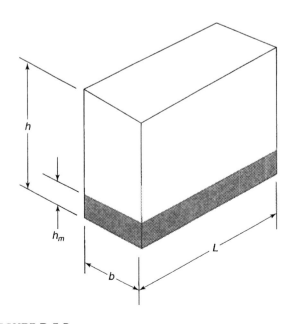

FIGURE P 5.3

beam on an elastic foundation. The darkly shaded part is metal; the rest of the beam is polyethylene. Determine the following:

(a) The location of neutral axis with respect to the *bottom* of the beam in terms of the ratio h_m/h.

(b) The structural stiffness (structural rigidity) in bending of the beam as a function of the ratios h_m/h and E_m/E_p, where the subscripts refer to metal and the polyethylene, respectively.

5.4   Consider an idealized vertebral body, as shown in Figure P 5.4, under a uniaxial compressive load, which is applied through loading platens that remain perfectly horizontal. The damaged region (right) amounts to $1/2$ the area (i.e., $A_2 = A_1 = A/2$), and the modulus is $E_2 = 0.08E_1$, where E_1 is the undamaged modulus.

(a) Calculate the stresses in each region after damage ($\sigma_{damage\text{-}1}$, $\sigma_{damage\text{-}2}$) in terms of the original (no damage) stresses (σ).

(b) If the strength of the damaged bone is $\sigma_{y\text{-damage}} = 0.70\sigma_y$ (i.e., 70% of the original strength σ_y), calculate the risk factor RF (functional stress/strength) in each region before ($RF_{intact\text{-}1}$; $RF_{intact\text{-}2}$) and after ($RF_{damage\text{-}1}$; $RF_{damage\text{-}2}$) partial damage occurs. Compare these answers with what you would get if the strength reduction with damage was exactly equal to the modulus reduction (i.e., $\sigma_{y\text{-damage}} = 0.08\sigma_y$ after damage).

(c) If these modulus and strength reductions were due to spatially nonuniform age-related density loss within the vertebral body (instead of damage), what would be the clinical implications in terms of vertebral fracture etiology?

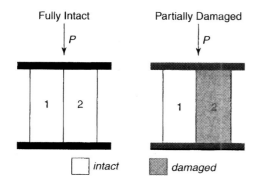

Fully Intact   Partially Damaged

□ intact   ▨ damaged

FIGURE P 5.4

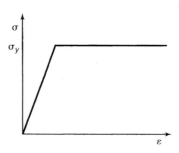

FIGURE P 5.5

5.5   Derive an expression for the moment required to cause fully plastic behavior of a beam (such as a machined specimen of cortical bone) in terms of the yield stress of the beam for

(a) equal tensile and compressive yield stresses;

(b) compressive yield stress = 1.5 × tensile yield stress.

For each case, assume elastic–perfectly-plastic (Figure P 5.5) behavior of the beam material.

5.6   When analyzing the behavior of a beam fabricated of traditional engineering materials such as steel, we often calculate the stress distribution across the section from the simple formula $\sigma = My/I$, where $y =$ distance from neutral axis, $M =$ applied moment, and $I =$ moment of inertia about the neutral axis. Also, we describe the local curvature by using the formula $1/\rho = M/(EI)$, where $\rho =$ radius of curvature, and $E =$ modulus of elasticity.

(a) Discuss the limitations of this approach for bones analyzed as beams in terms of the assumptions about material and geometric properties.

(b) Describe the approach you would take to develop the appropriate equations for the revised assumptions.

5.7   A bone is instrumented with strain gages at a cross section and loaded in bending about the x axis, as shown in Figure P 5.7. The applied bending moment is 10 newton-meters at the cross section where the three strain gages are located. The gage locations on the perimeter of the bone cross section are measured and the strains recorded. Use the data, along with the assumption of a linear strain distribution, to determine the angle between the neutral axis of bending and the x axis.

x, mm	y, mm	strain, mm/mm
13.1	0.0	3.07E-04
0.0	10.8	9.05E-04
−7.2	−7.2	0.09E-04

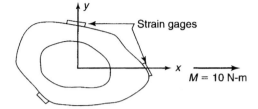

FIGURE P 5.7

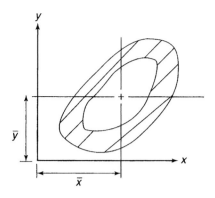

FIGURE P 5.9

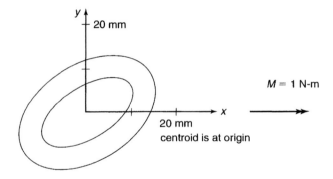

FIGURE P 5.8

5.8 A bone cross section is subjected to a bending moment about the x axis as shown in Figure P 5.8. The area moments and products of inertia about the mass center are $I_{xx} = 34{,}780$ mm^4, $I_{yy} = 40{,}520$ mm^4, $I_{xy} = 16{,}290$ mm^4. A bending moment of 1 newton-meter is applied about the x axis.

(a) Determine the orientation of the neutral axis of bending, and sketch it on the cross section.

(b) Identify the approximate point on the cross section where the maximum stress occurs, and calculate a corresponding stress value.

5.9 For the bone cross section in Figure P 5.9, the centroid is located at the values $\bar{x} = 1.67$ cm, $\bar{y} = 1.22$ cm. The measured area of the bone is 3.53 cm^2,

and the moments and product of inertia with respect to the (x, y) axes shown are $I_{xx} = 5.83$ cm^4, $I_{yy} = 10.76$ cm^4, $I_{xy} = 7.49$ cm^4.

Determine the principal centroidal moments of inertia of the bone cross section, and sketch the principal axes.

5.10 A proximal femur is loaded as shown in Figure P 5.10. The neck at A–A is comprised of a circular cortical shell (diameter D_C, modulus E_C) and a concentric circular trabecular core (diameter D_t, modulus E_t).

(a) Write out expressions for the maximum tensile stress in the trabecular *and* cortical bone at the cross section A–A (shear stresses can be neglected). Express your answer in terms of J, θ, β, L_{ne}, D_t, E_t, D_C, and E_C.

(b) Calculate the changes in the maximum tensile stresses in each of the cortical and trabecular bone compartments at section A–A for the following cases:

 (i) 50 percent decrease in modulus for only the trabecular bone;

 (ii) 50 percent decrease in modulus for only the cortical bone;

(iii) 50 percent decrease in modulus for both the trabecular and cortical bone.

(c) On the basis of your results, what can you say about the importance of the magnitude and distribution of bone loss in the femoral neck with respect to fracture risk for the hip?

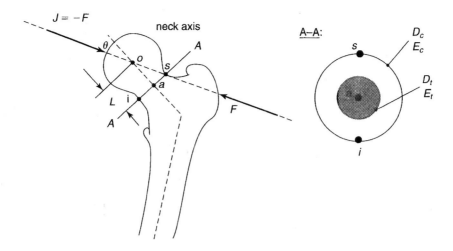

FIGURE P 5.10   Model of proximal femur with fall loading, and assumed circular cross section of the neck composed of cortical and trabecular bone. Assume the following values in any calculations: $J = 4*BW = 2800$ N; $\theta = 30°$ $L = 25$ mm; $D_t = 23$ mm; $E_t = 1000$ MPa; $D_C = 28$ mm; $E_C = 17,000$ MPa.

Note: Values of J and β are largely unknown for a fall to the side of the hip; values of D_t are also uncertain, due to the lack of clear boundary between cortical and trabecular bone in femoral neck.

5.11   A simple elliptical model of the vertebral body is shown in Figure P 5.11. Assume the following dimensions: $D_1 = 46$ mm, $D_2 = 32$ mm, $h = 26$ mm. Assuming that a compressive force $P = 2000$ N is applied centrally and distributed uniformly via a rigid plate (a common *in vitro* mechanical testing protocol),

(a) Derive an expression for the strain in the vertebral body as a function of the applied force P, the major and minor cortical diameters (D_1 and D_2, respectively), the moduli E_1 and E_2, and the cortical thickness t.

(b) Plot a graph of the strain ε vs. cortical thickness t (in the range 0.1–3.0 mm) for various ratios of E_1/E_2 (in the range 0.001–0.10). Assume that $E_2 = 13,000$ MPa.

(c) What are the implications of overestimating the thickness of the cortical shell regarding the strength of vertebral bodies? What are the implications regarding fracture risk prediction of vertebral bodies?

5.12   Assuming that the femoral diaphysis is a hollow tube with endosteal and periosteal diameters of 15 mm and 30 mm, respectively, calculate the maximum and minimum principal stresses and their directions with respect to the diaphyseal axis for a frontal bending moment of 140 Nm, a torque of 60 Nm, and a compressive axial force of 850 N for the following situations (ignore all other load components):

(a) Each load component is acting separately.

(b) All loads are superimposed.

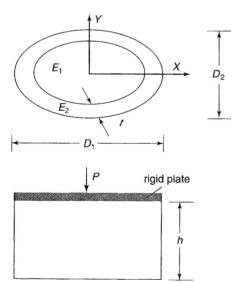

FIGURE P 5.11

(c) According to these results, which load components dominate the magnitudes and directions of the principal stresses in the femoral diaphysis during gait?

5.13   The transverse component of the resultant force at the hip joint is often neglected in stress analyses of the femoral diaphysis. Considering only loads in the frontal plane during the single-legged-stance phase of gait, discuss the validity of such an assumption with respect to maximum tensile stresses on the periosteal bone surface for a typically sized femur.

5.14   Consider a femur with a screw hole (diameter = d) in the femoral diaphyses, as shown in Figure P 5.14. The axis of the screw hole is oriented at 45 degrees from the medial–lateral (z) axis. Assume that the bone has a circular cross section and that the screw hole

cross section is rectangular, with width = d and height = $t = (D_o - D_i)/2$. D_o and D_i are the outer and inner diameters of the bone, respectively.

(i) The femur is subjected to a pure moment about the medial–lateral axis, M_z. Determine the stress in the bone at the edge of the screw hole (Point C), assuming a stress concentration factor of 3. *Hint: Resolve M_z about the axis of the screw hole (z'), and invoke symmetry about that axis.*

(ii) Determine the ratio of the stress at Point C when the hole is present to the stress at Point C when the hole is *not* present. Discuss the clinical implications of your findings.

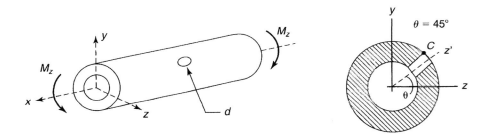

FIGURE P 5.14   (Left) A schematic showing the location of a screw hole in the femoral diaphysis. (Right) The cross section of the femur at the screw hole. Anatomical directions: x = distal–proximal, y = anterior–posterior, z = medial–lateral.

Structural Analysis of Musculoskeletal Systems: Advanced Topics

As we stated earlier, all levels of models, from the simplest to the most complex, can be used to provide important insights if used within their capabilities. For example, the stresses in a fixation stem of a bone–cement–stem system can be determined from composite beam theory. If, however, more detailed information about load transfer from the stem to the bone through the cement is desired, beam on elastic foundation theory is the least complex model that can be used. If information about the interface stresses are needed for cemented or cementless fixation stem systems, then one must resort to detailed finite element models.

Torsional stress analysis of long bones is another problem that involves somewhat more complex models. If one can assume that the cross section is essentially a circular cylinder, the simple formulas from basic strength of materials apply. However, bone cross sections are typically not circular, so more complex models are needed. With the application of methods from advanced strength of materials, elastic analysis of noncircular sections yields useful analytical solutions for several simple shapes, to be described.

Contact between natural and artificial joint surfaces is a nonlinear problem that can also be approached at several levels. Simple models based on Hertz theory, which assume that both surfaces deform, can provide a *qualitative* picture of contact and help to identify important parameters affecting performance of bearing surfaces. For artificial joints, however, that incorporate metal on polyethylene contact, the metal component acts as an indenter of the much less stiff polyethylene, and models that incorporate those features must be used to *quantify* stresses due to contact.

In summary, structural analysis of the skeletal system and its modifications requires an artful matching of the questions being asked with the capabilities of the models available. In this chapter, we will present a set of analysis methods (beyond the simple beam models of the previous chapter) that are useful for understanding the structural behavior of bones, bone-implant systems, and contact between articulating surfaces. Typically, these methods involve more complex differential equations, but the concepts are essentially extensions of earlier ideas. Along the way, a few applications of the methods will be presented. Applications will be considered in greater detail in later chapters of the text.

6.1 | Beams on Elastic Foundation

In the previous chapter, composite beam theory was introduced for the analysis of bone-implant systems. In general, composite beam theory and simple beam theory only apply away from abrupt changes in geometry, material properties, or loading. Consequently, the primary use of composite beam theory in the analysis of bone-implant systems is to determine how loads are shared between the components of the system at locations away from abrupt changes in the structure.

However, in addition to load sharing, it is often important to know more detail about how the loads are transferred from one component of the composite structure to another. In a bone–cement–stem system (Figure 6.1), it may be important to know how loads are transferred from the fixation stem, through the cement, to the endosteal surface of the bone. Beam on elastic foundation theory provides a means for determining these load distributions. Or, for example, one may want to know the distribution of stress on the bone at the interface between a tibial component for total knee replacement and the supporting cancellous bone (Figure 6.1).

In the case of the tibial component, loading due to contact with the femoral component causes deformation of both the tibial component (the beam) and the cancellous bone (the elastic foundation). In the case of a bone–cement–stem fixation system, two beams and an elastic foundation are involved. Loads applied to the fixation stem (one beam) cause deformation in both the cement (the elastic foundation) and the bone (the other beam). In both cases, the loading applied to the foundation by the beam is a function of the displacement of the beam. It is the distribution of this loading and the resulting distribution of internal loads in the beams that are of primary interest in these composite structures.

Tibial Components

Many contemporary tibial components for total knee replacements are fundamentally plates supported by the cancellous bone (Figure 6.2). Beam on elastic foundation theory

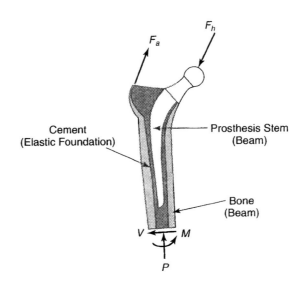

FIGURE 6.1 The proximal femur with prosthesis. The composite structure consists of the bone, the cement layer, and the fixation stem. The bone and the stem are two beams that are connected by an elastic foundation, the cement.

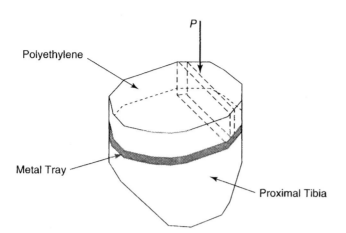

FIGURE 6.2 Proximal tibia with prosthesis. The anterior–posterior slice may be modeled as a beam on an elastic foundation.

can be used to analyze a slice of such systems, Figure 6.3, to determine the fundamental behavior of the composite structure. The slice may be in either the anterior–posterior direction, as shown in Figure 6.2, or in the lateral–medial direction.

It is then seen that three or four distinct materials make up the structure: the polyethylene, the metal (if a metal tray is used), the cement (for cement fixation), and the cancellous bone. We have some choices to make regarding our models of this composite structure. For the system shown in Figure 6.4, the beam can be considered to be a composite of polyethylene and metal, and the foundation to be a combination of cancellous bone and cement. An alternative would be to consider the beam to consist of polyethylene, metal, and cement, and the foundation to be cancellous bone only.

In either case, portions of the model representing the implant can be considered to be a composite structure that can be analyzed with composite beam theory. The structural stiffness of the beam, *EI*, is just the sum of the structural stiffnesses of the components of the beam,

$$EI = \sum_{i=1}^{n} E_i I_i$$

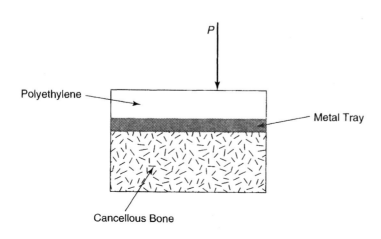

FIGURE 6.3 An idealized model of an anterior–posterior slice of a tibial component for a total knee replacement.

FIGURE 6.4 A schematic of a finite-length beam on an elastic foundation loaded by a concentrated load P.

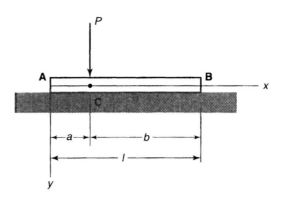

where EI is the bending stiffness of the composite beam, and E_i and I_i are the elastic modulus and second moment of area of the Ith component of the beam, respectively. Note again that I_i is computed with respect to the neutral axis of the composite beam.

The governing equation for this system is, then,

$$EI\frac{d^4v}{dx^4} + kv(x) = p(x)$$

where $v(x)$ is the displacement of the beam in the y direction, $p(x)$ is a distributed load (force/length) applied to the beam, $kv(x)$ is the distributed load (force/length) applied to the beam by the foundation, and k is the foundation modulus.

This equation may be derived by considering a section of the beam of Figure 6.4, which has thickness, dx, in the x direction and whose left face is a distance x away from the origin (Figure 6.5). This portion of the beam has the external load, $p(x)$, the foundation load, $q(x)$, internal shear force, V, and internal bending moment, M, acting on it. The forces $p(x)$ and $q(x)$ have units of force per unit length. The displacement of the beam, $v(x)$, is also the displacement of the foundation, and k is the foundation modulus. The sign convention is that positive internal forces and moments acting on a positive face are considered positive, as are negative forces and moments acting on a negative face.

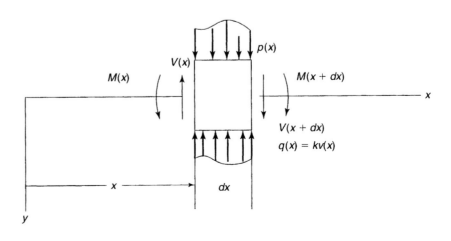

FIGURE 6.5 Section of a beam on an elastic foundation.

Our goal is to obtain an equation that relates the displacement of the beam, $v(x)$, to the applied load, $p(x)$. Summing forces in the y direction, we obtain

$$V(x + dx) - V(x) + p(x)dx - q(x)dx = 0$$

Dividing by dx, we get

$$\frac{V(x + dx) - V(x)}{dx} + p(x) - q(x) = 0$$

Taking the limit as $dx \to 0$ and rearranging yields

$$\frac{dV}{dx} = -p + q$$

Similarly, for equilibrium,

$$\sum M_{x+dx} = 0$$

which leads to

$$M(x + dx) - M(x) + V(x)dx + qdx\frac{dx}{2} - pdx\frac{dx}{2} = 0$$

Again, dividing by $dx \to 0$ gives

$$\frac{dM}{dx} = -V$$

If we now take a derivative of this expression and substitute for $\frac{dV}{dx}$, we obtain

$$\frac{d^2M}{dx^2} + q = p$$

From beam theory, we know that

$$M = EI\frac{d^2v}{dx^2}$$

and we also know that

$$q = kv$$

which gives us the governing differential equation

$$\frac{d^2}{dx^2}\left(EI\frac{d^2v}{dx^2}\right) + kv = p$$

and relates the displacement of the beam (and foundation) to the applied load $p(x)$. This equation is then solved, with appropriate boundary conditions, for $v(x)$. Then the loading on the beam due to the foundation is given by $q(x) = kv(x)$.

The strategy for determining the bending stresses in the beam is as follows. Calculate the bending moment from

$$M(x) = EI\frac{d^2v}{dx^2}$$

Then use $\sigma = -\dfrac{My}{I}$ to determine stress.

EXAMPLE 6.1 Infinite Beam on an Elastic Foundation

Question   An infinite beam, with constant cross section, is loaded by a concentrated force P at its center. What is the displacement $v(x)$ of the beam?

Solution   If we take the origin just to the right of the load, the governing equation is

$$EI\frac{d^4v}{dx^4} + kv = 0$$

The displacement and the slope of the beam at infinity must both be zero, and the slope under the load at $x = 0$ must also be zero. This leads to the following boundary conditions.

$$v(\infty) = v'(\infty) = 0$$
$$v'(0) = 0$$

In addition we know that force of the foundation on the right half of the beam must be $P/2$. Therefore the internal shear force just to the right of the load must also be $P/2$. This leads to the additional boundary condition required to solve the problem.

$$V(0) = \frac{-P}{2} = EI\frac{d^3v}{dx^3}$$

The general solution to the governing equation contains four arbitrary constants, which are determined using the boundary conditions. When this is done, we obtain

$$v(x) = e^{-\lambda x}(\cos \lambda x + \sin \lambda x)$$

where $\lambda = \sqrt[4]{\dfrac{k}{4EI}}$

Note that the solution oscillates about $v = 0$, so that for some portions of the beam the force $q(x)$ is compressive, and for others it is tensile. Note also that the magnitude of $v(x)$ decays to zero as $x \to \infty$.

The beams we encounter in bone-implant systems are typically not long enough to be modeled as infinite beams. The solution of the governing differential equation for a finite-length beam (Figure 6.4) produces the following equations for the deflection, slope, bending moment, and shearing force in the AC portion of the beam, where $x < a$ and $\lambda = \sqrt[4]{k/4EI}$:

$$
\begin{aligned}
v = {}& \frac{P\lambda}{k}\frac{1}{\sinh^2 \lambda l - \sin^2 \lambda l}\{2 \cosh \lambda x \cos \lambda x \\
& (\sinh \lambda l \cos \lambda a \cosh \lambda b - \sin \lambda l \cosh \lambda a \cos \lambda b) \\
& + (\cosh \lambda x \sin \lambda x + \sinh \lambda x \cos \lambda x) \\
& [\sinh \lambda l(\sin \lambda a \cosh \lambda b - \cos \lambda a \sinh \lambda b) \\
& + \sin \lambda l(\sinh \lambda a \cos \lambda b - \cosh \lambda a \sin \lambda b)]\}
\end{aligned}
$$

$$
\theta = \frac{2P\lambda^2}{k}\frac{1}{\sinh^2 \lambda l - \sin^2 \lambda l}\{\cosh \lambda x \cos \lambda x
$$

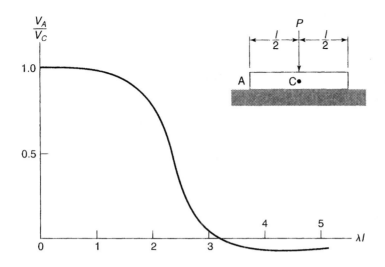

FIGURE 6.6 The ratio of end displacement to center displacement for a centrally loaded finite-length beam on an elastic foundation.

$$
\begin{aligned}
& [\sinh \lambda l(\sin \lambda a \cosh \lambda b - \cos \lambda a \sinh \lambda b) \\
& + \sin \lambda l(\sinh \lambda a \cos \lambda b - \cosh \lambda a \sin \lambda b)] \\
& - (\cosh \lambda x \sin \lambda x - \sinh \lambda x \cos \lambda x)(\sinh \lambda l \cos \lambda a \cosh \lambda b \\
& - \sin \lambda l \cosh \lambda a \cos \lambda b)\}
\end{aligned}
$$

$$
\begin{aligned}
M = {} & \frac{P}{2\lambda} \frac{1}{\sinh^2 \lambda l - \sin^2 \lambda l} \{2 \sinh \lambda x \sin \lambda x \\
& (\sinh \lambda l \cos \lambda a \cosh \lambda b - \sin \lambda l \cosh \lambda a \cos \lambda b) \\
& + (\cosh \lambda x \sin \lambda x - \sinh \lambda x \cos \lambda x) \\
& [\sinh \lambda l(\sin \lambda a \cosh \lambda b - \cos \lambda a \sinh \lambda b) \\
& + \sin \lambda l(\sinh \lambda a \cos \lambda b - \cosh \lambda a \sin \lambda b)]\}
\end{aligned}
$$

$$
\begin{aligned}
Q = {} & P \frac{1}{\sinh^2 \lambda l - \sin^2 \lambda l} \{(\cosh \lambda x \sin \lambda x + \sinh \lambda x \cos \lambda x) \\
& \cdot (\sinh \lambda l \cos \lambda a \cosh \lambda b - \sin \lambda l \cosh \lambda a \cos \lambda b) \\
& + \sinh \lambda x \sin \lambda x[\sinh \lambda l(\sin \lambda a \cosh \lambda b - \cos \lambda a \sinh \lambda b) \\
& + \sin \lambda l(\sinh \lambda a \cos \lambda b - \cosh \lambda a \sin \lambda b)]\}
\end{aligned}
$$

The same equations can be used for the BC section of the beam, where $x < b$, by measuring x from end B and replacing a by b and b by a.

It is interesting to look at the case where the load is applied at the center of the beam. The equation for v can be used to determine the deflection under the load, v_C, and the deflection at the end of the beam, v_A. If the ratio v_A/v_C is plotted against λl, the graph shown in Figure 6.6 results.

When $0 \le \lambda l \le 1$, the end deflection and the center deflection are very nearly the same; the beam behaves as a stiff structure. When $\lambda l > 3$, the end deflection is very small compared with the deflection at the center; the beam behaves as a very flexible structure. It should be noted that the structural stiffness is a function of k, EI, and l. A change in any of these quantities will affect the structural behavior of the beam on the elastic foundation.

Fixation Stems

When the articulating surfaces of the hip joint become damaged due to disease or wear and tear, the surfaces of the femoral head and the acetabulum are replaced by a total joint replacement. The femoral head and neck are removed, and a prosthetic femoral head is attached to the femur by means of a fixation stem, which is inserted into the medullary cavity of the bone (Figure 6.2). In most contemporary designs, the femoral component is a metal. The means for attaching the stem to the bone differs.

A common procedure is to fill the space between the bone and the metal with bone cement (polymethylmethacrylate). This material, as it is usually used in surgery, does not adhere to either the bone or the metal stem, but rather depends upon mechanical interlock for interface strength. The resulting bone–cement–stem system can be considered to consist of two beams (the bone and the stem) separated by an elastic foundation (the cement).

In cementless fixation, the prosthesis is initially held to the bone by a precise press fit. In some designs, a porous layer is provided on a portion of the prosthesis. Bone or soft tissue can grow into this layer to enhance fixation of the device to the bone. When no porous layer is employed, there will frequently be a thin layer of soft tissue interposed between the device and the bone. As in the case of cemented systems, the bone–interface–stem system can be viewed as consisting of two beams (the bone and the stem) and an elastic foundation (the interface layer). The interface layer may have the properties of soft tissue or some combination of properties such as soft tissue and porous metal or bone and porous metal.

As can be seen from Figure 6.2, the bone–interface layer–stem system will be subjected to both bending and axial loads. The bending is due to both applied moments and transverse loading. A schematic of the resulting beam on elastic foundation system is shown in Figure 6.7. A section of this system for analysis due to bending is shown in Figure 6.8, from which the governing equations follow:

$$E_b I_b \frac{d^4 v_b}{dx^4} + C_t(v_s - v_b) = 0$$

$$E_s I_s \frac{d^4 v_s}{dx^4} - C_t(v_s - v_b) = 0$$

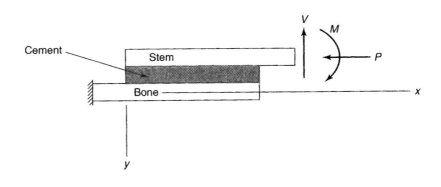

FIGURE 6.7 Schematic of a beam on elastic foundation model of a bone–cement–stem system.

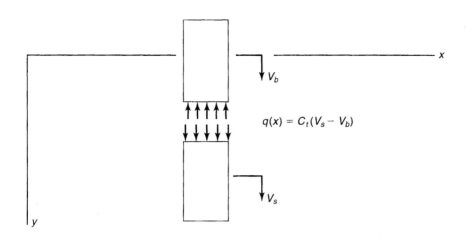

Here,

v_s is the displacement of the stem in the y direction,
v_b is the displacement of the bone in the y direction, and
C_t is the transverse stiffness of the interface layer.

The transverse stiffness of the interface layer is the foundation modulus of the interface layer (foundation) between the stem and the bone. C_t may be related to the material properties and geometry of the interface layer (e.g., cement) in a bone–interface layer–stem composite structure by the equation

$$C_t = \frac{4\left(\dfrac{r_s}{r_m}\right)E_c(1 - \nu_c)}{\left(1 - \dfrac{r_s}{r_m}\right)(1 + \nu_c)(1 - 2\nu_c)}$$

where

E_c is the elastic modulus of the interface layer,
ν_c is the Poisson's ratio of the interface layer in the transverse direction,
r_s is the radius of the fixation stem, and
r_m is the radius of the medullary cavity.

It can be shown that the general solutions for v_s, v_b, and $C_t(v_s - v_b)$ are given by

$$v_s = e^{\lambda_r x}D_1(x) + e^{-\lambda_r x}D_2(x) + \sum_{i=0}^{3}a_i x^i$$

$$v_b = -\frac{E_s I_s}{E_b I_b}e^{\lambda_r x}D_1(x)$$

$$-\frac{E_s I_s}{E_b I_b}e^{-\lambda_r x}D_2(x) + \sum_{i=0}^{3}a_i x^i$$

$$C_t(v_s - v_b) = C_t\left[1 + \frac{E_s I_s}{E_b I_b}\right][e^{\lambda_r x}D_1(x) + e^{-\lambda_r x}D_2(x)]$$

FIGURE 6.9 Schematic of a "long" bone–elastic layer–stem structure. The moment M is applied to the stem at the right-hand end. The left end of the bone is fixed (zero displacement and rotation).

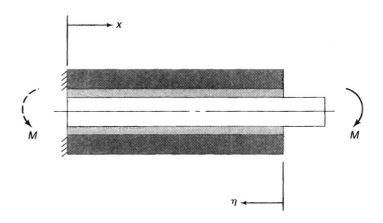

where

$$D_1 = A_1 \cos \lambda_t x + A_2 \sin \lambda_t x$$

$$D_2 = A_3 \cos \lambda_t x + a_4 \sin \lambda_t x \text{ and}$$

$$\lambda_t = \sqrt[4]{\frac{C_t}{4}\left(\frac{1}{E_s I_s} + \frac{1}{E_b I_b}\right)}$$

When $\lambda_t \geq \pi$, the composite beam is a "long" beam (Figure 6.9), and the following equations apply, where x is measured from the end of the system away from where the load is applied to the stem:

$$M_b(x) = M \frac{E_s I_s}{E_s I_s + E_b I_b}\left\{\frac{E_b I_b}{E_s I_s} + e^{-\lambda_t x}(\cos \lambda_t x + \sin \lambda_t x)\right\}$$

$$M_s(x) = M \frac{E_s I_s}{E_s I_s + E_b I_b}\left\{1 - e^{-\lambda_t x}(\cos \lambda_t x + \sin \lambda_t x)\right\}$$

$$q(x) = M\frac{1}{2}\frac{C_t}{\lambda_t^2}E_b I_b e^{\lambda_t x}(\sin \lambda_t x - \cos \lambda_t x)$$

Here,

M_s is the moment on the stem,
M_b is the moment on the bone,
M is the total moment on the bone–stem–cement system, and
q is the force per unit length of the foundation (the cement) on the stem and bone.

Note that these equations are based on x being measured from the end of the structure away from where the load is applied to the stem. Since these equations are based upon an infinitely long beam, M_s, M_b, and q will asymptotically approach a constant value as x becomes large.

To apply these equations to the end of the structure where the load is applied to the stem, replace x by η and switch the subscripts s and b. If this is done, the following set of equations is obtained:

$$M_b(\eta) = M\frac{E_b I_b}{E_s I_s + E_b I_b}\left\{\frac{E_s I_s}{E_b I_b} + e^{-\lambda_t \eta}(\cos \lambda_t x + \sin \lambda_t x)\right\}$$

$$M_s(\eta) = M\frac{E_b I_b}{E_s I_s + E_b I_b}\{1 - e^{-\lambda_t \eta}(\cos \lambda_t \eta + \sin \lambda_t \eta)\}$$

$$q(\eta) = M\frac{1}{2}\frac{C_t}{\lambda_t^2}E_s I_s e^{-\lambda_t \eta}(\cos \lambda_t \eta + \sin \lambda_t \eta)$$

6.2 | Torsion of Noncircular Sections

When a uniform, solid, or hollow circular shaft is subjected to a torque about its long axis, the shear stresses vary linearly with the radius. The angle of twist per unit length and the maximum stress at the outer boundary are given by

$$\theta = \frac{T}{GJ}; \qquad \tau_{\max} = \frac{Tc}{J},$$

where θ = the angle of twist per unit length and $\tau_{\max}$ = maximum shear stress, which occurs on the outer radius. T is the applied torque, G is the shear modulus for the material, and J is the polar moment of inertia of the cross section. However, bones are not circular in cross section, and the solution for the shear stresses due to torsional loading becomes considerably more complex. The difficulty arises because, unlike circular cross sections, noncircular cross sections do not remain plane under torsional loading. For this problem, the solution can be cast in terms of finding a particular function that describes this out-of-plane warping of the cross section. Unfortunately, there is no good way to get to the solution without retreating to the basic differential equations that represent the local stress equilibrium and the definition of strains. The good news is that the procedure turns out to be fairly straightforward, although a little messy. In what follows, we introduce the procedure for deriving for the warping function and its complementary function, the stress function, and we summarize some of the results that are most useful to our purposes.

General Solution

Figure 6.10 shows a bar with one end fixed and a torque T applied about the long axis, z, of the bar. The bar is assumed to be straight and prismatic, and the material in the bar is assumed to be homogeneous and elastic. We allow for the possibility that any point in the cross section can move in all three directions, and designate the x, y, and z displacements by $u(x, y, z)$, $v(x, y, z)$, and $w(x, y, z)$, respectively.

We also make the following additional assumptions in the stress analysis:

1. The material is isotropic, or at worst transversely isotropic, with the material axis of symmetry aligned with the bar's axis.

FIGURE 6.10 Prismatic bar under torsional loading. The left end of bar is fixed. A line on the right end rotates through an angle $\alpha = \theta L$, where L = length of the bar, and a longitudinal line along the bar rotates through an angle γ.

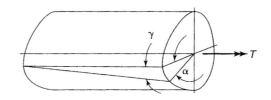

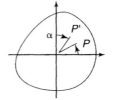
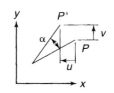

2. Deformations are small.

3. The distortion of any transverse plane due to the torsional load w is not a function of the position along the bar—that is, $w = w(x, y)$.

We define the total twist α, as at any cross section, as

$$\alpha = \theta z$$

where θ = the (constant) angle of twist per unit length and z = distance along the bar from the fixed end. In addition to the displacement of any point on the cross section, the twisting of the section causes the point P on the cross section to move to P':

$$P(x, y, z) \rightarrow P'(x + u, y + v, z + w)$$

On the basis of the second assumption, the three components of displacement of P are

$$u = r \cos(\beta + \alpha) - r \cos \beta \cong -y\alpha = -\theta yz$$
$$v = r \sin(\beta + \alpha) - r \sin \beta \cong x\alpha = \theta xz$$

According to the third assumption, that w is a function of x, y only, we have

$$w = \theta\psi(x, y)$$

where the function $\psi(x, y)$ is known as the warping function, because it describes the out-of-plane warping of the cross section. Using the standard definitions of strain in terms of the derivatives of the displacements, we have the following expressions for strain in terms of the angle of twist per unit length, θ, and the warping function ψ:

$$\varepsilon_x = \frac{\partial u}{\partial x} = 0, \quad \varepsilon_y = \frac{\partial v}{\partial y} = 0, \quad \varepsilon_z = \frac{\partial w}{\partial z} = 0$$

$$\gamma_{xy} = \frac{\partial u}{\partial y} + \frac{\partial v}{\partial x} = -\theta z + \theta z = 0$$

$$\gamma_{yz} = \frac{\partial w}{\partial y} + \frac{\partial u}{\partial x} = \theta\left(\frac{\partial \psi}{\partial y} + x\right)$$

$$\gamma_{xz} = \frac{\partial w}{\partial x} + \frac{\partial u}{\partial z} = \theta\left(\frac{\partial \psi}{\partial x} - y\right)$$

Differentiating the first of the preceding equations by x and the second by y and then subtracting them yields

$$\frac{\partial \gamma_{xz}}{\partial y} - \frac{\partial \gamma_{yz}}{\partial x} = -2\theta$$

This relationship is a *compatibility condition* that must be satisfied by the two shear strain components on the cross section if the stated assumptions about the behavior, particularly the warping of the sections, is to hold.

It is possible to go ahead and formulate all the necessary problem equations in terms of the warping function to get to a solution. However, it is convenient to introduce the stress function, which satisfies the equations of equilibrium exactly. To do so, we note that all of the stress components are zero except those which match the two strain components—that is, τ_{xz}, τ_{yz}. As a consequence, the only equilibrium equation that is not satisfied identically is the z direction equation:

$$\frac{\partial \tau_{xz}}{\partial x} + \frac{\partial \tau_{yz}}{\partial y} = 0$$

A function $\phi(x, y)$ would satisfy this equation identically if the stresses were given by

$$\tau_{xz} = \frac{\partial \phi}{\partial y}; \quad \tau_{yz} = -\frac{\partial \phi}{\partial x}$$

Thus, the problem now can be expressed in terms of finding the function ϕ that satisfies the compatibility equation on the strains that was previously derived, and satisfying the necessary boundary conditions for the given cross-sectional shape.

If we now substitute the stress–strain and the stress function definitions into the foregoing compatibility equation, we arrive at the following differential equation for ϕ:

$$\frac{\partial^2 \phi}{\partial x^2} + \frac{\partial^2 \phi}{\partial y^2} = -2G\theta$$

This differential equation describes the necessary behavior of the function ϕ on the cross section of the bar. In addition, there are boundary conditions to satisfy. One boundary condition is that the lateral surface of the bar is stress free. Expressed mathematically, the stress vector must be zero. We introduce a unit vector $\vec{\nu}$, which defines the normal direction to the surface S, and the stress vector $\vec{T}^{(\nu)}$, which defines the stress at any point on the lateral surface S. We can write the unit normal vector on the lateral surface as

$$\vec{\nu}(S) = l\hat{i} + m\hat{j} + n\hat{k} = l\hat{i} + m\hat{j} + 0\hat{k}$$

The components of the unit vector, $l = \cos(x, \nu)$, $m = \cos(y, \nu)$, and $n = \cos(z, \nu)$, are the direction cosines of the normal to the surface with respect to the x, y, and z axes, respectively. (Note that $n = 0$ because the lateral surface is parallel to the z axis). The vector $\vec{T}^{(\nu)} = 0$, or in terms of components,

$$T_x^{(\nu)} = 0 = \sigma_x l + \tau_{xy} m + \tau_{xz} n$$

$$T_y^{(\nu)} = 0 = \tau_{xy} l + \sigma_y m + \tau_{yz} n$$

$$T_z^{(\nu)} = 0 = \tau_{xz} l + \tau_{yz} m + \sigma_z n$$

The first two of these equations are satisfied identically. Substituting for the stresses in terms of the stress function in the third equation yields

$$\frac{\partial \phi}{\partial y} l - \frac{\partial \phi}{\partial x} m = 0$$

This equation reduces to a very simple result, given the following information: The direction vector tangent to the local surface (see Figure 6.11) can be written as

$$\vec{\tau} = \frac{dx}{ds}\hat{i} + \frac{dy}{ds}\hat{j} = -m\hat{i} + l\hat{j}$$

where $s = $ distance along the boundary. So, substituting $l = dy/ds$, $m = -dx/ds$ into the preceding equation for ϕ yields

$$\frac{\partial \phi}{\partial x}\frac{dx}{ds} + \frac{\partial \phi}{\partial y}\frac{dy}{ds} = \frac{d\phi}{ds} = 0$$

or $\phi = $ constant on the boundary.

So, now the solution for ϕ is the function that satisfies the previous differential equation and is equal to a constant on any boundary. This is a very important and useful result. Although a closed form solution is available for only a few cases, a numerical solution for any shape can be found by a variety of methods.

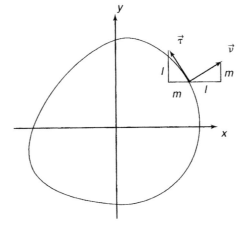

FIGURE 6.11 The contour of the cross section with unit normal vectors and unit tangent vectors. The direction cosines of the mutually perpendicular vectors are related as shown.

We note that the relationship between the stress function ϕ and the warping function ψ can be expressed by the stress–strain relations for a linear elastic material— that is, $\tau_{xz} = G\gamma_{xz}$, $\tau_{yz} = G\gamma_{yz}$—and the relationship between the strains and the warping function, namely,

$$\frac{\partial \phi}{\partial x} = -G\theta\left(\frac{\partial \psi}{\partial y} + x\right), \quad \frac{\partial \phi}{\partial y} = G\theta\left(\frac{\partial \psi}{\partial x} - y\right)$$

To satisfy the global equilibrium requirement, the moment of the shear stresses across any transverse face must equal the applied torque T. This requirement can be expressed as the following integral:

$$T = \iint_A (x\tau_{yz} - y\tau_{xz})\, dx\, dy$$

$$= -\iint_A \left(x\frac{\partial \phi}{\partial x} + y\frac{\partial \phi}{\partial y}\right) dx\, dy$$

This latter integral can be integrated by using Green's theorem from calculus to yield

$$T = 2 \iint_A \phi\, dx\, dy$$

This result can be interpreted as follows: The total torque across a section is equal to the volume under the surface $\phi(x, y)$. This result also leads to the very useful membrane analogy discussed next. We also note another useful result of applying the other function, the warping function ψ. By substituting the relationship between the two functions, we arrive at the following expression:

$$T = G\theta \iint_A \left(x^2 + y^2 + x\frac{\partial \psi}{\partial y} - y\frac{\partial \psi}{\partial x}\right) dx\, dy$$

If we let

$$J^* = \iint_A \left(x^2 + y^2 + x\frac{\partial \psi}{\partial y} - y\frac{\partial \psi}{\partial x}\right) dx\, dy$$

we can then write

$$T = GJ^*\theta \qquad \theta = \frac{T}{GJ^*}$$

This looks like the familiar equation relating torque to twist for a circular cross section; the difference is that the polar moment of inertia J has been replaced by the more complicated expression J^*. Note that if ψ is a constant, then $J^* = J$; hence, for a circular section, this must be the case.

Specific solutions are as follows:

(i) Circular cross section:

A function that will fit the boundary condition is $\phi(x, y) = C\left(\dfrac{x^2 + y^2}{a^2} - 1\right)$, where a is the radius of the circle. To find the unknown constant C, we can integrate the equation for the applied torque:

$$T = 2 \iint_A C\left(\frac{x^2 + y^2}{a^2} - 1\right) dx\, dy \Rightarrow T = \frac{2C}{a^2} \iint_A (x^2 + y^2 - a^2)\, dx\, dy$$

Integrating yields $C = (-T)/\pi a^2$. If we use this result to calculate the maximum stress from the stress function, we obtain the familiar expression, $\tau_{max} = Ta/J$. It is also easy to show that the corresponding warping function $\psi = 0$, and that the twist per unit length is the familiar expression $\theta = T/GJ$.

(ii) Elliptical cross section:

Following the same line of thought as for the circular cross section, we choose

$$\phi = C\left(\frac{x^2}{a^2} + \frac{y^2}{b^2} - 1\right),$$

where a and b are the half axis lengths of the ellipse. By substituting this expression into the equation for the torque and integrating, we arrive at the result $C = -(T/\pi ab)$. The corresponding value of the torsional constant is

$$J^* = \frac{\pi a^3 b^3}{a^2 + b^2}$$

This is in contrast to the polar moment of inertia,

$$J = \frac{\pi a^3 b}{4} + \frac{\pi a b^3}{4} = \frac{\pi}{a^2 + b^2}\left(\frac{a^5 b + ab^5}{4} + \frac{a^3 b^3}{2}\right)$$

The difference, and therefore the error from using J instead of J^*, increases as the elliptical cross section becomes more elongated. The corresponding angle of twist as function of torque for the elliptical cross section is

$$\theta = \frac{T}{J^* G} = \frac{T(a^2 + b^2)}{\pi a^3 b^3 G}$$

The shear stress components can now be expressed as follows:

$$\tau_{yz} = \frac{2Tx}{\pi a^3 b}, \qquad \tau_{xz} = \frac{-2Ty}{\pi ab^3}$$

$$\tau = \sqrt{(\tau_{yz})^2 + (\tau_{xz})^2} = \frac{2T}{\pi a^2 b^2}\sqrt{\frac{b^2 x^2}{a^2} + \frac{a^2 y^2}{b^2}}$$

By this equation and the fact that $-a \leq x \leq a$, $-b \leq y \leq b$, we can see that the shear stress will be largest on the boundary of the cross section. We can substitute the following relationships for a point (x, y) on the boundary:

$$x = a \cos \beta, \qquad y = b \sin \beta$$

Here, β is the angle between the x axis and a line from the centroid through the point on the boundary. Then the total shear stress on the boundary is given by

$$\tau = \frac{2T}{\pi a^2 b^2} \sqrt{b^2 + (a^2 - b^2) \sin^2 \beta}$$

If we now assume that a is the major half-diameter (i.e., $a > b$), then the maximum shear occurs at $\beta = \pi/2$ (i.e., along the minor axis at the least distance from the centroid of the cross section) and has the value $\tau_{max} = 2T/\pi ab^2$.

This is contrary to the result implied by the classical solution for a circular section where the largest shear stress occurs at the farthest distance from the center of the section. In noncircular sections, the maximum shear stress due to torsion still occurs at the boundary of the section, but not at the distance farthest from the centroid of the cross section. Note that the actual warping (i.e., the out-of-plane displacement of the cross section) is

$$w = \theta\psi = \frac{T(b^2 - a^2)}{\pi a^3 b^3 G} xy$$

(iii) Hollow elliptical cross sections:

The major complication with long bones is that they are hollow. For most hollow cross sections, solutions are difficult to obtain. However, for a hollow elliptical cross section of one particular type, the solution is fairly straightforward. This is the case where the inner and outer contours are related by a single constant ratio k. Let the outer elliptical contour be defined as done previously, and let the inner contour be defined as

$$\frac{x^2}{(ka)^2} + \frac{y^2}{(kb)^2} = 1$$

where $k < 1$ defines the ratio of the inner to outer radii. Then the torsional stiffness J^*, the twist versus torque relationship, and the maximum stress versus torque are given by the following equations:

$$J^* = (1 - k^4)\pi \frac{a^3 b^3}{a^2 + b^2}$$

$$\theta = \frac{1}{G} \frac{T}{(1 - k^4)} \frac{a^2 + b^2}{\pi a^3 b^3}$$

$$\tau_{max} = \frac{2T}{\pi ab^2} \frac{1}{1 - k^4}$$

The maximum shear stress still occurs at the outer radius along the minor axis. This is a fairly good approximation for a number of bone cross sections, where the medullary canal is reasonably congruent to the periosteal surface rectangular cross sections.

(iv) Rectangular cross sections:

Unlike the previous cases, it is not possible to write ϕ as a closed form function for a rectangular cross section. The solution can be expressed as an infinite series, and a few terms can be used to get good approximate solutions for some special circumstances. For the case where one cross-sectional dimension is reasonably large compared with the other, the approximations that follow are acceptable. For the torsional constant, the following three-term expression, where h and w are the thickness and width of the plate cross section, is a good approximation for $w/h \geq 4$ or so:

$$J^* = \frac{wh^3}{16}\left[\frac{16}{3} - 3.36\frac{h}{w}\left(1 - \frac{h^4}{12w^4}\right)\right]$$

The maximum stress, which occurs at the midpoint of the longer sides of the section (the shortest distance from the centroid), is reasonably approximated by the following expression:

$$\tau_{max} = \frac{3T}{wh^2}\left[1 + 0.6095\frac{h}{w} + 0.8865\left(\frac{h}{w}\right)^2 - 1.8023\left(\frac{h}{w}\right)^3 \right. $$
$$\left. + 0.9100\left(\frac{h}{w}\right)^4\right]$$

(v) Thin rectangular sections(Figure 6.12):

Obviously, if the width to thickness ratio is increased, the latter terms in the previous expressions can be ignored, leading to a simple result for the torsional constant and the maximum stress: $J^* = wh^3/3$, and $\tau_{max} = 3T/wh^2$. As one can deduce from the membrane analogy that follows, the maximum stress occurs nearly everywhere along the longer sides of the cross section in this case.

(vi) Thin-walled open sections:

Many open sections, such as thin-walled channels, angles, and even open circular sections, can be approximated by the solution for a long, thin rectangular cross section.

FIGURE 6.12 Some thin-walled shapes for which the thin rectangular section formula could be used. For sections with uniform thickness, the total width w would be the total perimeter. In cases (a), (b), and (c), the perimeter would be the sum of the leg lengths. If the thickness h varied from leg to leg, the products in the preceding expressions would be summed accordingly.

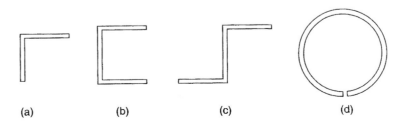

(a)   (b)   (c)   (d)

One interesting case in orthopaedic applications is the open circular section. One could estimate the effect of an open section for a bone with a significant defect or for a commonly used split intramedullary nail. The effect of an open section on strength and stiffness is dramatic. This comparison is left as an exercise for the student.

EXAMPLE 6.2 Torsional Characteristics of Square and Circular Bars

Question   Consider two bars with the same area and of circular and square cross sections. The square bar has width $2a$. The radius of a circular section with the same area would be $r = 2a/\sqrt{\pi}$. What is the torsional stiffness of each bar? What is the maximum shear stress due to a torque T for each bar?

Solution   For the square cross section, using the foregoing series expressions yields, for the torsional stiffness [i.e., torque/(twist per unit length)] and the outer fiber shear stress per unit moment,

$$T/\theta = \frac{(16Ga^4)}{16}(1 + .6095 + .8865 - 1.8023 + .91) = 2.253Ga^4$$

$$\tau_{max}/T = \frac{3}{8a^3}[1 + .6095 + .8865 - 1.8023 + .91] = \frac{.6014}{a^3}$$

where G is the shear modulus of the material. The corresponding values for the circular section would be

$$T/\theta = JG = \pi\frac{r^4}{2}*G = \frac{\pi}{2}\left[\frac{2a}{\sqrt{\pi}}\right]^4 *G = \frac{8}{\pi}a^4*G = 2.5465a^4*G$$

$$\tau_{max}/T = \frac{r}{J} = \frac{2}{\pi r^3} = \frac{2}{\pi\left[\dfrac{2a}{\sqrt{\pi}}\right]^3} = \frac{\sqrt{\pi}}{4a^3} = \frac{.4431}{a^3}$$

It can be seen that the circular section is more efficient in torsion. It is roughly 12 percent stiffer and roughly 35 percent stronger (35 percent less stress per unit torque) than for the square cross section. In fact, the circular cross section is the optimal shape of a solid section for resisting torsion. We note also that we used the series formula for calculating the twist and shear stress for the square cross section, even though the formula was said to be accurate for $w/t \geq 4$. A check with other approximations, such as tabulated values for constants in these equations, shows that these results are within 0.5 percent.

The Membrane Analogy

For most shapes, it is not possible to arrive at a closed form solution for ϕ, etc. If the shape is a polygon, there are solutions available in series form or through the use of conformal mapping using complex variables. However, there is a way of visualizing or even quantitatively predicting the torsional behavior of a prismatic bar of arbitrary cross section by using an analogy with the shape of a pressurized membrane. If a membrane is stretched across a hole that has the same shape as the cross section and then is inflated, the equilibrium of the membrane is represented by the same differential equation as the stress function ϕ if we let

$$\frac{P}{S} \Leftrightarrow 2G\theta$$

where

P = internal pressure behind the membrane and
S = tension in the membrane force/length.

Then the following analogies exist between the inflated membrane and the torsional stress distribution across the cross section of the bar:

The steepest slope of the membrane at any point $\Leftrightarrow$ magnitude of the shear stress.
The level contour line at any point $\Leftrightarrow$ direction of the total shear stress.
The volume under the membrane $\Leftrightarrow$ 1/2 the applied torque.

These analogies provide a convenient way for visualizing the shear stress distribution over any complex cross-sectional shape.

The membrane analogy can also be very helpful in dealing with hollow cross sections. In this case, a stress-free inner contour must also be at a constant value of ϕ. In the membrane analogy, the inner boundary must be parallel to the outer boundary, but displaced above it. Hence, to construct such a membrane model, it would be necessary to insert a rigid plate in the membrane that would elevate when the membrane is pressurized, but would remain parallel to the base. This idea is illustrated in Figure 6.13.

Also, recall that the density of the level contours (i.e., the slope of the membrane) defines the total stress at any point. This visualization suggests that, for a hollow section, the place where the stresses would be the highest correspond to the places where the wall thickness is least (Figure 6.13). This would correspond to the region where the contours are the closest together and the slope is the highest. Failure at the thinnest wall section is often observed when long bones are tested in torsion.

FIGURE 6.13 A membrane analogy for a hollow section. The interior region is represented as a rigid plate in the membrane model. The average membrane slope, corresponding to the average stress, would be greater at section B–B than at section A–A, because the wall is thinner.

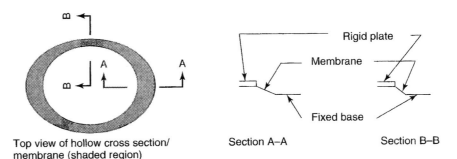

Top view of hollow cross section/ membrane (shaded region)

Section A–A

Section B–B

6.3 | Contact Stress Analysis

Joint replacements must provide motion while transmitting large forces across the joint. Consequently, they are similar to other contacting machine components such as rolling element bearings, gear teeth, and cams, where forces are transmitted across surfaces that are rolling or sliding with respect to each other. In many machines, the contacting elements have similar elastic moduli. This is also true in some joint replacements, where the bearing pairs are metal on metal or ceramic on ceramic. In such cases, both components deform in the region of contact. However, the most commonly used bearing pairs in joint replacements are metal on polyethylene, where the elastic modulus of the metal component is two orders of magnitude greater than the modulus of the polyethylene. When the moduli differ by such a large amount, the metal component functions as a rigid indenter of the polyethylene surface. To understand the mechanisms of damage that can occur in total joint replacements, we must be able to analyze the stresses and deformations associated with both types of contact.

For nonconforming contact such as occurs in many knee replacements, we realize intuitively that the maximum contact pressure or contact stress between two bodies increases as the contact area decreases. The contact area will decrease if the surfaces become less conforming or if the elastic moduli of the contacting components increase. Consequently, the maximum contact pressure generally increases with decreasing conformity and increasing elastic modulus. For conforming contact such as occurs in hip replacements, however, we will find that stresses become insensitive to modulus as conformity increases.

The contact pressures are not uniform across the contact area. For contact between spherical or toroidal surfaces, the maximum pressure occurs at the center of the contact area. But we will see that, for other geometries, the maximum contact stress occurs near the edges of contact.

We will also see that even frictionless contact produces normal stresses tangential to the surface and shear stresses beneath the surface. The situation is more complex if we include friction between the contacting components and nonlinear material properties. If we want to understand the mechanisms of damage in joint replacements, we will ultimately have to be prepared to include these factors in our analyses.

Therefore, it is clear that stress analysis of bodies in contact is a complex problem. The topic is often introduced in books on advanced strength of materials. It is helpful, therefore, to take a step-by-step approach to develop an understanding of the problem. Because the detailed derivations are fairly involved, we will omit much of that and concentrate on the relevant results. A good place to start is with Hertz theory for contact between elastic bodies with similar moduli. Hertz theory will provide good approximations to the stresses due to contact between metal on metal and ceramic on ceramic joints, and in the process we will learn some general characteristics of the contact problem that will give us insight into the behavior of rigid indenter contact as well. However, to understand the behavior of metal on polyethylene joints in more detail, we will need to take the next step and use approximate solutions from the theory of elasticity or the results from finite element analyses. Therefore, in the second part of this section, we will develop an approximate solution for elastic behavior when one of the contacting components can be considered to be rigid with respect to the other.

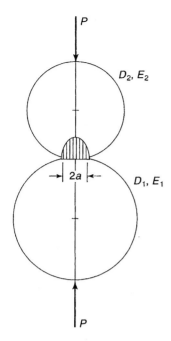

FIGURE 6.14 Contact between two spheres.

Contact Stresses: Hertz Theory

The basic assumptions for Hertzian contact are that the contact areas are small with respect to the size of the bodies in contact, that both surfaces deform, and that the elastic moduli of the contacting components are similar.

For two spheres in contact (Figure 6.14), the maximum pressure is given by

$$p_{max} = \frac{1.5P}{\pi a^2}$$

and the relative motion between the spheres along the axis of loading is given by

$$\delta = 1.04 \left(\frac{P^2 C_M^2}{C_G} \right)^{1/3}$$

where the radius of the contact area is

$$a = 0.721 (P C_G C_M)^{1/3}$$

The two parameters C_M and C_G account for the material properties of the contacting spheres (C_M) and the relative geometry of the contacting spherical surfaces (C_G). These parameters are given by

$$C_M = \frac{1 - \nu_1^2}{E_1} + \frac{1 - \nu_2^2}{E_2}$$

and

$$C_G = \frac{D_1 D_2}{D_1 + D_2}$$

For convex contact between spheres that have the same diameter D and are made of the same material with $\nu = .3$, these equations reduce to

$$a = .699 \left[\frac{PD}{E} \right]^{1/3}$$

and

$$p_{max} = .978 \left[\frac{PE^2}{D^2} \right]^{1/3}$$

We can see that both the contact area and the maximum contact pressure are nonlinear functions of load, modulus, and conformity, even though linearly elastic material behavior is assumed. All contact problems are inherently nonlinear. These relationships show us some fundamental characteristics of contact problems encountered in bone-implant systems. First, when the load increases, the contact area and the stress both increase. Second, if the diameter of the spheres decreases (contact is less conforming), the contact area decreases and the contact pressure increases. Finally, if the elastic modulus increases, then the contact area decreases and the maximum pressure increases.

The relationships for contact between spherical components are easily modified for two important cases. First, a sphere on a flat plate can be modeled by dividing the numerator and denominator of the expression for C_G by D_1 and then letting D_2 go to ∞, to obtain

$$C_G = D_2$$

If the contact is between a sphere and a spherical cup, as shown in Figure 6.15, C_G is given by

$$C_G = \frac{D_1 D_2}{D_1 - D_2}$$

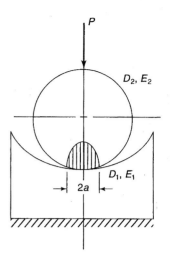

FIGURE 6.15 Contact between a sphere and a spherical cup.

EXAMPLE 6.3 Contact Stress in a Total Knee Replacement

Question The contact between femoral and tibial components in a total knee replacement can be approximated by contact between a metal sphere ($D_2 = 40$ mm) and a polyethylene cup ($D_1 = 80$ mm, $E_1 = 1$ GPa, $\nu_1 = .46$). How does the maximum pressure change if the metal component is made of CoCr alloy ($E = 200,000$ MPa, $\nu = .3$) instead of titanium alloy ($E = 100,000$ MPa, $\nu = .3$).

Solution Since the polyethylene cup is concave,

$$C_G = \frac{D_1 D_2}{D_1 - D_2} = \frac{80(40)}{80 - 40} = 80 \text{ mm}$$

The material parameter when CoCr alloy is used is given by

$$C_M = \frac{1 - \nu_1^2}{E_1} + \frac{1 - \nu_2^2}{E_2} = \frac{1 - .46^2}{1000} + \frac{1 - .3^2}{200,000} = 7.93(10^{-4})$$

Then

$$a = 0.721(PC_G C_M)^{1/3} = .721[(3000)(80)7.93(10^{-4})]^{1/3} = 4.15 \text{ mm}$$

and the maximum pressure is given by

$$p_{max} = \frac{1.5P}{\pi a^2} = \frac{1.5(3000)}{\pi(4.15)^2} = 83.2 \text{ MPa}$$

Similarly, for a titanium alloy sphere, we obtain

$$C_M = \frac{1 - \nu_1^2}{E_1} + \frac{1 - \nu_2^2}{E_2} = \frac{1 - .46^2}{1000} + \frac{1 - .3^2}{100,000} = 7.98(10^{-4}),$$

$$a = 0.721(PC_G C_M)^{1/3} = .721[(3000)(80)7.98(10^{-4})]^{1/3} = 4.16 \text{ mm, and}$$

$$p_{max} = \frac{1.5P}{\pi a^2} = \frac{1.5(3000)}{\pi(4.16)^2} = 83.0 \text{ MPa}.$$

We see that the maximum pressure is essentially the same, whether the contact occurs between CoCr alloy and polyethylene or titanium alloy and polyethylene. Most of the deformation takes place in the polyethylene; a metal sphere is basically a rigid indenter.

The maximum pressure for contact between two spheres with different radii is shown in Figure 6.16, where, for each case, $D_1 = 40$ mm. Note that when the load increases, the pressure also increases, but nonlinearly, because the contact area also increases with increasing load. Contact between a ball and flat can be modeled by making one of the radii infinitely large ($D_2 = 10,000$ mm in Figure 6.16). In Figure 6.17, the curve for $D_2 = -80$ represents the contact pressure between a 40 mm ball and an 80 mm socket, which might approximate contact between the femoral and tibial components of the knee joint. The curve for $D_2 = -41$ approximates contact between the ball and socket of the hip joint. $D_2 = 40$ or 80 could represent the convex–convex contact between the femoral and patellar components of a total knee replacement.

So far, we have considered only the maximum pressure due to contact. This is the stress acting normal to the contact surface, and for frictionless contact, it is the only surface traction between the contacting bodies. There are, of course, other

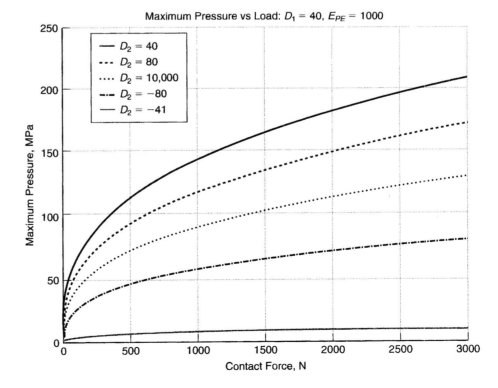

FIGURE   6.16 Maximum Hertzian contact pressure as a function of load. The indenter diameter (D_1) is 40 mm, and the modulus of the polyethylene is $E_{PE} = 1000$ MPa. The contact conditions range from convex–concave ($D_2 = -41$), to ball-on-flat ($D_2 = 10,000$), to convex–convex ($D_2 = 40$ mm).

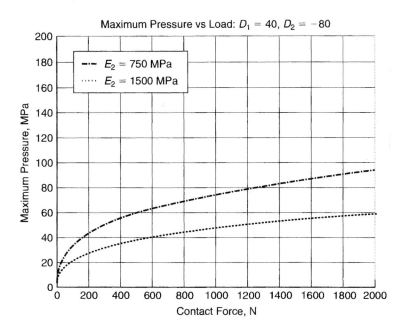

FIGURE   6.17 Maximum pressure as a function of load for two spherical surfaces in contact.

stresses acting within the material. In contact mechanics, it is important to know how these stresses vary near the surface and how they vary with depth beneath the surface.

The stresses due to contact across the contact area and beneath the center of the contact area are shown for two spheres in Figure 6.18. The spheres have the same diameter and the same material properties; the contact is frictionless; and the contact area is circular. The normal stress components at the surface are shown in the upper portion of the figure; the stresses below the center of the contact area are shown in the lower portion of the figure as a function of depth beneath the surface.

There are three important characteristics to notice. First, tensile stresses occur in a radial direction at the edge of the contact area. Second, at the center of the contact area, a nearly hydrostatic stress state occurs; if the material is incompressible ($\nu = .5$), the stress at the center of the contact area is hydrostatic. Finally, the maximum shear stress occurs below the center of the contact area at $z/a = 0.51$, and its magnitude is $\tau_{max} = 0.31 p_{max}$.

Note that the normal stress components shown in Figure 6.18 are principal stresses because the contact is frictionless. In the upper portion of the figure, the compressive (negative) stresses are plotted above the axis. Therefore, the maximum normal stress, σ_r/p_m, which acts at the surface and parallel to the surface, is compressive at the center of contact and tensile at the edge of contact. As noted previously, the maximum shear stress acts beneath the surface below the center of contact. We will see these same phenomena when we look at more detailed analyses based on the theory of elasticity and finite element methods.

At the surface, the stresses tangent to the surface, σ_r and σ_θ, at the center of the contact are compressive. This can be understood by considering a cylindrical column of material immediately under the load. When the load is applied, the column shortens and expands, but since the column is part of the larger component, its

FIGURE 6.18 Hertz stresses for two spheres in contact. In the figure p_m = average pressure = $P(\pi a^2)$, τ_1 = maximum shear stress.

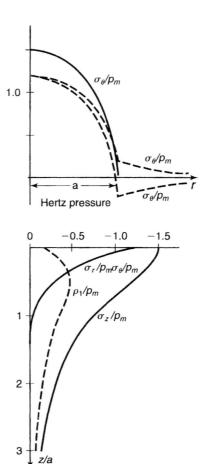

expansion is restricted by the material surrounding it, which induces a radial compressive stress acting on the column. Note also that the maximum shear stress occurs under the center of the contact area, but beneath the surface.

When the appropriate values for modulus and Poisson's ratio are substituted into these equations, we find that

$$\sigma_{max} = \frac{1.5P}{\pi a^2} \text{ or } a = a(P^{1/3})$$

$$\tau_{max} = \frac{\sigma_{max}}{3} \text{ at a depth } 0.51a$$

$$\sigma_{T_{max}} = \frac{(1 - 2\nu)\sigma_{max}}{3} \text{ at radius } a$$

Contact Stresses: Elasticity Solution

Consider the axisymmetric contact problem of a metal ball indenting a metal-backed polyethylene cup (Figure 6.19). The radius of the ball is r_b, the inside radius

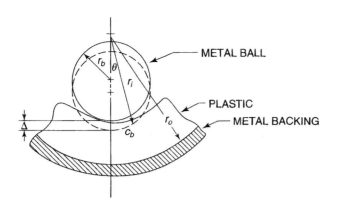

of the polyethylene liner is r_i, and the outside radius of the liner is r_b. The radial clearance is $r_i - r_b$. The ball acts as a rigid indenter. The metal backing is also rigid since, for dimensions typical of most implant applications, the backing may be assumed to be a thick shell. Consequently, it is structurally very stiff with respect to the polyethylene component. The system is axisymmetric, and displacement of the ball with respect to the cup is along the axis of symmetry.

The model is a good approximation of an acetabular cup, where the contact surfaces are nearly conforming. As will be shown, it can also be used to approximate less conforming surfaces, such as those found in certain metal-backed tibial components. Consequently, it may be employed to study a wide variety of design variables, including the effect of conformity on contact stresses.

Elasticity Solution

The displacement of the ball with respect to the cup along the axis of symmetry is Δ. This causes a radial displacement of the surface, b, along the line that makes an angle θ with the axis of symmetry. The surface displacement b is assumed to vary between a maximum value Δ along the axis of symmetry ($\theta = 0$) and zero at the edge of the contact zone ($\theta = \theta_{max}$).

The differential equations of equilibrium are written in spherical coordinates (r, α, θ) in terms of displacements $(u_r, u_\alpha, u_\theta)$. It is then assumed that the displacement in the radial direction, u_r, dominates, and that the displacements u_α and u_θ and the derivatives of all displacements with respect to α and θ may be neglected. This reduces the equilibrium equations to a single differential equation in terms of the radial displacement only:

$$\frac{\partial^2 u_r}{\partial r^2} + \frac{2}{r}\frac{\partial u_r}{\partial r} - 2\frac{u_r}{r^2} = 0$$

The general solution of this equation is

$$u_r = Ar + \frac{B}{r^2}$$

The parameters A and B are determined from the boundary conditions

$$u_r(r_i) = b(\theta), \quad u_r(r_o) = 0$$

where b is a known function of θ. Substituting the results into the general solution and writing the stresses as a function of the radial displacement u_r, we see that the contact stress may be written as a function of b:

$$\sigma_r = -\left[\frac{1}{1-2\nu} + \frac{2}{1+\nu}\frac{1}{(r/r_o)^3}\right]\left[\frac{1}{(r/r_o)^3 - 1}\right]E\frac{b}{r_i}$$

The radial displacement, b, is determined from the law of cosines,

$$r_b^2 = (r_i + b)^2 + (r_i - r_b + \Delta)^2 - 2(r_i + b)(r_i - r_b + \Delta)\cos\theta$$

This equation is a quadratic in $r_i + b$, so the following general expression for b can be obtained:

$$b(\theta) = \left[\cos\theta + \sqrt{\left(\frac{r_b}{r_i - r_b + \Delta}\right)^2 - \sin^2\theta}\right](r_i - r_b + \Delta) - r_i$$

The angle defining the limit of contact, θ_{max}, can be determined from the law of cosines equation by setting $b = 0$.

$$\theta_{max} = \cos^{-1}\left[\frac{r_i^2 - r_b^2 + (r_i - r_b + \Delta)^2}{2r_i(r_i - r_b + \Delta)}\right]$$

Therefore, the contact stress $\sigma_r(r_i)$ and the extent of contact are completely determined when Δ is known.

The relationship between the maximum radial deflection and the applied load P is obtained using from the equation

$$P = \pi\int_0^{\theta_{max}} \sigma_r(r_i + b)^2 \sin(2\theta)\, d\theta$$

and the expression for $r_i + b$ is determined from

$$b(\theta) = \left[\cos\theta + \sqrt{\left(\frac{r_b}{r_i - r_b + \Delta}\right)^2 - \sin^2\theta}\right](r_i - r_b + \Delta) - r_i$$

The value of Δ corresponding to a given applied load, P, was determined by solving the equation for P iteratively.

This approach was used to compute the values of contact stress as a function of thickness and conformity (Figure 6.20), and contact stress as a function of thickness and polyethylene modulus (Figure 6.21).

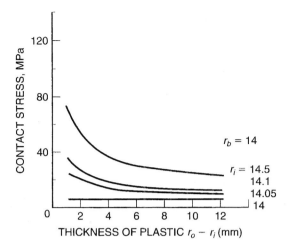

FIGURE 6.20   Contact stress as a function of thickness for various clearances.

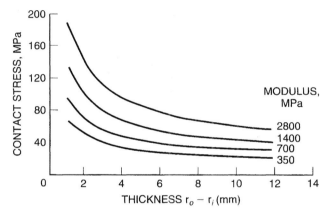

FIGURE 6.21   Contact stress as a function of thickness for various values of polyethylene modulus.

6.4 | Summary

A number of important structural mechanics problems in skeletal biomechanics do not yield to simple beam analysis. Beginning with the fundamental principles of elastic behavior of materials, one can address several of these problems with somewhat more complicated models represented by more complex differential equations. These models can still be used to efficiently examine basic behaviors and effects of material parameters without resorting to more sophisticated computer models.

Beam on elastic foundation theory is useful to examine the transverse load transfer of an implant against a bone, such as the load transfer between a hip stem and a femoral shaft and between a tibial component and the proximal tibia. The theory requires some knowledge of the elastic stiffness of the foundation representing the material adjacent to the femoral stem or tibial tray. The model shows that relatively short, stiff beams move into the substrate almost as a rigid body, whereas relatively long, flexible beams will tend to lift off at their ends under the loads.

Torsional analysis of long bones with noncircular cross sections yields differential equations that can be solved analytically for only a few simple shapes. Approximate solutions can be obtained for other shapes, which yield an insight into the significance of shape factors, for example. The peak stresses for irregular shapes do not occur at the greatest distance from the centroid of the cross section. For instance, an ellipsoidal or rectangular cross section receives the highest stresses at the outer surface closest to the centroid—that is, the minor diameter or the least width. This result cannot be anticipated from the simple torsional analysis of a circular cross section.

Basic features of the contact problem between articulating joint surfaces can be examined by Hertz theory if the contact area is small compared with the curvature of the contacting surfaces. Hertz theory yields the interesting result that the peak stresses in the contacting materials can occur at some depth below the contact surfaces. This is an important result in application to the design of articular joint replacements. Hertz contact theory allows the ready examination of geometric factors, especially component radius, on component stresses.

Many problems require even more complex models because the problem geometry or material behavior does not conform to the assumptions in these models. Often, these problems are attacked by the finite element method, a numerical method that has become a ubiquitous tool in structural analysis and other applications. However, the methods of this and the previous chapter have proven very useful in studying the fundamental structural behavior of the skeletal system. Further, they provide efficient tools to study the effects of various material and geometric factors on the performance of devices used to repair and reconstruct the system.

6.5   EXERCISES

6.1   A finite-length beam is supported by an elastic foundation. The 50-mm-long beam is made of polyethylene with modulus 1.0 GPa and has a cross section 8 mm high by 5 mm wide. It is supported by cancellous bone with modulus 800 MPa. Recall that $k \neq E$ for the foundation.

A 1000 N load is applied at the center of the beam. Determine the maximum stress in the beam and the loading on the foundation along the length of the beam.

6.2   Do Exercise 6.1 for the case where the beam is a composite beam. The cross section comprises a 2-mm-thick layer of CoCr alloy next to the cancellous

bone with a polyethylene component bonded to it, whose cross section is 5 mm × 6 mm.

6.3   The finite-length beam in Figure P 6.1 is subjected to a load that moves from the center, $x = 0.5L$, to a point $x = .9L$ along the length of the beam. By plotting the loading as a function of length for $x/L = 0.5$, 0.6, 0.7, 0.8, and 0.9, show how the loading on the foundation varies as the load moves.

6.4   For the finite-length beam in Figure P 6.1, plot the loading on the foundation as a function of x for changes in the modulus of the foundation, $E = 400$, 600, 800, 1000, 1200 MPa.

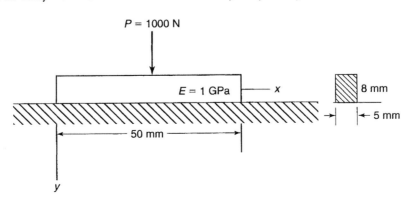

FIGURE P 6.1

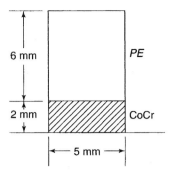

FIGURE P 6.2

6.5 For the finite-length beam in Figure P 6.1, plot the loading on the foundation as a function of x for changes in the structural rigidity, EI, of the beam. Use a range for EI that includes cross sections that are 5 mm wide, but that vary in height from 6 mm to 10 mm, and material properties varying from all polyethylene to all CoCr.

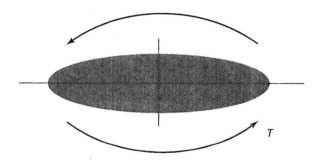

FIGURE P 6.6

6.6 A beam with an irregular cross section develops a much more complex distribution of torsional stresses than one with a circular cross section.

(a) Indicate where you expect the highest torsional stresses due to twisting of the bar with the cross section shown in Figure P 6.6.

(b) Provide a qualitative explanation for this difference.

6.7 The stress function for a torsional member with an equilateral triangular cross section is given by

$$\phi = k\left(x - \sqrt{3}y - \frac{2}{3}h\right)\left(x + \sqrt{3}y - \frac{2}{3}h\right)\left(x + \frac{1}{3}h\right)$$

where h is the height of the triangle and the origin of (x, y) is at the centroid.

(a) Determine the torsional rigidity parameter J^*.

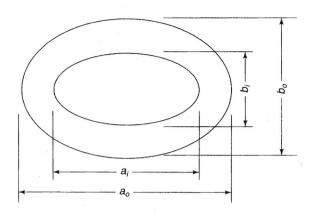

FIGURE P 6.8

(b) Compare J^* with the corresponding value of J^* for a circular cross section with the same area.

6.8 A bone cross section can often be approximated as an ellipse(Figure 6.8). The torsional rigidity of a cross section is defined by the product of shear modulus G and the torsional constant J^*, which is given as follows for a cross section defined by congruent ellipses.

(a) Compare the torsional rigidity of the section with that of a circular section of the same area and ratio of inner to outer diameter.

(b) Describe the location of the maximum shear stress for the elliptical cross section.

(c) Indicate whether the torsional strength of the elliptical cross section would be less than or greater than the circular case.

$$J^* = \pi\left\{\frac{a_o^3 b_o^3}{a_o^2 + b_o^2} - \frac{a_i^3 b_i^3}{a_i^2 + b_i^2}\right\} = \pi \frac{a_o^3 b_o^3}{a_o^2 + b_o^2}(1 - f^4)$$

$$\text{Area} = A = \pi(a_o b_o - a_i b_i) = \pi a_o b_o(1 - f^2)$$

$$\text{where } f = a_i/a_o = b_i/b_o.$$

6.9 Estimate the strength of the tibial cross section shown in Figure P 6.9. The section is about 50 mm below the tibial tuberosity; the largest dimension of the cross section is 40 mm.

6.10 Three cross sections of a tibia are shown in Figure P 6.10: 100 mm, 150 mm, and 200 mm below the tibial tuberosity. The 150 mm cross section is very near the isthmus of the tibia. Determine the relative torsional strength of these cross sections compared with that of the weakest section by approximating each cross section, using congruent, hollow elliptical geometry.

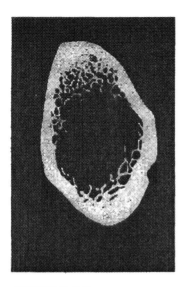

FIGURE P 6.9

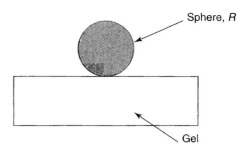

FIGURE P 6.11   A sphere placed on a gel. The elastic modulus of the gel can be estimated by measuring the amount the sphere sinks into the gel.

6.11   Cell deformation and motion are a function of the elastic properties of the substrate to which they are attached. The substrates for *in vitro* studies are typically quite thin. Thicker specimens of the substrate material can be used to estimate the elastic modulus by using Hertz contact theory. Figure P 6.11 shows a sphere of radius R and a gel substrate. Determine an expression for the elastic modulus of the gel in terms of the distance the sphere sinks into the gel and the size and weight of the sphere. Assume that the sphere is rigid with respect to the substrate and that the Poisson's ratio for the gel is $\nu = .45$.

6.12   Use Hertz theory to estimate the maximum contact pressure between a ball and a socket that are both made from Al_2O_3, with modulus $E = 300$ GPa. The ball is 28 mm in diameter, and the diametral clearance varies from 0.0 to 0.5 mm. Make a plot that shows how the maximum contact pressure varies with clearance.

6.13   Assume axisymmetric contact between CoCr and polyethylene components with spherical surfaces. The contact force is 1500 N, and the diameter, D_2, of the CoCr component is 40 mm. Show how the depth of the maximum shear stress in the polyethylene varies with the diameter of the polyethylene component for $D_1 = -41, -80, 10{,}000, 80, 40$. Recall that the negative signs indicate a concave surface.

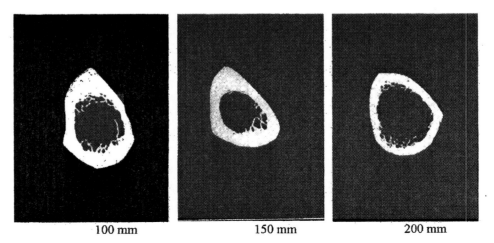

FIGURE P 6.10   Cross sections of a tibia at 100, 150, and 200 mm below the tibial tuberosity.

Bone-Implant Systems

Treatments for many orthopaedic disorders involve implants that are attached to bone. Examples include devices for fixation of bone fractures, joint replacements for arthritic joints (Figure 7.1), and devices to promote fusion of bony segments. When a device is attached to bone, the load transfer through the bone is altered. As we saw in Section 5.1 and 6.1, the magnitudes of the loads carried by the bone and the implant as part of the composite system depend upon the elastic modulus and geometry of the implant and the bone.

The geometry and the material properties of the implant and the bone determine not only how loads are shared between the bone and the implant, but also how the load is transferred from one to the other. Load transfer occurs at the interfaces between the bone and the implant and between the components of a modular implant. Often, this involves intermediate materials or devices. Examples include porous coatings on joint replacement components for bone ingrowth, the layer of polymethylmethacrylate used for cement fixation in joint replacements, the screws used to hold fracture fixation devices to bone, and the locking mechanisms in modular prostheses.

As we saw in Chapter 2, the loads acting on bones through the joints can be quite large. Therefore, we are not only interested in the elastic properties of the components; we have to be concerned about the strength of the components as well. Clearly, to understand the performance of implants, we need to know something about their mechanical properties; an overview is provided in the next section.

After an introduction to materials and how they are processed, the general concepts of bone-implant systems, fracture fixation devices, and joint replacements are presented in Sections 7.3 and 7.4. Although both involve the interaction of an implant with the bone to which it is attached, their functions are quite different. Fracture fixation devices are assistive devices and are in many cases removed after the fracture has healed enough to allow the bone to support functional loads. Joint prostheses replace the articulating surfaces of damaged joints and are intended, in most cases, to last the life of the patient. More detail about the mechanics and design of these important bone-implant systems is provided in subsequent chapters.

FIGURE 7.1 This knee replacement is made from metal and polyethylene. The femoral component is often made of CoCr alloy; the metal in the tibial tray and fixation stem component may be either CoCr or titanium alloy. The tibial component can also be made entirely out of polyethylene.

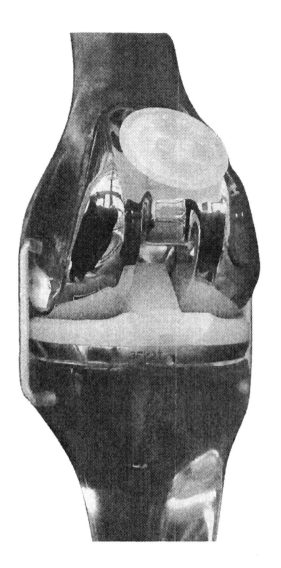

7.1 | Implant Materials

Materials that are used in the body are often called biomaterials, which include both engineered and natural materials. We have already encountered natural biomaterials in Chapters 3 and 4, where the hard and soft tissues of the musculoskeletal system were discussed. Engineered materials can further be divided into two classes—bio-inert materials and bioactive materials. Both types are used in bone-implant systems. The metal and polymeric components typically used for joint replacements are bio-inert, but portions of joint replacement components may be coated with bioactive materials to enhance bone response. For example, some devices are fixed to bone by bone ingrowth into a porous layer or by bone growth against a roughened surface. Bioactive materials can be used to enhance this process.

Bioactive materials may also be used for structural components. An internal fracture fixation device, such as plate or a screw, must be stiff enough and strong enough to enhance fracture healing initially, but may be surgically removed after healing has occurred to avoid stress shielding in the bone. An alternative approach is to make the device or screw from a bioactive material that is gradually resorbed by the body. This avoids the surgery required to remove components that are no longer necessary and allows the bone to take the entire load, instead of sharing it with an implant.

Tissue engineering is a field that is concerned with creating and modifying biological materials for specific purposes. For example, a tissue defect might be treated by filling it with a scaffold that has been seeded with cells. The scaffold can be made of material that initially provides the necessary structural function, allows the cells to reproduce the lost tissue, and gradually resorbs to allow the new tissue to take over the function entirely. These approaches will become increasingly important in the future.

Both bio-inert and bioactive materials used in the body must be biocompatible. That is, the body must not damage or impair the function of the implanted material, and the material must not damage the tissues of the musculoskeletal system. Biocompatibility is a two-way street.

Biocompatibility is determined by extensive testing before an implant is used in people. For commonly used implant materials, the biocompatibility of bulk components has been established for many years through *in vitro* and *in vivo* evaluation and clinical experience. Materials that pass the tests in bulk, however, may produce tissue reactions as small particles. For example, a polyethylene component may be biocompatible, but if the bearing surface of the component wears, particles are released that can trigger biological reactions when enough of them accumulate in the surrounding tissues. To a large extent, this is the response of the body to foreign particles regardless of material, but the material type and chemistry can also affect both the kind and degree of tissue reactions that occur.

The range of materials encountered in treating musculoskeletal disorders is broad, and the interactions of these materials with tissues are complex. Experts in this area of biomaterials must know the characteristics of the implanted materials and the reactions of these materials with the biological environment over scales ranging from the cellular level to tissue systems. The biological interactions involved in biocompatibility, bioactive materials, and tissue engineering are beyond the scope of this book. In this chapter, we restrict ourselves to a discussion of the structural properties of bio-inert metals and polymers to lay a foundation for understanding the structural interactions between implants and components of the musculoskeletal system that are discussed in the chapters that follow.

Typical Mechanical Properties of Implant Materials

The most commonly used metals and polymers for orthopaedic applications are stainless steels, cobalt–chromium alloys, titanium alloys, ultrahigh molecular weight polyethylene (UHMWPE), and polymethyl methacrylate (PMMA). Their typical mechanical properties, are presented in Table 7.1. The values in the table approximate medians of the ranges of values that one finds in the literature. The ranges can be surprisingly large, even for materials described by the same name and

TABLE 7.1

Typical Mechanical Properties of Implant Metals and Polymers					
Material	Condition	Elastic Modulus (GPa)	Yield Strength (MPa)	Ultimate Strength (MPa)	Endurance Limit (MPa)
Stainless Steels	Annealed	190	331	586	260
	30% cold worked	190	792	930	380
	Cold forged	190	1213	1351	820
Cobalt–Chromium Alloys	As cast/annealed	210	480	770	260
	Hot forged	210	1050	1500	750
Titanium	Pure titanium	97	175	240	200
	Pure 30% cold worked	110	485	760	300
	Alloy forged annealed	116	896	965	620
UHMWPE		1	25	45	22
PMMA	Tension	2.3	—	35	8
	Compression	2.7	—	98	—

condition. This suggests that small changes in production processes can result in relatively large changes in mechanical properties. The representative values in Table 7.1 are suitable for our studies of bone-implant systems. However, those who analyze or design systems with specific materials should not be satisfied with generic properties, but should establish the properties for the particular materials they are using.

We can make some interesting general observations from the table. For example, stainless steel and cobalt–chromium alloys have similar elastic moduli, which are about twice the modulus of titanium alloys, and an order of magnitude stiffer than the typical cortical bone (Chapter 3), which is in turn about an order of magnitude stiffer than either UHMWPE or PMMA. In addition, cobalt–chromium and titanium alloys are typically less ductile and stronger than stainless steels. We can also see that the processing conditions have large effects on static and fatigue strengths of the materials and that materials such as PMMA have properties that differ in tension and compression.

Metals

Stainless Steels   Stainless steels can be cast, forged, or extruded. The primary strengthening mechanism is cold working. They are primarily used for temporary implant devices, such as fracture plates (Figure 7.2), screws, and hip nails. Although they have been largely supplanted by cobalt–chromium and titanium alloys for permanent implants, stainless steels are still used in some joint replacement components. The properties of medical grade stainless steel provide a balance between high strength, ductility, and fatigue performance. Ductility is important for fracture fixation components, where, for example, bone plates are deformed in the operating room to conform to the bone curvature at the fracture site.

Corrosion resistance is an important consideration and is achieved in stainless steels by keeping the carbide content to a minimum and by including chromium.

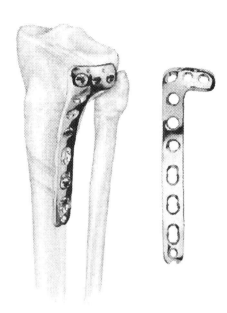

FIGURE 7.2 A stainless steel plate for fracture fixation of the proximal tibia. Ductility is important because the plate must be deformed in the operating room to conform to the bone. The fracture fragments are held in place with stainless steel screws. (Reproduced with permission of Synthes.)

Resistance to pitting and crevice corrosion is also important and typically increases with increasing contents of chromium, molybdenum, and nitrogen. When components are manufactured from stainless steel, a cobalt, chromium, and nickel oxide layer is formed by passivating the devices in a strong nitric acid bath. If the protective film is scratched in air, no serious problem results because the film reforms. This oxide layer improves the *in vivo* corrosion resistance by providing a passive layer between bodily tissues and the bulk material.

Cobalt–Chromium Alloys   The range of properties available for cobalt–chromium alloys (Table 7.1) and the ability to easily fabricate components from these alloys make them ideal for metallic components of joint replacements and fracture fixation devices. Cobalt–chromium alloys are also highly resistive to corrosion (particularly crevice corrosion), resistant to fatigue cracking caused by galvanic corrosion, and relatively ductile. The modulus of elasticity for cobalt–chromium alloys varies from 210 to 253 GPa (Table 7.1), which is higher than for stainless steel and titanium alloys. As with stainless steel, the chromium forms a strongly adherent oxide film that provides a passive layer shielding the bulk material from the environment. These alloys also have exceptional biocompatibility in bulk form.

There are two cobalt–chromium alloys commonly used for medical applications: a cobalt–chromium–molybdenum alloy (CoCrMo) and a cobalt–nickel–chromium–molybdenum alloy (CoNiCrMo). The predominant difference between the two is the process by which they are shaped. The CoCrMo alloy is difficult to forge and hard to machine. Therefore, parts are typically made by using investment (lost wax) casting procedures. In the investment casting process, a wax replica of the component is created and dipped into a ceramic slurry, which is then heated until the wax flows out (the wax is lost), leaving a ceramic mold into which molten metal is poured. The casting and cooling process is controlled to improve properties by insuring that the resulting microstructure has a small grain size and evenly distributed carbides; unacceptably large grain sizes compromise fatigue strength and can lead to clinical failures. The properties of the material can be further improved by using hot isostatic pressing to produce plastic flow of the alloy, which collapses voids and cavities in the material that might otherwise act as crack initiators within the material. Table 7.1 shows the improvement in strength that can be achieved with this process over cast material.

Components made from CoNiCrMo alloy are usually formed by hot forging processes. Post-processing procedures, including cold working and annealing, are applied to forged cobalt alloys to produce a very fine grain size that contributes to making this alloy one of the strongest and most fatigue resistant alloys for orthopaedic applications. The superior fatigue and ultimate tensile strength of the forged alloy make it suitable for applications that require long service life without fracture or fatigue. As with other alloys, however, increased strength is accompanied by decreased ductility.

Titanium Alloys   The titanium-based material most commonly used in orthopaedic applications is titanium–aluminum–vanadium alloy, Ti-6Al-4V. It was developed by the aerospace industry as a high strength-to-weight ratio material. Unalloyed pure titanium is sometimes used for implants where high stresses are not expected, such as fracture fixation devices for hands and wrists, because its tensile strength is low compared with stainless steel (Figure 7.3). If high strength is necessary, titanium alloys must be used.

An adherent passive layer of titanium oxide (TiO_2) provides corrosion resistance that significantly exceeds that of stainless steel and the cobalt alloys, even in saline solutions. The material also has excellent resistance to pitting, intergranular, and crevice corrosion. Furthermore, the oxide surfaces of titanium and its alloys provide outstanding interfaces with bone, which can grow right up to the surface without the substantial fibrous layer seen at other metal–bone interfaces.

The elastic modulus of titanium alloys is about half that of stainless steel or cobalt–chromium alloys. Thus, the structural rigidity of components that share load with bone can be reduced by half without changing the shape of the implant. As was seen in Chapters 5 and 6, loads in some bone-implant systems are shared according to the relative structural rigidity of the implant to the bone. In such cases, the bone will carry more of the load when a titanium implant is used instead of one made from stainless steel or cobalt–chromium alloys, and the risk of stress shielding may be reduced.

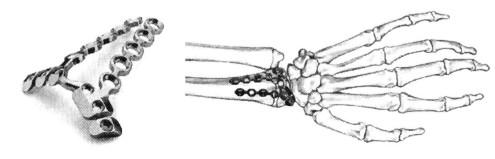

FIGURE 7.3 A pure titanium fixation plate for distal fractures of the radius. (Reproduced with permission of Synthes.)

Ti6Al4V alloy is a notch-sensitive material. As a result, titanium implants must be designed with care. This is particularly true when porous coatings (Figure 7.4) for biological fixation (beads or mesh) are employed. Sintering, which is often used to attach the coatings to the substrate, can produce changes in microstructure, along with sharp discontinuities (notches) where the coating is attached. As a result, the fatigue strength of the implant may be reduced (even when additional post-sintering heat treatment is done) to only about 200 MPa, which is well below the strength of titanium alloys without porous coating.

Without additional surface treatment, Ti6Al4V alloys have poor wear resistance relative to stainless steel and cobalt–chromium alloys. Scratching and wear have been observed clinically on titanium alloy femoral heads, particularly in the presence of particles that become interposed between bearing surfaces. As a result, the metal components for metal on polyethylene bearings in joint replacements are usually made from cobalt–chromium alloys.

Ultrahigh Molecular Weight Polyethylene (UHMWPE)

UHMWPE was first used in total hip replacements in the early 1960s. Other polymers have been tried, but UHMWPE remains the material of choice for polymeric bearing components in total joint replacements, due to its biocompatibility, high impact strength, toughness, and abrasive wear characteristics.

Polyethylene components, such as the glenoid components shown in Figure 7.5, can be machined from ram-extruded bars or compression-molded sheets. They can also be made by directly molding the resin into the shape of the implant (net shape molding). Further machining of the articular surfaces is unnecessary, but some machining may be required to create the locking mechanisms required for metal-backed polyethylene components.

Polyethylene is sterilized by using either ethylene oxide or, more commonly, gamma radiation. The effects of gamma radiation on the mechanical properties of polyethylene components depend upon the dose used and the environment in which the components are irradiated. In the irradiation process, gamma or electron beam radiation produces free radicals (unpaired electrons) in the UHWMPE, which in secondary chemical reactions leads to a combination of chain scission and crosslinking. When irradiation is conducted in the presence of oxygen, scission is predominant over crosslinking, and oxidative degradation occurs because some of the free radicals react with oxygen. Crosslinking can be beneficial, particularly for reducing wear, but chain scission and oxidation lead to a decrease in molecular

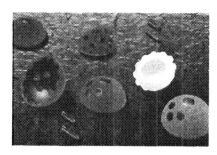

FIGURE 7.4 Various coatings can be used for bony ingrowth or ongrowth for cementless fixation. These include layers of porous sintered beads (as shown here), porous metal foams, and plasma coatings. (Reproduced with permission of Exactech Corporation.)

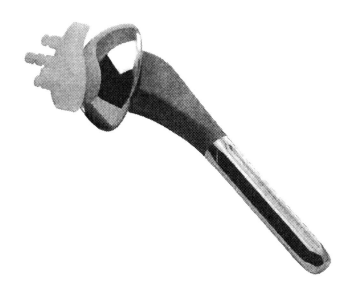

FIGURE 7.5 A shoulder replacement with an all-polyethylene glenoid. Other designs employ polyethylene inserts supported by a metal tray with a fixation peg. The humeral component is typically made from a CoCr alloy. In most metal on polyethylene bearings for joint replacements, the metal component is convex and the polyethylene component is concave, as shown here. (Reproduced with permission of Exactech Corporation.)

weight, with concomitant loss of wear resistance and mechanical properties. Crosslinking is predominant when irradiation is done in an inert environment, such as nitrogen. Increased crosslinking improves the abrasive and adhesive wear performance of UHMWPE, compared with conventional UHMWPE (noncrosslinked, or crosslinked at a low level during radiation sterilization). However, the presence of the crosslinks adversely affects ductility. Because crosslinking occurs primarily in the amorphous phase of UHMWPE, the amount of crosslinking and the corresponding decrease in ductility depend on the crystallinity of the UHMWPE. Unirradiated UHMWPE typically has a crystallinity of at least 50 percent, so approximately 50 percent of the material is amorphous in content and may be crosslinked during irradiation.

Since increased crosslinking generally increases the abrasive and adhesive wear resistance needed in hip replacements, it has the potential to improve their performance. As a consequence, crosslinked UHMWPE has seen increasing use in total joint replacements. However, crosslinking also generally decreases the fracture toughness and fatigue resistance of the material needed in less conforming joints, such as most knee replacements. In the 1990s and early 2000s, a number of processes were devised to increase the crosslinking without decreasing other desirable characteristics. In a typical process, most crosslinked UHMWPE components are subjected to a three-step process: an irradiation step to promote crosslinking, a thermal processing step to remove residual stresses and reduce free radicals (to prevent oxidative degradation), and a sterilization step. The final properties of UHMWPE implants can be substantially varied by modifying these processing steps.

It is apparent that the typical UHMWPE properties presented in Table 7.1 depend upon many factors, including the base resin used, the methods employed to form the components, and the irradiation and thermal processes utilized to sterilize the components and modify the material. As a result, the properties of UHMWPE can vary over a rather wide range. Long-term clinical experience is used, along with laboratory tests, to identify the best of these processes.

Finally, it should be noted that the stress–strain behavior of polyethylene components is viscoelastic–viscoplastic and nonlinear for the ranges of stresses and strains encountered *in vivo*. The elastic modulus in Table 7.1 is the initial modulus of the stress–strain curve; strictly speaking, the implied linear behavior only applies for low-stress, low-strain conditions, such as those found in highly conforming joints like hip replacements. For less conforming joints like knee replacements, the stresses due to contact will be overestimated if the initial modulus is used and linear behavior is assumed.

Bone Cement (PMMA)

Poly (methyl methacrylate), PMMA, or "bone cement," has been used to fix components to bone for about 50 years. PMMA has the same basic chemistry as Plexiglas® or Lucite®, but instead of being formed in a factory, part of the polymerization process is initiated in the operating room and completed *in situ*. Bone cement comes in two parts: a liquid monomer and a prepolymerized powder. These are mixed in the operating room; an initiator in the prepolymerized powder starts polymerization of the liquid monomer. When the material has reached the proper consistency, it is inserted into the bone. As an example, consider the process of fixing a medullary stem of the type used on femoral components for total hip replacements (Figure 7.6) and similar stemmed prostheses. The medullary cavity is machined to a shape consistent with the implant shape plus a cement mantle, a plug is inserted to keep the cement from extruding too far down the cavity, the cement is then inserted into the cavity by means of cement guns (like caulking guns) that allow the cavity to be filled from the bottom up, and, finally, the implant is inserted into the cement. Polymerization then occurs over a very short time (minutes), during which the implant must not be moved with respect to the bone. Any cement extruded by this process must be trimmed and removed from the joint space. Otherwise there is an increased risk of cement particles becoming trapped between the articulating surfaces of the prosthetic components, which in turn increases the risk of damage to these surfaces.

As the material polymerizes, it gives off heat that theoretically has the potential to damage bone. But the heat of polymerization is transferred in part to the implant

FIGURE 7.6 A Charnley Cobra stem implanted with cement in a cadaveric femur from an elderly donor (note the porosity of the cortical bone). (a) A cross section at the level of the lesser trochanter just below the collar of the prosthesis. The cement has penetrated into the cancellous bone, providing excellent interlock with the bone at the bone–cement interface. (b) A cross section in the distal third of the stem. At this section, there is much less cancellous bone, but cement penetration into the available cancellous bone can be seen, as well as into the general roughness of the endosteal surface of the femur.

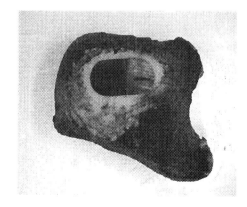
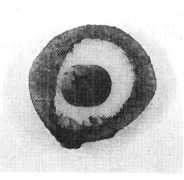

and the bone, and any damage to the bone is minimal at most. The long-term success of this method of implant fixation demonstrates that the heat generated does not affect the performance of the joint replacement.

Bone "cement" is a misnomer, because PMMA does not chemically bond to either bone tissue or implant materials, except possibly very weakly. It is best thought of as a grout that fills the space between the implant and the bone. Fixation at the PMMA–implant interface is accomplished by providing undercuts or textured surfaces where the PMMA can interlock with the component. Fixation at the PMMA–bone interface is provided by forcing the material into the interstices of the bone, using pressure applied before implant insertion, as a by-product of inserting a tapered stem into the cavity, or after the stem is in place.

It is possible to get PMMA to chemically bond to metal implants, but only under controlled conditions during implant manufacture. PMMA precoating has been used on the proximal portions of femoral stems for total hip replacements. The idea behind the process is that the cement, which does not bond to the metal during surgery, will bond to the coating. However, the success of this approach has been mixed. Lack of success may be due to inadequate bonding of the coating to the metal, concomitant changes in design of the implant, surgical technique, or a combination of these factors.

Typical mechanical properties of PMMA are provided in Table 7.1. The material is brittle, weak in tension, and strong in compression and has a low endurance limit. The *in vivo* properties can vary with the chemical formulation of the material, bone preparation, cement handling, and cement delivery. Various formulations of the basic material are available. In addition, either $BaSO_4$ or ZrO_2 is added to the cement to make it visible on radiographs. It is also possible to add antibiotics to PMMA that leach out over time to minimize the risk of infection or to deal with infection that may be present at the time of implantation. These additives can be incorporated without substantially affecting the mechanical properties of the material.

Handling and delivery involves four phases: mixing, waiting, application, and setting. The time from initial mixing to complete polymerization varies from 5 to 13 minutes, depending upon the cement formulation. In addition, the curing time is highly dependent on the ambient temperature, with higher temperatures requiring less time to complete the polymerization process. The liquid monomer and prepolymerized powder can be mixed by hand or machine. Some formulations have high viscosity from the start of mixing; others are less viscous. The less viscous cements lend themselves to machine mixing using a vacuum mixer or centrifuge.

Shrinkage of PMMA cement during polymerization causes pores to be formed in the cement mass. The conversion of monomer to polymer results in a loss in volume, generally on the order of 6–7 percent. Consequently, some void formation will occur, regardless of how the cement is mixed. Vacuum mixing or centrifugation decreases the number of voids in the cement, compared with the number generated during hand mixing, but porosity can never be completely eliminated. Some studies have indicated that this porosity reduction improves the static and fatigue properties of the material, but others show no apparent correlation between porosity and the mechanical properties of the material.

The apparent increase in mechanical properties of the *material* may be due in part to the fact that the *structural* properties of test specimens made from the same material with the same nominal geometry can vary with porosity. Test specimens are structures, and specimens with less porosity will have greater structural rigidity and increased apparent material properties because more material is enclosed within the same nominal volume.

Furthermore, it is not obvious that fatigue resistance of the cement layer is necessarily improved by reducing the internal porosity of the material. First, pores can be either crack initiating or crack arresting sites, depending upon their location and the nominal stress state. Second, internal pores are not the only types of voids in resulting bone–cement–implant systems. When the cement is inserted into the bone, gaps (i.e., voids) also occur at the cement–stem and cement–bone interfaces. Furthermore, the cement–bone interface, particularly for trabecular bone, may have sharp changes in geometry due to the local shape of the cortical or trabecular bone in contact with the cement. Consequently, reducing internal porosity may not increase the fatigue strength of the mantle if other sites in the construct are more likely to be locations of crack initiation.

Even given these confounding factors, one might expect that decreasing the internal porosity of the material would have some overall positive effect clinically. This has not been the case. Data from a large number of clinical cases have shown a significant increase in the short-term risk of loosening for patients who have received vacuum mixed cement, compared with those who have received hand-mixed cement.

These clinical results emphasize that, during surgery, a *structural* element, the cement layer, is created from a *material*, PMMA. The mechanical properties of the material (Table 7.1) can be used to estimate the structural role of the PMMA layer in cemented bone-implant systems. But one must always keep in mind that the structural properties of the cement layer depend upon the geometry of the layer, including the distribution of gaps and pores; the chemical formulation of the PMMA; the mixing, handling, and delivery of the cement during surgery; and complex interactions between these factors.

7.2 | Fracture Fixation Devices

As described in Chapter 6, fracture healing requires an environment that permits the biology of repair to proceed through a series of stages successfully. Some fractures can be treated conservatively with splints, casts, or traction devices that allow some movement at the fracture site. In these cases, a successful process may involve early callus formation and gradual transformation of this primitive tissue to bone like the original bone. For other fractures, devices may be required that will stabilize the fracture more securely, which may result in more rapid healing and repair processes that can even skip some of the early stages. This can be achieved by a variety of more or less complex devices that have been developed for fixing fractures, including screws, wires, internal plates fixed to the bone fragments with screws, intramedullary rods (IMR's), and external fixation frames, also known as external fixators (EF's). A few examples of the great variety of devices that have been developed for fracture fixation are shown next.

Screw Fixation

An example of a fracture that is fixed with screws alone is shown in Figure 7.7. The fragment is held to the remaining portion of the tibia with two screws that can all be inserted through one incision. Note that the two screws have threads only near the tip, so that the fragment can be pulled tightly against the remaining bone, which produces the interfragmentary pressure necessary for healing. The threads are coarse to get good purchase in the low-stiffness, low-strength trabecular bone. When the fracture divides the articular surface, it is extremely important to get the surfaces fragments aligned properly.

Plates, Intramedullary Rods, and Nails

When a fracture occurs in a portion of the shaft of a bone, like the tibial and fibular fractures shown in Figure 7.8, the bone can no longer withstand bending loads. Structures such as plates (Figure 7.8), intramedullary rods (Figure 7.9), or hip nails (Figure 7.10) are used to hold the fracture surfaces in apposition and provide bending resistance. The plates are held to the bone by screws with much finer threads than those shown in Figure 7.7. With the plate temporarily held in

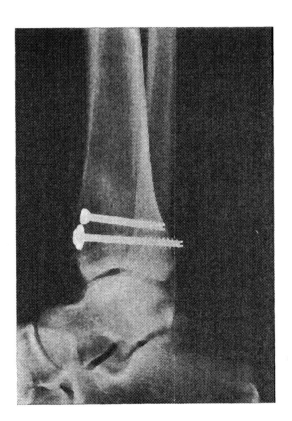

FIGURE 7.7 A fracture of the distal tibia fixed with lag screws through the fragments. (Reproduced with permission of Synthes.)

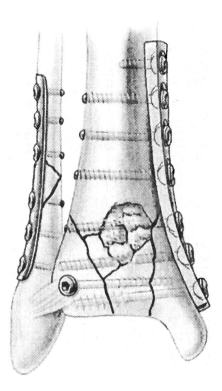

FIGURE 7.8 A fracture of the distal tibia and fibula fixed by a single plate on each bone. (From Müller et al., *Manual of Internal Fixation*. Springer-Verlag, Berlin and New York, 1970.)

position, holes are drilled into the bone and then tapped (threaded) to accept the threaded screws.

External Fixators

Complex fractures can also be treated with a variety of external fixators (i.e., fixation devices with external frames fixed to the bone fragments with transcutaneous pins; see Figure 7.11). Particular circumstances, like spinal segment fixation or fixation of facial bones, require very specialized devices, such as small fixation frames or very small plates or screws.

Analysis and Design of Fracture Fixation Devices

The basic design criteria for fixation devices are similar to those for other orthopaedic implants. The device must be sufficiently strong and stiff to provide the support and stability of the bone-device construct under conditions that range between normal loading and loads decreased by rehabilitation restrictions, walking aids, etc. The device must be compatible with the biological system. Internal devices must be nontoxic and resistant to corrosion. All the biocompatibility criteria for any musculoskeletal implant must be met. In addition, there may be design goals that are unique to fracture fixation devices. For example, tuning the device to the changing biological state of the healing fracture is highly desirable. Specifically, it would be desirable to decrease the rigidity of the fixation device as the fracture heals, to allow the skeletal segment to pick up an increased portion of the load, as it is able to do so.

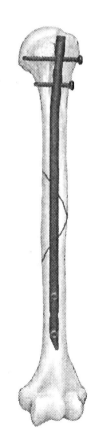

FIGURE 7.9 A fracture of the humeral shaft fixed by a locked intramedullary rod. The locking is achieved by the transverse screws through holes in the ends of the rod. (Reproduced by permission of Synthes.)

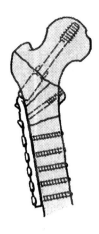

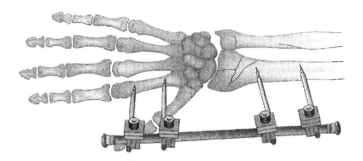

FIGURE 7.11   External fixator for a fracture of the distal radius. (From Müller et al., *Manual of Internal Fixation*. Springer-Verlag, Berlin and New York, 1970.)

FIGURE 7.10 *A femoral neck fracture fixed with a sliding hip nail. (From Müller et al., Manual of Internal Fixation. Springer-Verlag, Berlin and New York, 1970.)*

This increased bone load stimulates bony remodeling and avoids the risk of decreased bone mass due to abnormally low stresses and strains. A variety of schemes have been developed to pursue this goal, including resorbable plates and external fixation frames that allow loosening of some degrees of freedom.

While in most cases the detailed mechanics of the bone-fixator structure are fairly complex, there are some basic principles of behavior that can be derived with methods of mechanics of materials. These serve to guide both the development of design concepts as well as the clinical application of the devices. In the use of fixation devices, there are two issues of interest: the mechanical behavior of the device alone and the mechanics of the bone and fixator composite structure. The performance of the isolated fixation device is important if the device must carry the load without any contribution of the bone. The combined performance is important for understanding how the application might take advantage of bone-implant load sharing, as well as for understanding the potential for stress-shielding.

Obviously, one important factor in the analysis of these devices is the knowledge of the actual loads that are expected. In some circumstances, these loads may be known from measurements or from rigid body analyses like those developed in Chapter 2. However, it is often possible to design the devices in light of the knowledge of the bony structure itself. For example, if a rod or plate is to be used to stabilize a femoral fracture, the strength and stiffness of the femur itself can provide good guides for the required strength and stiffness of the implant.

7.3 | Joint Replacements

Joint replacement is a surgical procedure where the articulating surfaces are replaced to restore function to joints that have become damaged and painful due to trauma or disease. Arthritis, either osteoarthritis or rheumatoid arthritis, is the most common reason for joint replacement. The characteristics of these two broad categories of arthritic joints are distinct. Consequently, the design requirements for prosthetic components may differ.

Osteoarthritis commonly affects isolated joints such as the hip, knee, or elbow and may be due to normal wear and tear during the lifetime of the patient or may be secondary to joint trauma. For example, repetitive loading of elbows and wrists when using impact tools can eventually result in osteoarthritis, as can sports injuries to knees and ankles. The resulting pain is due to the destruction of the articular cartilage, which is still irreparable, although considerable research is being done to develop procedures for biological repair. In most cases, the damage is restricted to the articular surfaces and the bone tissue is generally normal and can provide good support for an implant. The disease itself does not generally attack the soft tissue structures around the joint. However, structures such as the cruciate ligaments and the menisci in the knee may be absent due to previous injury, and if the replacement is to function as a normal joint, the constraints usually provided by these anatomical structures will have to be furnished by the prosthesis itself.

Rheumatoid arthritis, on the other hand, is a systemic disease that often affects multiple joints in the body. In addition to damaging the articulating surfaces, the disease also compromises bone tissue and the soft tissue structures around the joint. For example, the sheaths that constrain the tendons in the hand to pass over the joints may be lost, resulting in deformities and loss of function. Some types of fixation may be more difficult to achieve in the rheumatoid patient, and the prosthesis may have to provide functional constraints that are unnecessary for patients with osteoarthritis.

Hundreds of thousands of joints are replaced each year worldwide. The hip and knee joints are the most common, because it is important to provide mobility for the patient. But upper extremity joints are also frequently replaced, since they are essential for activities of daily living, such as dressing, grooming, and eating. In most cases, total joint replacements are used; that is, both surfaces of a joint pair are replaced. The most common exception is hemiarthroplasty of the hip, where the natural socket in the pelvis is retained and only the ball portion of the joint on the femur is replaced.

A total knee replacement is shown in Figure 7.12. The tibial component consists of a polyethylene insert and a metal tray. The tibial components for some total knee replacements are made entirely of polyethylene. The component shown has an upper constraint spine that engages a cam in the femoral component to provide a functional substitute for the posterior cruciate ligament. The patellar component is made from polyethylene.

Successful total joint replacement designs involve both functional and structural considerations. The artificial joint must provide the normal range of motion while transmitting joint forces that are generally several times body weight. The resulting bone-implant system is a composite structure consisting of several components that should last for the lifetime of the patient. This is a challenging design problem that must account for the strength of the prosthetic components, damage to the articulating surfaces, the strength of the interfaces between the implanted materials and the bone, and the potential adaptation of the bone due to altered loading.

In addition to being structurally sound, the implanted components must be biocompatible in a hostile environment; they must not harm the body, and the body must not harm them. The interaction of prosthetic components with the biological environment occurs at all scales, ranging from the cellular for biocompatibility and tissue adaptation to the system level, where functional interactions with soft-tissue structures and load sharing between implant and bone are a concern.

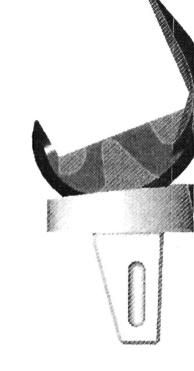

FIGURE 7.12 Cross-sectional view of a total knee replacement. The metal femoral component is in contact with the UHMWPE articulating surfaces of the patellar and tibial components. The posterior cam of the femoral component contacts the upper constraint spine of the tibial component during flexion to provide substitute posterior cruciate function; the anterior cam provides a hyper extension stop

Function

As just mentioned, the function of a joint involves force transmission coupled with kinematics. The motion of a natural joint is determined by the geometry of the joint surfaces; constraint provided by the ligaments, the joint capsule, and other soft tissue structures; and the active muscle forces acting across the joint. The kinematic constraint that must be provided by the prosthesis depends upon the severity of the damage that has occurred to the soft tissue structures. For example, the constraint that must be provided by an artificial knee joint depends upon the extent to which the stability normally supplied by the collateral and cruciate ligaments has been compromised. In addition, it is sometimes advantageous to deliberately eliminate a ligament, such as the posterior cruciate ligament in the knee, to obtain other advantages—for example, surgical exposure. If this is done, the constraint provided by the ligament must be provided by the prosthetic components if normal function is to be achieved.

Joint loads are large, because the muscle forces act close to the center of rotation, so their moment arms with respect to the joint center are small. Consequently, the muscle forces must be large to equilibrate the large moments produced by the functional loads acting on the skeleton. Joint loads of three to ten times the functional loads are not uncommon. Joint loads must be known to design the articulating surfaces and the fixation of the components to the bone. It is difficult to get precise values for the contact forces between articulating surfaces because the system is indeterminate, but reasonable approximations can be obtained by the methods explained in Chapter 2.

One of the most intriguing aspects of joint function is that the kinematics and the joint forces are coupled: Changing one will change the other. An interesting case in point is the knee, which is constrained by soft tissue structures and, as a result, has substantial laxity. The points of contact between the articulating surfaces and the rotation of the tibia with respect to the femur may all be affected by the type and location of the external loads applied to the shank or foot. For example, the position of the pad on the lower leg in a knee exercising machine can influence the direction of the anterior–posterior component of the joint force (Figure 7.13). The functional load in this case is the force, R, of the pad on the leg. If the pad is placed near the ankle, the fore–aft component of the joint force, J, at the knee is directed posteriorly; if the pad is placed near the knee, the joint force, J, is directed anteriorly. Therefore, the resulting relative motion between the condyles and the tibial plateau will be in opposite directions for these two cases. In the first case, the anterior cruciate ligament will be loaded; in the second, it will be the posterior cruciate ligament.

The kinematics created during total joint replacement surgery can also influence the joint loads. In a total hip replacement procedure, the surgeon can choose the location of the femoral head with respect to the femur and the location of the acetabulum with respect to the pelvis. As a result, the relative motion between the proximal femur and the pelvis can be altered, and as a consequence, both the magnitude and direction of the hip joint force may be affected. The change in relative motion between the femur and the pelvis has further implications. The distance between the origin and insertion of a muscle may be lengthened or shortened when the geometry of the systems is changed. This in turn causes changes in muscle force capabilities because of the force–length relationship for muscle.

Structure

Fixation   Total joint replacements fall into two broad classes: those which replace only the articulating surface and those which replace the surface and a substructure of the bone. Acetabular cups for total hip replacements, glenoid components for total

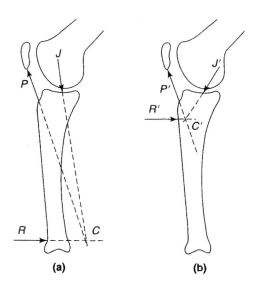

(a)   (b)

FIGURE 7.13 The position of the tibial pad in a knee exercising machine affects the loading on the cruciate ligaments. When the pad is placed distally, the anterior cruciate ligament is loaded. When the pad is placed proximally, the posterior cruciate ligament is loaded. From Otis, *J Sports Med* 13:254–258.)

shoulder replacements, and femoral and tibial components of total knee arthroplasty are examples of surface replacements. The goal is to transfer the joint loads to the underlying cancellous bone similar to the way it is done in the normal joint.

Femoral components for artificial hips, humeral components for shoulder replacements, and loose hinges for elbow prostheses (Figure 7.14) are examples of total joint replacements where a substantial portion of the bone is also replaced. In hips a new femoral head, and in shoulders a new humeral head, replaces the natural head. Such components are typically fixed to the bone by means of a fixation stem that extends into the medullary canal. Fixation stems or pegs may also be used to augment fixation of surface replacements to bone. The most common example is in the knee

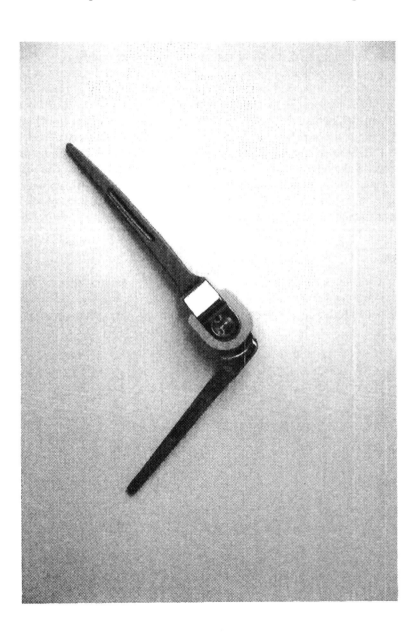

FIGURE 7.14 This total elbow replacement is a loose hinge. The articulating surfaces are metal–polyethylene pairs. Humeral and ulnar stems provide fixation.

joint, where prostheses intended to provide substitute collateral ligament function often incorporate long fixation stems as well. Load transfer in designs that employ stems may be quite different from load transfer to bone in natural joints—much of the joint load may be transferred through the fixation stem into the endosteal surface of the bone.

Surface replacements have also been used for femoral components of total hip replacements and components for total elbow replacements. The success of elbow and hip arthroplasties, where surface replacements have been used to replace both of the contacting surfaces, has been modest at best.

Components of artificial joints are most commonly fixed to bone with either PMMA (polymethyl methacrylate, bone cement) or cementless techniques. Bone cement is created by mixing a polymer and monomer in the operating room; the mixture polymerizes *in situ*. "Bone cement" is a bit of a misnomer because, when used under operating room conditions, it is not an adhesive; there is negligible chemical adhesion between either the cement and the bone or the cement and the prosthesis (see Section 7.1). Bone cement can adhere to metal if the surface is treated properly as part of the manufacturing process; a thin layer of PMMA can be used to precoat portions of the fixation stem. The cement used during surgery then bonds to the precoating, and a strong interface can be created. Only a portion of the stem, however, is bonded to the cement. In regions outside the precoated areas, the strength of the interface is minimal at best. Therefore, the transition between the bonded and unbonded interface regions may be a region of stress concentration.

In the absence of precoating, the cement is basically a grout, which fills the space between the implant and the bone. Consequently, the strengths of the cement–implant and cement–bone interfaces, which are critical to the integrity of the bone-implant system, primarily depend upon mechanical interlock. At the cement–bone interface, the PMMA interlocks with the roughness of the bone; at the cement–implant interface, grooves and undercuts or roughened surfaces are often employed to provide interlock between the implant and the cement.

The primary disadvantage of PMMA is that it has relatively low tensile fatigue strength. Consequently, the bone-implant system must be designed so that stresses in the cement and the interfaces are within safe limits. Well-designed cemented systems have performed extremely well. Nevertheless, cement is considered by many to be the weak link in the bone–cement–implant system, particularly in younger, more active patients. As a result, considerable work has been done on finding methods for fixing the implants to bone without using cement. One approach is to simply use a press-fit prosthesis and to depend upon the shape of the fixation stem to safely transfer the loads from the prosthesis to the bone, without depending upon tensile or shear strength at the interface. A second approach is to provide tensile and shear load transfer at the interface through biologic fixation.

The most common way for achieving biologic fixation is to coat portions of the prosthesis with a porous layer of material (Figure 7.4). For example, layers of metal beads or mesh may be sintered to a substrate of the same material. The cavity in the bone is then shaped so that an interference fit between the implant and the bone will occur for short-term fixation. Ingrowth of the bone into the porous layer then provides the long-term fixation of the device. (See Figure 7.17). Roughened surfaces can also be created by techniques such as plasma spraying. In this case, there are no interconnecting pores, so bone ingrowth cannot occur. As a result, the

FIGURE 7.15 This device is designed for fixation by bone ingrowth. The fixation stem is coated with layers of beads that provide interconnecting pores into which bone can grow. The distal 30 percent of the stem is uncoated. This design is symmetric, so that the same device can be used for both right and left legs.

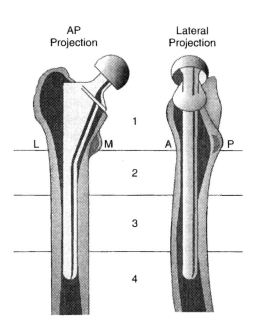

interface has limited, if any, tensile strength. Bone ongrowth onto the roughened surface, however, can provide interface shear strength.

The Composite Structure: Load Transfer The bone-implant structure created at surgery is a multicomponent system that replaces the bone alone, which is itself a composite structure consisting of cortical and cancellous bone. The new composite structure consists of cortical and cancellous bone, the implant, and usually an interface layer such as bone cement. Interface layers also occur between the implant and the bone in cementless joint replacements. These interfaces are complex and vary from point to point. In some regions, there may be simple bony contact, allowing only compressive loads and shear transfer through friction, as long as separation doesn't occur. In other regions, bone ingrowth may provide transfer of tensile, compressive, and shear loads (Figure 7.15). In still other regions, there may be fibrous tissue interposed between the implant and the bone that provides a weaker, less stiff connection between the bone and the implant.

The new structure must be able to withstand the forces applied to it due to contact between the articulating surfaces of the total joint replacement. Failure may occur within the prosthetic materials themselves, at the interfaces between implant materials and bone, or in the bone. Therefore, it is important to understand how the loads are transferred from the prosthetic components to the bone.

Implant materials must have sufficient strength to function for long periods without failure, and they must be compatible with the biological environment. Because biological materials are living, minor damage (cracks or small tears) are often repaired (Sections 3.9 and 4.1). However, cracks or flaws in implant materials do not heal and may be propagated with repeated loading. Consequently, the fatigue behavior of metals and polymers used for prosthetic replacements is an important concern. To determine the stresses associated with failure, the load distributions within the components of the composite structure must be known.

Bone fracture in the presence of an implant can occur, but the more important consideration is the bone adaptation that takes place in the presence of an implant. The loading applied to the bone tissue by the prosthesis may be substantially different from the loading applied to the same tissue without an implant in place. This is a very important consideration, because bone remodels when the loading environment is changed. If the loading on bone tissue is increased, both the mechanical properties and the volume of the bone may be increased. When an artificial joint is used, the load previously carried by the bone alone is now shared by the bone and the implant. Consequently, the amount of load carried by the bone generally is decreased, and the bone will remodel to meet the requirements of the new loading situation. It is not unusual in such cases to see radiographic evidence of changes in volume and density (material properties), except for local areas of high stress or strain near abrupt changes in geometry or structural characteristics of the bone-implant system.

In composite systems with parallel load paths, load is shared according to the relative stiffness of the components in the composite structure. If, when the implant is in place, the stiffness of the bone decreases due to decreased load, the relative stiffness of the implant with respect to the bone will increase, the load carried by the prosthesis may increase, that carried by the bone may decrease, and a further decrease in stiffness of the bone may occur. Thus, there is the possibility of a vicious cycle, in stemmed components, for example, in which the strength of the bone and the amount of bone may decrease to the point where the structural integrity of the system is in jeopardy and the risk of failure of both the bone and the stem is increased. It is also important to recognize that bone–prosthesis interface characteristics can also evolve with time due to biological and mechanical influences. Interface changes over time provide yet another way in which the loads on the bone may be modified to produce bone adaptation.

Articulating Surfaces

The second major structural consideration is the surface damage that occurs due to contact between the articulating surfaces (Figure 7.16). This will be discussed in detail in Chapter 11. Here we only note that well-designed components generally do not wear out, but debris is liberated. The particles from the damaged surfaces collect in the surrounding soft tissue. When sufficient debris accumulates, the biological response of the body can lead to increased risk of infection and increased risk of loosening. This often happens after years of excellent service and is probably the factor that has the greatest effect on the life of the joint replacement.

The mechanisms by which surface damage occurs are complex and difficult to delineate. In hip joints abrasive wear is thought to dominate, whereas in knee joints surface damage is most often due to pitting and delamination. One goal is to reduce the stresses that are associated with the observed damage modes; another is to use materials or manufacturing processes that increase the resistance to damage. Both experimental and theoretical methods may be used to determine the stresses due to contact between the articulating surfaces. Design analyses, along with analyses of retrieved components, can be used to determine the effects of design on stresses, and mechanical simulators can be used to evaluate materials and functional performance in particular designs.

FIGURE 7.16 Surface damage of a polyethylene tibial component. The *in vivo* damage shown is severe and includes pitting, delamination, and radial cracks propagating from the edge of the component. Damage of this type has become rarer because of increased attention to manufacturing, sterilization, and storage methods. Well designed and manufactured components show only modest pitting of the articulating surfaces after many years of use.

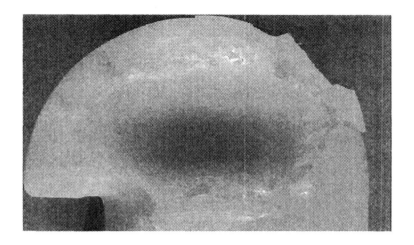

Modular Components Structural issues must also be addressed when modular components are used. Modularity provides flexibility at the time of surgery. For example, several modular heads can be used with the same femoral fixation stem to produce different neck lengths in a total hip replacement. Modularity is also used in acetabular components of total hip joints and tibial components of total knee replacements. In knees, two types of modularity are employed. Polyethylene may be attached to a metal backing (Figure 7.1), and stems of various lengths may be added to the inferior surface of the component to improve the fixation of the device. In hips, a polyethylene liner may also be used in conjunction with a metal backing for the acetabular component. In addition to giving the surgeon more choices at the time of surgery, metal backings provide a substrate for a porous surface at the metal–bone interface to improve cement fixation or to enhance bony ingrowth.

Custom Designs As the success with conventional implants has grown, custom implants designed for particularly difficult replacement problems have been developed. These may be required to correct congenital problems or replace failed conventional prostheses. In addition, custom implants are being used as an alternative to limb amputation for patients with bone tumors. For example, when a bone tumor occurs above the knee, the knee joint may be replaced, along with segments of the femur and the tibia.

7.4 | Design of Bone-Implant Systems

Factors Influencing Performance

In this book, we are primarily concerned about how to design implants for structural performance. Our basic premise is that joint replacements fail structurally because stresses have exceeded the strength of components, interfaces, or articulating surfaces. As can be seen in Figure 7.17, the performance of the system is affected by implant, patient, and surgical factors. Each factor (and its interactions with other elements of

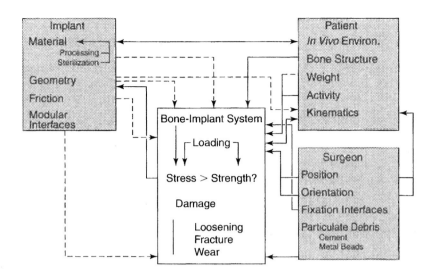

FIGURE 7.17 Factors influencing the design of a bone-implant system.

the system) can have a substantial effect upon the structure and must be taken into account by the design engineer. The surgical factors are particularly important. Variations in the position and orientation of components affect the loading, kinematics, and interfaces directly, because they alter the basic characteristics of the bone-implant system. Position and orientation can also affect the system indirectly, because they may alter patient behavior. Therefore, surgical instrumentation (Figure 7.18) is an important aspect of design for total joint replacement surgery. Engineering designers, in collaboration with surgeons, must develop the jigs and fixtures that are used

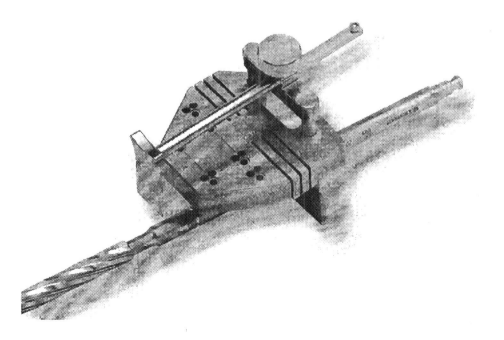

FIGURE 7.18 A joint line reference instrument for knee replacement surgery. The tools and fixtures necessary for implantation are an important part of the engineering design of total joint replacements. (Reproduced with permission of Exactech Corporation.)

by the surgeon to get consistent position and orientation and good fixation of the implant to the bone.

The major factors shown in Figure 7.17 may be divided into design variables, which are under the control of the designers, and environmental variables, over which the designers have little or no control. The variables associated with the implant (material, geometry, manufacturing processes, etc.) are design variables. The patient variables (bone structure, weight, activity, etc.) are clearly environmental variables. The variables introduced at surgery are more difficult to classify. On the one hand, the procedures and instrumentation are designed to achieve particular positions and orientations. On the other, variations in these positions and orientations occur even for the most experienced and competent surgeons. Therefore, surgical variables are in part design variables and in part environmental variables. A goal is to design the composite system so that it is robust—insensitive to both patient and surgical environmental variables.

Evaluation of Implant Performance

Total joint replacements are evaluated with long-term follow-up studies of patients, survival analyses, and retrieval analyses. Clinical studies are the most subjective and must be constructed with care to obtain reliable information. Survival analyses involve statistical methods to determine the probability of survival of replacements involving specific designs at particular times post-surgery. These analyses are useful for determining which prosthetic systems and surgical procedures lead to the best clinical results, but give little information regarding the design features that are responsible for good or bad performance. Retrieval analyses, the examination of devices removed during revision surgery or at autopsy, are the best source for evaluating *in vivo* performance of the structural aspects of the system. Failure modes may be identified, and alterations to material properties may be determined. This information is essential if improvements to designs are to be made.

It would be advantageous to be able to evaluate the performance of new prosthetic designs before a component was ever implanted into a patient. This concept is called preclinical evaluation. To do it accurately would require the ability to predict the performance of all aspects of the bone-implant system, including the long-term remodeling of the bone, while taking into account intra- and interpatient environmental variables and surgical variations. Until this is possible, we must rely on a combination of experiments and computer analyses to predict performance. *In vivo* human studies of new designs or procedures are only justified when the benefits to the patients outweigh the risks. Custom devices for patients with unusual needs sometimes provide an opportunity to use new technology when conventional approaches are insufficient. However, such opportunities are rare. As a result, preclinical evaluation is usually limited to a combination of computer simulations and *in vitro* experiments to evaluate bone-implant performance. In some cases, limited *in vivo* animal studies are used in conjunction with computer analyses and *in vitro* tests when there is no other way to get essential information.

Given the relatively long experience with joint replacement surgery, most design changes are incremental extrapolations from proven designs and should result in little if any increased risk to the patient. Even so, when new designs are introduced, they are first tried on a limited basis by a few skilled surgeons and then used more broadly in multicenter trials by a broader group of surgeons before they are released for general use. The FDA has established the procedures that must be followed. These precautions are essential because there have been a number of examples of design variations, which seemed to be minor modifications of existing designs, that for one reason or another proved to be unsatisfactory when evaluated clinically.

7.5 | Summary

As noted in the introduction to this chapter, a broad range of materials is used in musculoskeletal reconstruction. Here we have considered only those materials that are most commonly used in total joint replacements and fracture fixation components. This somewhat limited approach provides the groundwork necessary for later chapters that explore how material choices can influence function, load sharing, and longevity of these bone-implant systems. Because of this focus, we have not discussed bone inductive or conductive materials, ceramics, coatings for fixation or wear resistance, or resorbable materials, all of which have the potential for playing increasing roles in joint replacement and fracture fixation.

To minimize the risk of failure of bone-implant systems, either the *in vivo* stresses must be reduced or the strength (resistance to fracture, fatigue, and wear) must be increased. Material enhancement is an ongoing goal of the biomaterials community. Therefore, Table 7.1 is at best a snapshot in time of *representative* mechanical properties of implant materials that are continually being improved. Ultimately, the designer is concerned with the strength of the system (the loads at which the system fails). Design analysis and evaluation depend critically upon knowledge of the specific values of the materials used in the system. Because implant materials continue to be developed and improved, and because considerable variations in mechanical properties can occur due to changes in composition and manufacturing processes, designers and analysts should not be satisfied with representative values, but should determine the properties that are appropriate for the particular materials being used.

7.6 EXERCISES

7.1 What concerns must be addressed when considering the biocompatibility of orthopaedic implant materials?

7.2 What are the relative advantages and disadvantages of titanium and CoCr alloys for metal components used in joint replacement prostheses?

7.3 How do the characteristics of metals for fracture fixation devices differ from metals for joint replacement components?

7.4 Many components of bone-implant systems are subjected to cyclic loading. In what ways might the design and fatigue strength requirements differ for porous coated fixation stems, compared with those for cemented fixation?

7.5   What factors affect the durability of ultrahigh molecular weight polyethylene components?

7.6   What are the advantages and disadvantages of all-polyethylene components and metal components with polyethylene inserts?

7.7   In what ways would you expect surgical technique to affect the performance of cemented and cementless joint replacements?

7.8   Would you expect surgical technique to be more important for cemented or cementless joint replacements?

7.9   What are the primary factors that must be considered when designing an implant for function and structure?

7.10   How do the functional requirements for hip replacements differ from those for knee replacements?

7.11   What are the pros and cons of cemented versus cementless fixation?

7.12   How might the patient's disease (rheumatoid arthritis versus osteoarthritis) affect the design of prosthetic components for function and structure?

7.13   Write down several examples of patient variables and how you think they might vary over the population of patients receiving joint replacements.

7.14   Compare the roles of fracture plate fixation and external fixation.

Fracture Fixation Devices

Bone fractures represent a structural failure of the primary load-carrying apparatus of the body. The uniquely biological aspect of a skeletal structure is its capability to repair itself; bone fractures can heal without intervention. On the other hand, they sometimes fail to heal successfully, at least in a timely way, without treatment. The primary purpose of fracture treatment devices is to provide the initial structural reinforcement that is necessary for the healing process to occur as quickly and uneventfully as possible.

To understand the effects of structural interventions, the process of natural healing and the relationships between biology and biomechanics must be appreciated. The process of fracture healing is discussed in this context in the next section. With this background, the basic concepts of common fracture treatment methods, such as internal fixation plates, intramedullary rods, and external fixation frames, can be addressed. The focus is on long-bone fractures, which are the most common fractures requiring treatment, but the basic principles apply to other bones as well.

We will use methods of mechanics of materials to study the performance of intramedullary rods, plates, and external frames in comparison to the stiffness and strength characteristics of intact long bones; composite beam theory will be used to examine the combined performance of these bone-implant systems. We will also briefly address some of the more complex problems that may come into play, as well as some of the techniques that have been proposed for stimulating healing mechanically.

8.1 | Fracture Repair

Biology of Fracture Healing

The biological process of fracture healing involves the development of tissue at the fracture site that reinforces and eventually welds the bone fragments together. This tissue is called callus. Callus is a term which actually describes a number of different

FIGURE 8.1 The stages of fracture healing.

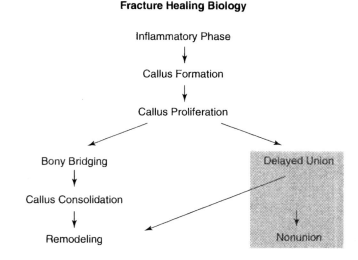

tissue types that may appear during the healing process. The biological stages of normal fracture healing are shown in the left branch of Figure 8.1.

Following a fracture, there is inflammatory phase, and initially much of the space around the fracture site may be filled with hematoma. The callus that forms in this space is typically a very poorly organized fibrous tissue. If healing progresses appropriately, the callus begins to develop into a more mature tissue. In natural healing without other intervention, the amount of callus may become quite large. The proliferating callus begins to develop cartilaginous characteristics in the center of the fracture gap, and bony characteristics adjacent to the major bone fragments. This is partly due to strictly biological factors, including local blood supply, and partly to the mechanical environment. In successful healing, bone eventually bridges the fracture gap and is followed by the maturation and eventual remodeling of the bony callus tissue. In children, the remodeling process may obliterate any evidence of the fracture site. In adults, the evidence of the fracture site may persist throughout life.

Failure of the natural healing process is essentially a failure of the callus material to stabilize the fracture site effectively. Failure of natural healing involves a divergence from the normal healing sequence to produce a delayed union or a nonunion (right branch of Figure 8.1). These are clinical terms used to describe a healing process that is either excessively long or never fully completed.

Fracture Treatment Concepts

A primary goal of fracture treatment is to provide the initial mechanical stability required to achieve successful and rapid fracture healing. The traditional approach has been to stabilize the fracture sufficiently so that the normal healing process can occur with the use of splints and casts. This is still the option of choice in simple fractures.

One school of thought in modern fracture treatment, called functional bracing, is based upon the idea that the introduction of function (weight bearing and motion) results in stimulation of vascularity and proliferation of periosteal (on the external bone surface, literally around the bone) callus. The idea is to enhance the natural healing process so that it occurs rapidly and successfully. While this approach has the advantage that it is noninvasive, it has been mostly limited to femoral and tibial fractures. Furthermore, it is difficult to predict the amount of bracing (stability) that represents a proper compromise between adequate callus stimulation and excessive fragment motion leading to nonunion.

It is also possible to essentially bypass the process of callus formation. A second school of thought uses the concept of "rigid" fixation and "primary healing," healing via direct bony bridging without any significant external callus formation. This can be accomplished by fixation, usually employing internal fracture plates. In its most successful form, this healing process is essentially reduced to the process of normal bone remodeling. In this case, the biological process responsible for the normal turnover of healthy bone provides a direct bony connection across the fracture site, and the healing process can be very rapid. This has been a popular treatment technique for long-bone fractures.

It, too, however, has potential problems. First, there are the obvious problems of morbidity and risk of infection due to the surgery involved. Second, very precise fragment positioning may be required to allow primary healing. Also, at the latter stages of healing, there is actually a loss of bone tissue under the plate. This may come in part from the stress-shielding effect, whereby the presence of the bone plate reduces the normal loads in the bone. The bone then responds by reducing its mass. This capability of bone to adapt to functional requirements is discussed in Section 3.9. It is also possible that a major amount of this bone resorbtion occurs because the plate rides directly on the bone and prevents the normal revascularization of the bone. In either event, it is often true that the bone fails to return to normal biological and mechanical function, unless the plate is removed.

The concepts of functional cast bracing and rigid internal fixation represent the extremes of a spectrum of possible treatment techniques for fractures. A graphical description of the relationship between relative motion of the fracture fragments and type of treatment is shown in Figure 8.2, along with the relationship between the type of treatment and the amount of callus formation. By a particular choice—for example, internal plates, intramedullary rods, or external fracture fixator frames—one can allow more or less interfragmentary motion and produce more or less callus. The

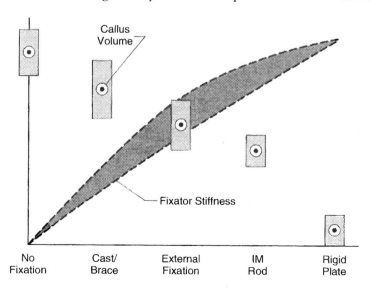

No Fixation   Cast/Brace   External Fixation   IM Rod   Rigid Plate

FIGURE 8.2 Callus volume and stiffness of various fixators. The greatest callus volume occurs when the stiffness at the fracture site is least. The shaded area and boxes show that the stiffness and callus volume are variable, depending on patient factors and the nature of the fracture.

FIGURE 8.3 Tensile properties of biological tissues. Bone tissue can survive only if the strains are small.

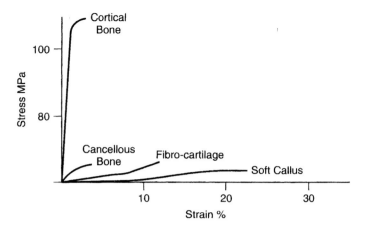

question of what choice is best is controversial. Often, other issues or the personal preferences of the clinician will be the deciding factor.

Interfragmentary Strain

One of the major contributions in understanding biology versus biomechanics in fracture healing was that healing is not successful unless interfragmentary strains (the motion between fragments at the fracture site) are reduced enough to permit the development and survival of each type in the sequence of tissues that form at the fracture site. This has both mechanical and biological implications. If a tissue fails mechanically (yields, ruptures, or sustains unacceptable damage) at a particular amount of deformation or strain, it is obviously necessary that strains remain below that level if the tissue is to survive. It is possible that even lower strains may be required for the biology involved in the tissue differentiation and maturation to proceed successfully.

Figure 8.3 describes qualitatively the strain behavior in tensile loading of several possible callus tissues. This figure illustrates that, for the more mature tissues (e.g., cancellous or compact bone) to survive, the tissue strains must be reduced to relatively small values. The body's way of reducing the strains is to produce enough callus volume to do the job. The physician's intervention is designed to guarantee that this will happen or to obviate the need for it to occur.

EXAMPLE 8.1 Bending Stiffness of Callus Versus Bone

Question Consider an idealized long bone with a fracture callus as shown in Figure 8.4. What callus diameter is required to match the bending rigidity of the bone?

Solution The bending rigidity of the bone is given by the product of the moment of inertia and elastic modulus $E_b I_b$. For a cylindrical cross section, the moment of inertia is

$$I = \frac{\pi}{4}(r_o^4 - r_i^4)$$

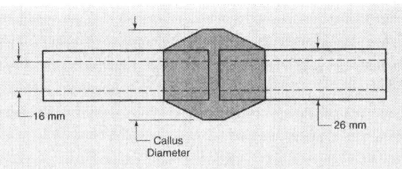

16 mm

26 mm

Callus
Diameter

FIGURE 8.4   A simple model of bone healing.

TABLE 8.1

**Callus Diameter to Match
Bending Rigidity of Intact Bone**

$E_{callus}E_{bone}$	Callus Diameter/ Bone Diameter (mm)
0.01	3.04
0.05	2.04
0.10	1.72

for periosteal callus that has the same nominal inside diameter and an outside diameter of sufficient size to match the bending rigidity of the intact bone (i.e., $E_c I_c = E_b I_b$). It then follows from the definition of I_c and I_b, that the outer radius must be

$$r_c = \left\{ \frac{E_b}{E_c}(r_o^4) + \left(1 - \frac{E_b}{E_c}\right)r_i^4 \right\}^{1/4}$$

The necessary ratios of callus diameter to bone outer diameter for several different values of callus elastic modulus are shown in Table 8.1. Since the moment of inertia changes as the fourth power of the diameters, it is not difficult to produce sufficient callus, even if it has a fairly low modulus, to stabilize the fracture by limiting bending strain at the fracture site.

Biomechanical Stages of Repair

The biomechanical behavior of a healing long bone parallels the biological process. Based on torsional tests of animal bones, four stages have been identified (Table 8.2). Stage 1, during which the torsional stiffness and strength of the healing bone are low, corresponds to the early callus formation stage. When bony callus bridges the fracture gap, then the structural stiffness increases substantially (Stage 2). If a very large volume of callus is formed, it is possible for the stiffness to be fairly high without significant bony bridging, but normally there is a significant increase in stiffness when bony bridging occurs. As healing progresses, the maturation of the bone at the

TABLE 8.2

Four Biomechanical Stages of Fracture Healing Determined from Torsional Tests of Animal Bones			
Stage	Stiffness	Strength	Failure
1	Low	Low	Fracture site
2	High	Low	Fracture site
3	High	Medium	Partial fracture site
4	High	High	Parent bone

fracture site results in a substantial increase in strength, and the fracture site begins to approach the strength of the parent bone (Stage 3). Often, in long-bone fractures in animals that are healing, the stiffness and strength exceed the parent bone, and failure in torsional testing will occur in the parent bone adjacent to the fracture site (Stage 4).

8.2 | Mechanics of Intramedullary Rods

The IMR is a commonly used device in long-bone fractures, particularly in the lower limb. It provides the advantage that it can often be implanted in "closed fashion" through a small incision, without significant surgical exposure. To simplify the model, we assume that a cylindrical bone shape with a solid circular rod is placed inside that fills the intramedullary cavity. Given these assumptions, the basic mechanics of this device can be examined relatively easily.

In general, a long bone is subjected to bending, torsional, and axial loads. The isolated performance of the bone and IMR can be compared by considering their relative strength and structural stiffness in each of these modes. Recall from the analysis of beams in Chapter 5 that the structural stiffness in bending (or bending rigidity) is given by the product EI, and the axial rigidity is given by the product EA. For the torsional rigidity, a similar expression relating the torque to the twist per unit length can be written as GJ^*, where G is the elastic shear modulus for the material, and J^* is sometimes called the torsional constant. For a circular, cylindrical cross section, J^* is just equal to the polar area moment of inertia, J. For noncircular shapes, J^* is more complicated. To compare strength, the maximum allowable stress for the material can be used to calculate the maximum allowable load.

At the fracture site, the rod alone may carry the loads, unless some compressive load is transferred across the fragments. Away from the fracture site, the rod and bone can act as a unit if the purchase between rod and bone is sufficient. To compare behaviors, we can calculate the axial rigidity, bending rigidity, torsional rigidity, and bending strength of the rod alone and the bone plus rod. Since, in this simple model, the rod and bone are concentric, the combined rigidities are just the sums of the individual rigidities. The ratio of the axial stiffnesses of the intramedullary rod to the bone can be defined as

$$\rho_A = \frac{E_D A_D}{E_B A_B}$$

where E_D and E_B are the modulus of the device and the bone, respectively, and the areas of the device and bone are

$$A_D = \pi(r_m^2)$$

and

$$A_B = \pi(r_o^2 - r_m^2)$$

in which r_o and r_m are the outer radius of the bone and the radius of the device (equal to the medullary canal radius). If we designate the ratio of the radii as $\beta = r_m/r_o$, the ratio ρ_A becomes

$$\rho_A = \left(\frac{E_D}{E_B}\right)\left(\frac{\beta^2}{1 - \beta^2}\right)$$

Obviously, as β goes to zero (r_m approaches zero), the axial stiffness ratio ρ_A goes to zero, and as β goes to unity (r_m approaches r_o), ρ_A becomes infinite. For the stiffness of the plate to match the stiffness of the bone, ρ_A must be unity—that is, $E_D\beta^2$ must equal $E_B(1 - \beta^2)$. As will be shown, usually rods are not solid, but for metal rods, it is easy to match or exceed the axial stiffness of the bone with a solid rod.

Since the stress in pure axial loading is just the load per unit area, we can express an axial strength ratio in terms of the areas and the allowable stresses as

$$\mu_A = \frac{S_D A_D}{S_B A_B} = \left(\frac{S_D}{S_B}\right)\left(\frac{\beta^2}{1 - \beta^2}\right)$$

where S_B and S_D are the maximum allowable stresses in the bone and rod, respectively.

For the case of pure bending, the ratio of stiffnesses can be expressed as

$$\rho_I = \frac{E_D \bar{I}_D}{E_B \bar{I}_B}$$

where the centroidal moments of inertia for the device and bone are, respectively,

$$\bar{I}_D = \frac{\pi}{4}(r_m^4) = \frac{\pi}{4}r_o^4\beta^4$$

and

$$\bar{I}_B = \frac{\pi}{4}(r_o^4 - r_m^4) = \frac{\pi}{4}r_o^4(1 - \beta^4)$$

The stiffness ratio now becomes

$$\rho_I = \left(\frac{E_D}{E_B}\right)\left(\frac{\beta^4}{1 - \beta^4}\right)$$

The strength ratio in bending can be expressed as the ratio of the maximum allowable bending moments for the IMR and the bone. The maximum allowable bending moment is given by

$$M_{max} = S\left(\frac{\bar{I}}{c}\right) = SZ$$

where S is the maximum allowable stress and $Z = \bar{I}/c$ is the section modulus (c is the outer radius of the bone or of the rod). For the bone with intramedullary rod, we can write the section modulus as

$$Z_B = \frac{\pi}{4} r_o^4 (1 - \beta^4)/r_o = \frac{\pi}{4} r_o^3 (1 - \beta^4)$$

$$Z_D = \frac{\pi}{4} r_o^4 \beta^4 / r_o \beta = \frac{\pi}{4} r_o^3 \beta^3$$

Then the ratio of strengths can be written as

$$\mu_I = \frac{S_D Z_D}{S_B Z_B} = \left(\frac{S_D}{S_B}\right)\left(\frac{\beta^3}{1 - \beta^4}\right)$$

Comparing this result with the previous result for the stiffness ratio, we can see that the elastic moduli are replaced by the maximum allowable stresses, and the numerator is β^3 instead of β^4. For a strength ratio of one, the ratio of maximum allowable stresses must equal $(1 - \beta^4)/\beta^3$. Thus, we see that matching the bending strength of the rod to the bone means that the bending stiffness will *not* be matched. We will see, throughout the following, that it is not possible to match all properties between the rod and the bone without introducing some new degrees of freedom, for example, by using a hollow rod.

The torsional rigidity and torsional strength ratios can be worked out in a similar fashion. For a circular cross section, the torsional rigidity ratio can be expressed as

$$\rho_T = \frac{G_D J_D}{G_B J_B} = \left(\frac{G_D}{G_B}\right)\left(\frac{\frac{\pi}{2} r_o^4 \beta^4}{\frac{\pi}{2} r_o^4 (1 - \beta^4)}\right) = \left(\frac{G_D}{G_B}\right)\left(\frac{\beta^4}{1 - \beta^4}\right)$$

where G_D and G_B are the shear moduli for rod and bone. The strength ratio is

$$\mu_I = \frac{S_D^T Z_D}{S_B^T Z_B} = \left(\frac{S_D^T}{S_B^T}\right)\left(\frac{\beta^3}{1 - \beta^4}\right)$$

where S^T signifies the maximum allowable shear stress and $Z^T = J/c$. The analogy to the bending behavior is obvious. If the ratio of shear moduli is similar to the ratio of elastic moduli, and if the ratio of max allowable shear stresses is similar to the ratio of max allowable bending stresses, the comparisons will come out the same for torsion as for bending.

With high-modulus materials, such as implantable metals, it is possible to design a solid intramedullary rod that actually has a bending rigidity and bending strength comparable to the bone. It is also easy to see that when the bending stiffness is matched, the axial stiffness of the rod will significantly exceed that of the bone. In practice, solid rods are not used for several reasons; one is that the combined behavior of the rod and bone greatly reduces the stresses in the bone.

One common design is an open-section, thin tube in one or another shape. The open section allows for some deformation of the rod when it is placed and enhances the contact between the rod and the bone. However, introducing an open section greatly reduces the torsional strength and stiffness. Consider the two rod designs shown in Figure 8.5.

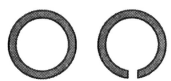

FIGURE 8.5 Closed and open cross sections for intramedullary rods with the same outside radius, r_m, and inside radius, r_i.

For the closed section, the torsional rigidity is given by the product of the polar moment of inertia and the shear modulus:

$$GJ = G\frac{\pi}{2}(r_m^4 - r_i^4)$$

$$= G\frac{\pi}{2}(4r^3t + rt^3)$$

Here,

$$r = \frac{r_m + r_i}{2}$$

and

$$t = r_m - r_i$$

For the open section, the torsional rigidity is no longer given by a simple expression, but can be approximated by the expression (see Section 6.2)

$$GJ^* = G\frac{2\pi}{3}rt^3$$

If we define the ratio of inner to outer radii for the rod to be $\beta_r = (r_i/r_m)$, we can write

$$r = r_m\left(\frac{1 + \beta_r}{2}\right); \qquad t = r_m(1 - \beta_r)$$

The ratio of stiffnesses then becomes

$$\frac{GJ^*}{GJ} = \frac{G\frac{2\pi}{3}r_o^4\left(\frac{1 + \beta_r}{2}\right)(1 - \beta_r)^3}{G\frac{\pi}{2}r_o^4(1 - \beta_r^4)} = \frac{2(1 - \beta_r)^2}{3(1 + \beta_r)^2}$$

For a tubular rod with $t = .25r$, we find that the opening of the section, even without significant loss of material, leads to a drop of 92 percent in the torsional rigidity. The comparable drop in torsional strength is on the order of 91 percent. Note that, on the basis of I_D and A_D values, the bending and axial properties would be comparable for the two designs.

EXAMPLE 8.2 Comparison of an IM Rod and Bone

Question   A bone with an outer diameter of 36 mm and an inner diameter of 20 mm is to be fixed by a hollow IMR made of stainless steel and with an outer diameter of 20 mm and an inner diameter of 18 mm. (a) How do the bending stiffness and torsional stiffness of the rod compare with the bending stiffness of bone? (b) How much is the torsional stiffness of the rod reduced if it is split longitudinally to create an open section?

Solution The bending stiffness is just the product of the moment of inertia and the modulus for each. Assuming a Young's modulus for bone $EB = 20$ GPa and for the stainless steel $ED = 190$ GPa, we get

$$E_B I_B = (17,000)\frac{\pi}{4}(18^4 - 10^4) = 1268 \times 10^6 \text{ N-mm}^2$$

$$E_D I_D = (190,000)\frac{\pi}{4}(10^4 - 9^4) = 513 \times 10^6 \text{ N-mm}^2$$

Using $G_B = 3.3$ GPa for shear moduli for bone, and $G_D = 75$ GPa for the stainless steel, we get

$$G_B J_B = (3300)\frac{\pi}{2}(18^4 - 10^4) = 492 \times 10^6 \text{ N-mm}^2$$

$$G_D J_D = (75,000)\frac{\pi}{2}(10^4 - 9^4) = 405 \times 10^6 \text{ N-mm}^2$$

Although the torsional stiffness comes close, neither bending nor torsional stiffness of the rod reaches that of the bone.

If the rod is slit and becomes an open section, the torsional rigidity becomes

$$G_D J_D = (75,000)\frac{2\pi}{3}\left(\frac{10 + 9}{2}\right)(10 - 9)^3 = 1.5 \times 10^6 \text{ N-mm}^2$$

The split rod has almost no torsional stiffness, compared with the bone or closed section rod.

8.3 | Combined Behavior of Bone and Rod

If we assume that the intact bone and rod act as a unit, then we can analyze the behavior by using methods of composite beams, as developed in Chapter 5. For the assumed simple geometry of a cylinder within a cylinder, the combined properties are just the sum of the two. For example, the bending stiffness is given by

$$K_I = E_B I_B + E_D I_D$$

Similar expressions can be written for the axial and torsional stiffness. Note that this simple result holds only because the rod and bone are concentric. As will be seen in Section 8.5 on plates, when this is not true, the relationship becomes more complex. The maximum bending stresses in the bone and in the rod are given by

$$\sigma_B = \frac{E_B M r_o}{E_B I_B + E_D I_D}; \qquad \sigma_D = \frac{E_D M r_m}{E_B I_B + E_D I_D}$$

Note that, to determine the strength of the composite structure, it will be necessary to check both these equations to identify which yield strength determines the maximum allowable moment.

We can write a similar expression for the torsional stresses versus an applied torque T as follows.

$$\tau_B = \frac{G_B T r_o}{G_B J_B + G_D J_D}; \qquad \tau_D = \frac{G_D T r_m}{G_B J_B + G_D J_D}$$

Before going on to the somewhat more complex problem of a plate on a bone, we note several things. First, *in vivo* loads are not as simple as a pure axial load, a pure moment, or a pure torque acting individually. Real loads involve all three in combination. As long as the linear elastic behavior we have previously assumed holds, the stresses from each load component can be superimposed. In particular, the axial stresses due to axial and bending loads can be summed. If there are combined torque and axial loads, the stress state involves both normal stresses and shear stresses. In some circumstances, the strength of a material under combined loading can be described by a surface in stress space that provides bounds on the allowable combined stresses. This is a subject beyond the scope of the present text, but is one that has been addressed.

Also, we have examined the behavior for the two extreme cases, where the rod acts alone and where the rod and bone act as though they are tightly bonded together. It is entirely possible that the rod–bone interface is not a perfect bond, but involves some degree of slip. In that case, it is possible that the bending behavior is not greatly modified (since the rod is forced to bend inside the bone), but the axial and torsional behavior is much less tightly coupled. Allowing axial load transfer across fragments may in fact be desirable to achieve better load sharing and less stress shielding in the bone. However, in most cases, torsional coupling is desirable to prevent excessive motion of the fragments. A number of IMR designs try to enhance torsional coupling by increased interference, the use of longitudinal flutes, or the use of locking screws at the ends of the rods.

EXAMPLE 8.3 Bone with Intramedullary Rod

Question   What are the axial, bending, and torsional stiffness and strength properties for the combined IR and bone of Example 8.2? Compare the results with the individual IR and bone values.

Solution   Assume the following properties for the device and bone: For the bone, $E_B = 17$ GPa, $G_B = 3.3$ GPa, strength in axial or bending loading $= S_{BN} = 100$ MPa, strength in torsional shear $S_{BT} = 40$ MPa. For the device, $E_D = 190$ GPa, $G_D = 75$ GPa, strength in axial or bending loading $= S_{DN} = 790$ MPa, strength in torsional shear $= S_{DT} = 440$ MPa. Recall that the dimensions of the bone are 36 mm OD and 20 mm ID, and of the rod are 20 mm OD and 18 mm ID.

Shown in Table 8.3 are the results for the calculations based on the various formulas previously given for combined stiffness and strength.

TABLE 8.3

Comparison of Structural Properties of an Intramedullary Rod–Bone System.[1]

Property	Bone	Rod	Bone + Rod
Axial rigidity, N	11.9×10^6	11.3×10^6	23.3×10^6
Axial strength, N	70,400	47,160	137,000
Bending rigidity, N-mm^2	1268×10^6	513×10^6	1781×10^6
Bending strength, N-mm	414×10^3	213×10^3	582×10^3
Torsional rigidity, N-mm^2	492×10^6	405×10^6	897×10^6
Torsional strength, N-mm	331×10^3	237×10^3	604×10^3

[1]Strength (lower failure load for bone or device) is determined by maximum stress in the bone in all cases.

8.4 | Mechanics of Bone Plates

First we consider an idealization of a bone-implant system consisting of a plate attached to a long bone, which is regarded as a hollow, circular cylinder, as shown in Figure 8.6. In general, the *in vivo* loading on a bone-plate system is complex and includes axial, bending, torsional, and shear loads. The structural characteristics of the bone and the plate are also complex. For example, the cross-sectional shape of long bones and the material properties of the bone tissue vary along the length. Additionally, the plate cross section is generally not rectangular, because the long edges of the cross section are slightly curved (see Figure 8.6) to conform approximately to the circumferential shape of the bone. Also, the plate is often deformed plastically (twisted and bent) in the operating room to better conform to the bone along its length. Finally, the plate is not bonded to the bone, but is attached at discrete points with screws.

The purpose of the plate in the near term is to hold the fragments in apposition as the bone heals, while providing the load-carrying capabilities lost because of the fracture. During this time, the behavior of the construct is further complicated by any small gaps that exist between the fragments. As the bone-plate system is loaded, these gaps can close (or open), which adds further complexity to the structural analysis problem.

In the short term and in the long term, there may be situations where the plate carries the lion's share of the load. This occurs in the short term if the fracture is so severe that the load in the bone cannot be transferred across the fragments of the fracture. In the long term, stress shielding may cause the structural rigidity of the bone to decrease with respect to the plate, which can further decrease the stresses in the bone and further decrease the structural rigidity of the bone. The potential exists for the process to enter a vicious cycle until, eventually, the plate itself is taking the load. The concern then is that the plate may be at risk of failure.

We have already described the strength and stiffness properties for the bone treated as a circular tube. The plate can be approximated by a rectangular cross section; the area moments of inertia about the two axes are the well-known expressions

$$I_{zz} = \frac{wh^3}{12}; \qquad I_{yy} = \frac{w^3h}{12}$$

FIGURE 8.6 Idealized model of a bone plate attached to an intact bone. Here it is assumed that these loads have been reduced to an equivalent axial load, which acts at a distance αr_o from the centroidal axis of the bone. The neutral axis of the composite structure is located a distance $\hat{y}$ from the centroidal axis of the bone, and the centroid of the device is located at a distance $\bar{y}_D$ from the centroidal axis.

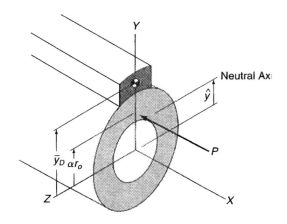

TABLE 8.4

w/h	κ	κ₁
Values of Torsional Constants for Rectangular Cross Section of Dimensions (2a) × (2b)		
1	2.250	1.350
2	3.664	1.860
4	4.496	1.994
10	4.992	2.000

Source: Wang, C.T., *Applied Elasticity*. McGraw-Hill, New York, 1953.

where the h is the smaller dimension and w is the larger dimension of the cross section of the plate shown in Figure 8.6. The expression for the torsional constant of a rectangular cross section is more complicated, but can be approximated by the expression

$$J^* = \kappa \frac{wh^3}{16}$$

where the parameter κ is a shape factor that gives good approximation to the exact value, which is determined from a series solution for the torsion problem. Some values for κ are given in Table 8.4.

Similarly, the maximum shear stress for a rectangular cross section is given approximately by

$$\tau_{max} = \kappa_1 \frac{T(h/2)}{J^*}$$

where T is the applied torque, J^* is as previously defined, and some values of a second parameter κ_1 are also given in Table 8.4. We can express the torsional strength (maximum allowable torque) as

$$T_{max} = \left[\frac{J^*}{\kappa_1(h/2)}\right](S_D)_T$$

where $(S_D)_T$ is the maximum allowable shear stress. Recall that the maximum shear stress occurs at the midpoint of the longer side, which is the shortest distance from the plate centroid to the surface (see section 6.2). This rather counterintuitive fact seems contrary to the result for the circular section, but is an important feature of torsion of noncircular sections.

8.5 | Combined Behavior of Bone and Plate

In the long term, after healing has occurred, the plate may become something of a liability. The bone becomes capable of carrying the entire load itself, but must share the load with the attached plate. Our goal is to understand the fundamental behavior of bone–plate systems after healing has occurred. As mentioned earlier, if the plate carries a substantial part of the *in vivo* load, less bone tissue is needed than when it carried the entire load, and it may change both its density and geometry due to the stress shielding of the device.

To analyze this situation, we assume that the plate is attached firmly to the bone and behaves generally as a composite beam. We will assume elastic behavior of both the bone and plate, and use the results for composite beams from Chapter 5 to describe the mechanics of the combined plate and bone. The best case for the bone is that it has the properties of the intact bone, which is what we will assume.

In Figure 8.6, the bone and the plate have a common plane of symmetry. Therefore, according to the results of Chapter 6, the axis along this plane of symmetry (y axis in Figure 8.6) and a perpendicular axis through the modulus-weighted centroid of the composite (parallel to the z axis in Figure 8.6) are principal axes of bending. The bending behavior can be described by the sum of bending in the plane of symmetry and in the plane perpendicular to this plane. The more complex situation, where the system is unsymmetric, is addressed in an example problem later in the chapter.

Bone plates are usually applied to the bone on the tensile side, where the tensile stresses are the hightest. The load will be represented by a single eccentric axial load, which is applied in the plane of symmetry, as shown in Figure 8.6. The bone and plate are assumed to act as a single unit; that is, the bond between the two is perfect, and stresses due to torsion can be neglected. Here we focus on the bone because of the potential for stress shielding and bone resorption.

The analysis of bone stress that follows may be generalized by writing the equations in terms of the following normalized structural stiffnesses and normalized geometry:

$$\rho_I = \frac{E_D \bar{I}_D}{E_B \bar{I}_B}$$

$$\rho_A = \frac{E_D A_D}{E_B A_B}$$

$$\beta = \frac{r_m}{r_o}$$

and

$$\gamma = \frac{\bar{y}_D}{r_o}$$

In these equations,

> r_m is the radius of the medullary cavity;
> r_o is the outside radius of the bone;
> $\bar{I}_D$ and $\bar{I}_B$ are the are moments of inertia of the device and the bone, respectively, with respect to their centroidal axes;
> A_D and A_B are the cross-sectional areas of the device and the bone, respectively; and
> E_D and E_B are the moduli of elasticity of the device and the bone, respectively.

From composite beam theory (see Chapter 5), the stress in the bone at a distance t_B from the neutral axis of the composite structure may be written as

$$\sigma_B = -\frac{PE_B}{E_B A_B + E_D A_D} - \frac{E_B M t_B}{E_B I_B + E_D I_D}$$

where the first term represents compressive stress due to the axial compressive load, and the second term represents the bending due to the axial load being applied at a point away from the centroidal axis of the bone.

The moment about the neutral axis M may be expressed as

$$M = P(\alpha r_o - \hat{y})$$

and the location of the neutral axis of bending $\hat{y}$ is given by

$$\hat{y} = \frac{\rho_A}{1 + \rho_A} \gamma r_o$$

Using these relationships, we may write the moment as follows:

$$M = P\left(\alpha r_o - \frac{\rho_A}{1 + \rho_A} \gamma r_o \right)$$

The stress in the bone may be written

$$\sigma_B = -\frac{P}{A_B}\left[\frac{1}{1 + \rho_A} + \frac{\left(\alpha - \dfrac{\rho_A}{1 + \rho_A} \gamma \right)\dfrac{t_B}{r_o}}{\dfrac{1}{4}(1 + \beta^2)(1 + \rho_I) + \gamma^2\left(\dfrac{\rho_A}{1 + \rho_A} \right)} \right]$$

A similar expression could be derived for the stress in the plate.

To compute the largest values of bending stresses in the bone, t_B must be known. The largest value of t_B in the positive y direction (immediately beneath the plate in Figure 8.6) is given by

$$t_B = r_o - \hat{y} = r_o - \frac{\rho_A}{1 + \rho_A} \gamma r_o$$

or

$$\frac{t_B}{r_o} = 1 - \frac{\rho_A}{1 + \rho_A} \gamma$$

The largest value of t_B in the negative y direction (farthest away from the plate in Figure 8.6) is given by

$$t_B = -(\hat{y} + r_o) = -\left(r_o + \frac{\rho_A}{1 + \rho_A} \gamma r_o \right)$$

or

$$\frac{t_B}{r_o} = -\left(1 + \frac{\rho_A}{1 + \rho_A} \gamma \right)$$

EXAMPLE 8.4

Question: For the simple bone-plate system in Figure 8.6, assume that the load is applied at the centroid of the bone, $\alpha = 0$, the centroid of the device is given by $\bar{y}_D/r_O = 1.11$, and the ratio of inner and outer radii of the bone is $\beta = 0.615$. How does the stress immediately beneath the plate (stress in the bone with plate, divided by the stress in the bone without plate) vary as the plate stiffness increases?

Solution: The result can be calculated for any bending stiffness ratio ρ_I using the preceeding equations. The result is shown in Figure 8.7 as a function of normalized axial stiffness. Curves for two values of normalized bending stiffness ($\rho_I = 0.1$ and $\rho_I = 1.0$) are shown. The case for an intramedullary rod that fills the medullary cavity of the bone is also shown for comparison.

The first thing to note in the preceding example is that bending is induced when the plate is added, even though the load produced only compression in the intact bone. It should also be noted that when a plate is used, the stress is not very sensitive to the relative bending stiffness of the plate with respect to the bone. The stress is very sensitive, however, to the relative axial stiffness of the plate with respect to the bone, because this ratio determines the location of the neutral axis. When the plate is applied to the bone, the neutral axis moves from the centroid of the bone to a location close to the plate; and the load, which was axial with respect to the bone alone, now produces a bending moment with respect to the neutral axis of the bone–plate system. When the intramedullary rod is used, the neutral axis of the bone–rod system remains at the centroid of the bone (for the model shown in Figure 8.7). As a result, the stress in the bone is much less sensitive to the normalized axial stiffness of the rod with respect to the bone than when a plate is used.

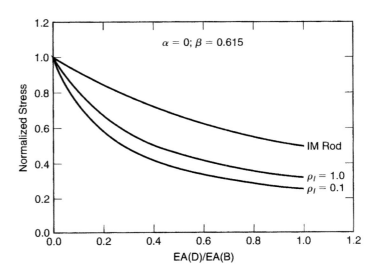

FIGURE 8.7 Normalized stress in the bone for two different plates and an intramedullary rod as a function of normalized axial stiffness.

Figure 8.7 suggests that ρ_A and ρ_I are independent variables. This is indeed the case. It is possible to design bone plates that have specified values for these ratios. For example, for a one-material, rectangular plate, it is possible to keep the cross-sectional area constant, but change its height–width ratio to obtain a specified bending stiffness. Two-material plates have also been proposed to provide the necessary bending stiffness, but reduced axial stiffness, compared with a one-material plate.

The ratio ρ_A can also be considered independent of ρ_I in another way. As discussed previously, fixation devices may be coupled stiffly to bone in bending, but not coupled perfectly to the bone axially. In some situations, this is desirable. The degree of coupling can be represented in the general equation for bone stress as

$$\sigma_B = -\frac{P}{A_B}\left[\frac{1}{1+\rho_A} + \frac{\left(\alpha - \dfrac{\rho_A}{1+\rho_A}\gamma\right)\dfrac{t_B}{r_o}}{\dfrac{1}{4}(1+\beta^2)(1+\rho_I) + \gamma^2\left(\dfrac{\rho_A}{1+\rho_A}\right)}\right]$$

by varying the value ρ_A while keeping ρ_I constant.

It should also be noted that this equation depends only upon the location of the centroid of the device, as well as the area and the area moment of inertia of the implant. Therefore, it can be used to describe the behavior of the bone-implant system for a variety of fracture fixation devices, as long as the system satisfies the basic assumptions in the derivation.

8.6 | Plate Fixation: Other Considerations

For the cases where the loading on the bone–plate system is being carried mostly by the plate, the assumptions and methods of basic strength of materials can be used, and the stresses in the plate due to axial, bending, and torsional loads combined, to determine the risk of failure of the plate. Materials that are easily deformed plastically in the operating room to shape the plate to the bone generally have low fatigue strength, compared with less ductile materials. Consequently, both the engineer and clinician must be aware that in some cases there may be a race between bone healing and plate failure.

Therefore, successful plate fixation must be concerned with both structural stiffness and strength of the plate. As was stated previously, important insight can be obtained by comparing the structural properties of the plate with those of the bone. A comparison of a specific bone and plate are given in Table 8.5 for axial, bending, and torsional behavior. Except for the combined torsional stiffness, all values are calculated from the equations in this section. The determination of the torsional properties of the bone plus plate is complex and beyond the scope of this text.

The results for this example show that the plate falls well short of the bone in terms of its bending and torsional rigidity and strength. It would be possible to

TABLE 8.5

Comparison of Structural Properties of a Plate–Bone System.[1]			
Property	Bone	Plate	Bone Plus Plate
Axial rigidity, N	4.95×10^6	10×10^6	14.95×10^6
Bending rigidity, N/mm²	288×10^6	21×10^6	880×10^6
Bending strength, N/mm	148×10^3	38.8×10^3	247×10^3
Torsional rigidity, N/mm²	231×10^6	23×10^6	*
Torsional strength, N/mm	177×10^3	33.8×10^3	*

[1]For the bone, $r_o = 13$ mm, $r_m = 8$ mm. The axial and bending properties for the bone and plate are $E_B = 15,000$ N/mm², $E_D = 200,000$ N/mm², $S_B = 100$ MPa, $S_D = 930$ MPa. The torsional (shear) moduli and strength properties of the bone and plate are $G_B = 6000$ N/mm², $G_D = 80,000$ N/mm², $(S_B)_T = 60$ N/mm², $(S_D)_T = 550$ N/mm². The plate is assumed rectangular, with width = 10 mm and height = 5 mm. Bending rigidity and strength are calculated about the plate's least stiff axis (the neutral axis for combined bone and plate; see Figure 8.6).
*Calculating the combined torsional properties is beyond the scope of this text.

make a plate thick enough or of sufficient material strength to actually achieve comparable rigidity. However, its cross-sectional dimensions would make it very difficult to use because of its size. This limitation can be overcome by using two plates, either at 90 degrees or at 180 degrees with respect to each other. These two-plate configurations can be analyzed as well by means of composite beam theory; this is left as an exercise for the reader.

The importance of placing the plate on the "opening" side of the fracture under normal loads (tensile side of a bone in bending) is shown in Figure 8.4. When this is done, the bone fragments are allowed to close on each other, and the effective stiffness and strength across the fracture site can be as great as or greater than the parent bone (Figure 8.8). Also, it is obvious that for most properties, except possibly torsion, the combined behavior of the bone and plate is in fact much stiffer and stronger than the original parent bone by itself. As we have already noted, this actually causes reduced stresses in the bone when the bone and plate work together. This is the so-called stress-shielding problem, which results in bone loss because the

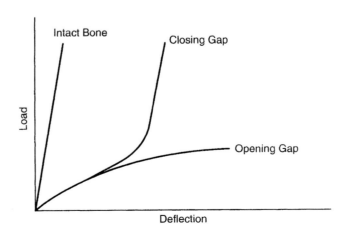

FIGURE 8.8 Stiffness of the bone–plate system at the fracture site.

stresses in the bone fall below their normal values. It also may be responsible for slowed maturation of the new bone at the fracture site.

8.7 | Irregular Bone Cross Section with a Plate

So far, we have dealt with idealized systems where the bone was modeled as a concentric circular cylinder. Real bones are not perfectly straight circular cylinders, and the resulting bone–plate systems generally do not have a plane of symmetry. However, using the ideas of composite beams from Chapter 5, we can find the bending stresses for any cross section and any plate position, as long as we can treat the bone as a straight beam. This is usually a quite acceptable assumption for diaphyseal fractures of long bones. The general approach for determining the structural stiffness and stresses for a bone–plate system where the bone has an irregular cross section is illustrated in the next example, which demonstrates all the detailed calculation that is necessary to handle the combination of a bone with an irregular cross section and a plate that is applied at an arbitrary angle with respect to the chosen reference frame.

EXAMPLE 8.5 Unsymmetric Bending of Bone with Plate

Question   What is the stress distribution for the applied moment for the bone cross section with a plate attached, as shown in Figure 8.9?

Solution   We will assume that the bone is rigidly fixed to the plate. A bending moment of 1000 N-mm is applied about the z axis.

To calculate the stress and strain distribution with the use of composite beam theory, we will choose the centroid of the bone cross section as our reference point. About the bone centroid, the area properties are given as

$$A_B = 276 \text{ mm}^2; \; I_{Byy} = 3990 \text{ mm}^4; \; I_{Bzz} = 4170 \text{ mm}^4; \; I_{Byz} = -335 \text{ mm}^4$$

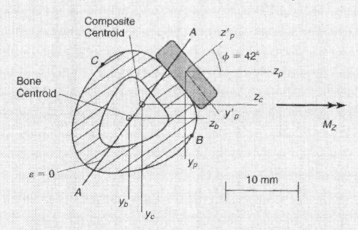

FIGURE 8.9   A bone cross section with an attached plate.

The centroid of the rectangular plate is located at $y_b = -6.4$ mm, $z_b = 7.4$ mm, with respect to the centroid of the bone cross section, and the plate is oriented at $42°$ with respect to the z axis. The dimensions of the plate are 4 mm $\times$ 10 mm, and the elastic modulus of the plate is $E_P = 120$ GPa. We will take the modulus of the bone to be $E_B = 15$ GPa.

To determine the properties of the composite section, we will first calculate the location of the composite centroid and then calculate the composite area moments and products of inertia about the composite centroid. We can then use these properties to calculate the orientation of the neutral axis and the stress and strain distributions across the section. We begin by calculating the y- and z-oriented area properties of the plate about its own centroid. About the y'_p and z'_p axes, which are principal axes for the plate, the moments and products of inertia are

$$I_{Py'y'} = \frac{(4)^3 10}{12} = 53.3 \text{ mm}^4; \quad I_{Pz'z'} = \frac{4(10)^3}{12} = 333 \text{ mm}^4.$$

We can transform the moments and product of inertia from these principal axes to the y and z axes by using the following equations (note that these are the inverse of the transformations to the principal axes given in Chapter 5):

$$
\begin{aligned}
I_{Pzz} &= \frac{I_{Pz'z'} + I_{Py'y'}}{2} + \frac{I_{Pz'z'} - I_{Py'y'}}{2} \cos(2 \cdot \phi) \\
&= \frac{333.3 + 53.3}{2} + \frac{333.3 - 53.3}{2} \cos(-84) = 208 \text{ mm}^4 \\
I_{Pyy} &= \frac{I_{Pz'z'} + I_{Py'y'}}{2} + \frac{I_{Pz'z'} - I_{Py'y'}}{2} \cos(2 \cdot \phi) \\
&= \frac{333.3 + 53.3}{2} - \frac{333.3 - 53.3}{2} \cos(-84) = 179 \text{ mm}^4 \\
I_{Pyz} &= \frac{I_{Pz'z'} - I_{Py'y'}}{2} \sin(2 \cdot \phi) = \frac{333.3 - 53.3}{2} \sin(-84) = -139 \text{ mm}^4
\end{aligned}
$$

The weighted centroid (neutral axis) of the composite section is given by

$$
\begin{aligned}
\bar{y}_c &= \frac{E_B A_B y_B + E_P A_P y_P}{E_B A_B + E_P A_P} = \frac{(0) + (120{,}000)(32)(-6.4)}{(15{,}000)(276) + (120{,}000)(40)} = -3.43 \text{ mm} \\
\bar{z}_c &= \frac{E_B A_B z_B + E_P A_P z_P}{E_B A_B + E_P A_P} = \frac{(0) + (120{,}000)(32)(7.4)}{(15{,}000)(276) + (120{,}000)(40)} = 3.97 \text{ mm}
\end{aligned}
$$

The moments and product of inertia of the bone about the centroid of the composite are obtained by using the parallel axis theorems:

$$
\begin{aligned}
\bar{I}_{Byy} &= I_{Byy} + (\bar{y}_B - \bar{y})^2 A_B = 3990 + (0 + 3.43)^2 276 = 7240 \text{ mm}^4 \\
\bar{I}_{Bzz} &= I_{Bzz} + (\bar{z}_B - \bar{z})^2 A_B = 4170 + (0 - 3.97)^2 276 = 8520 \text{ mm}^4 \\
\bar{I}_{Byz} &= I_{Byz} + (\bar{y}_B - \bar{y})(\bar{z}_B - \bar{z}) A_B = -335 + (0 + 3.43)(0 - 3.97)276 \\
&= -4090 \text{ mm}^4
\end{aligned}
$$

Similarly, for the plate, we get

$$\bar{I}_{Pyy} = I_{Pyy} + (\bar{y}_P - \bar{y})^2 A_P = 179 + (-6.4 + 3.43)^2 40 = 532 \text{ mm}^4$$

$$\bar{I}_{Pzz} = I_{Pzz} + (\bar{z}_P - \bar{z})^2 A_P = 208 + (7.4 - 3.97)^2 40 = 679 \text{ mm}^4$$

$$\bar{I}_{Pyz} = I_{Pyz} + (\bar{y}_P - \bar{y})(\bar{z}_P - \bar{z})A_P = -139 + (-6.4 + 3.43)(7.4 - 3.97)40$$

$$= -546 \text{ mm}^4$$

We can now calculate the total weighted moments and products of inertia for the plate and bone as

$$\bar{I}^*_{yy} = E_B\bar{I}_{Byy} + E_P\bar{I}_{Pyy} = (15{,}000)(7240) + (120{,}000)(532) = 172 \times 10^6 \text{ N-mm}^2$$

$$\bar{I}^*_{zz} = E_B\bar{I}_{Bzz} + E_P\bar{I}_{Pzz} = (15{,}000)(8520) + (120{,}000)(679) = 209 \times 10^6 \text{ N-mm}^2$$

$$\bar{I}^*_{yz} = E_B\bar{I}_{Byz} + E_P\bar{I}_{Pyz} = (15{,}000)(-4090) + (120{,}000)(-546)$$

$$= -127 \times 10^6 \text{ N-mm}^2$$

Now the strain distribution in the bone and plate is given by

$$\varepsilon = \frac{(M_y I^*_{zz} + M_z I^*_{yz})z - (M_y I^*_{yz} + M_z I^*_{yy})y}{I^*_{yy}I^*_{zz} - I^{*\,2}_{yz}}$$

$$= \frac{(1000 \cdot -132 \times 10^6)z - (1000 \cdot 178 \times 10^6)y}{178 \times 10^6 \cdot 214 \times 10^6 - (-132 \times 10^6)^2}$$

$$= -6.40 \times 10^{-6}z - 8.67 \times 10^{-6}y$$

and the bending stresses at any point in the bone and plate can be calculated as

$$\sigma_B = E_B\varepsilon; \qquad \sigma_P = E_P\varepsilon.$$

We could use these equations to calculate the stress distribution across the bone and plate. To determine the location of the peak stress, it is most convenient to determine the orientation of the neutral axis of bending. This is found by setting ε in the previous equation to zero, leading to

$$\varepsilon = \frac{(M_y I^*_{zz} + M_z I^*_{yz})z - (M_y I^*_{yz} + M_z I^*_{yy})y}{I^*_{yy}I^*_{zz} - I^{*\,2}_{yz}} = 0$$

$$z = \frac{(M_y I^*_{yz} + M_z I^*_{yy})}{(M_y I^*_{zz} + M_z I^*_{yz})}y = \frac{1000(178 \times 10^6)}{1000(-132 \times 10^6)}y = -1.35y$$

This is a line at $\theta = \arctan(-1.35) = -54°$ from the y axis, which is shown as line AA in Figure 8.9. By inspection, we see that the greatest perpendicular distance from the neutral axis is at point B on the compressive side and point C on the tensile side of the bone. These points are at approximately ($y = 4.4$ mm, $z = 6.8$ mm) and ($y = -5.6$ mm, $z = -5.2$ mm), respectively. The stresses at these two points are, respectively, $\sigma = -1.31$ MPa and $\sigma = +1.22$ MPa per N-m of applied moment.

The preceding example demonstrates that the analysis of the combined behavior involves a considerable amount of calculation. The calculation of torsional stresses for the composite section is considerably more complicated and is usually achieved only by using numerical models, such as the finite element method.

8.8 | External Fixators

External fixators have become widely used to stabilize fractures with major soft tissue injuries. They are now commonly employed not only for long-bone fractures, but also for pelvic fractures and a variety of other complex fractures. External fixators are quite versatile and can be configured in many different ways.

To determine how fixator parameters relate to the effective stiffness of the bone-device system, we will consider a simple example of a planar frame. In this case, pins are placed through the major fracture fragments above and below the fracture site in a single plane. These pins are connected to the side bars or rods by clamps, as illustrated in Figure 8.10. Since the side bars and clamps can be made quite stiff, and the bone is relatively large and stiff compared with the pins, the primary deformations that occur in the fixator are in the pins.

We will examine the axial stiffness of the assembly by calculating the ratio of the axial deflection at the fracture gap to an applied axial load. The portion of each pin between the bone and the side bar can be modeled as a beam with one end (side bar) fixed and the other end (bone) guided. From the theory of elastic beams, the deflection of the ith pin at the bone due to an applied axial load, P, acting on the bone is given by

$$\Delta_i = \frac{P_i}{12E_iI_i}s_i^3$$

where P_i is the share of the load P applied to the ith pin and s_i, I_i, and E_i are the length, cross-sectional moment of inertia, and elastic modulus, respectively, of the pin.

We will assume that s, E, and I are the same for each pin, that each pin carries an equal load on either side of the fracture, and that half of the gap closure is

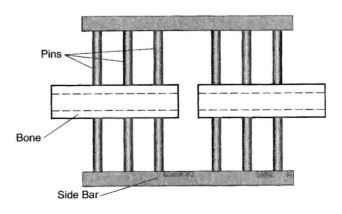

FIGURE 8.10 A schematic of an external fixator. The pins may go through the bone and may be attached to one or both side bars.

attributable to the deflections of the pins on either side of the fracture gap. On this basis, we arrive at the following expression for the stiffness of the fixator system:

$$K = \frac{P}{\Delta}$$

$$\approx 6\left(\frac{n_s n_P E_P I_P}{s^3}\right)$$

Here,

n_s is the number of side bars,
n_P is the number of pins on each side of the fracture,
E_P is the pin modulus,
$I_P = \pi d^4/64$ (d is the pin diameter), and
s is the pin length between the bone and the side bar.

From this relation, it is clear that the primary contributors to the axial stiffness of the single-plane fixator are the diameters of the pins and the side bar separation distance. Increasing the pin diameter by 50 percent will increase the stiffness by a factor of approximately five. Decreasing the side bar separation distance by 50 percent will increase the stiffness by a factor of eight.

EXAMPLE 8.6 Effects of Pin Parameters on Fixator Stiffness

Question   Consider a 6-pin, double-sided configuration, as shown in Figure 8.6. What are the effects of going from a 4 mm pin diameter to a 6 mm pin diameter and decreasing the side bar offset from 50 mm to 40 mm? Assume stainless steel with a modulus of 190 GPa for the pins.

Solution   Using the foregoing equation and calculating the results for each of the preceding cases, we obtain the results in Table 8.6.

TABLE 8.6

Comparison of External Fixator Stiffness Versus Pin Diameter and Offset

d_p, mm	s, mm	Stiffness, N/mm
4	50	687
4	40	1343
6	50	3481
6	40	6799

It is obvious that the offset and pin diameter have a dramatic effect on the fixator stiffness. This simple expression helps to guide these choices and to identify the merit of fixator parameter changes. As usual, changing out the material simply modifies the stiffness in a linear fashion, at least to first order approximation. In practice, other factors come into play, which tend to diminish the theoretical stiffness of the bone-fixator construct. For example, the pin anchorage in the bone is often not sufficient to justify the assumption of a fixed-end condition at the bone. Also, the side bars can bend, and the resulting bending deflections may contribute to the compliance of the system.

The simple planar fixator is not often used. A half-plane fixator with a single side bar is more common, because it is much easier for the surgeon to assemble. In order to improve the out-of-plane bending stiffness, it is often combined with a second half-plane fixator to provide a more rigid three-dimensional structure.

8.9 | Controlling Callus Strains

Modern fracture fixation techniques, particularly the use of external fixators, have provided the opportunity to actually control callus strains. One approach is to periodically change the stiffness of the fixator by changing side bars. For example, one could introduce a relatively high stiffness side bar in the early stages and then change to a lower stiffness side bar to provide greater fracture-site loading as healing progressed. There is considerable controversy over which stiffness regimen works best. There have been valid arguments offered for a high initial fixator stiffness followed by a lower stiffness, or alternatively, a low initial fixator stiffness followed by a higher stiffness. Long-term clinical outcome studies will help identify the best procedures.

More aggressive approaches to controlling callus strains have also been introduced. One is an external fixator system that allows for axial pistoning of the fixator side bar. This method, called dynamization, has been championed by several investigators.

An even more aggressive approach has been to directly impose callus strains by providing a load on a pistoning external fixator frame. Investigators using this technique have found improved rates of healing in animal studies and evidence of improved rates of healing in humans under controlled loadings. This is carrying the concept of strains versus tissue differentiation to its logical limit. Again, clinical studies will be important in determining whether there is a sufficient decrease in morbidity and in the risk for failed unions to merit the use of these considerably more complex and aggressive treatment approaches.

The external fixator also provides a possible means of tracking the healing. Fixator deflections or loads measured over time have been used to estimate the changing characteristics of the fracture callus. As the fracture healing progresses, the loads carried by the external fixator are expected to diminish. Therefore, by measuring deflections (or loads), one can follow this process. One of the most sophisticated approaches is to introduce a complex load cell into the fixator system. In this case, direct measurements of fixator loads, combined with a model of the fixator system, bone, and callus, make it possible to predict the actual callus stiffness properties.

8.10 | Bone Screws and Effects of Holes

The simple issue of introducing holes into bones has been studied to a considerable extent. Theoretical analyses of stress concentrations due to introducing a hole suggest that the local strength of the bone should be reduced by approximately a factor of 3. (For a small hole in an infinite sheet of material, the limiting value for the stress concentration is 3.) Experimental studies indicate that the introduction of small holes has relatively little effect on the torsional strength of long bones. This is no doubt because bone has many local stress risers occurring naturally. As the size of the hole is increased from approximately 10 percent to 50 percent of the diameter of the bone, the torsional strength decreases approximately linearly to about 40 percent. Larger holes amount to reducing the bone to an open section rather than a tube with a stress concentration. The presence of a pin or screw in the hole creates minimal improvement in the strength. However, over a period of several weeks, a considerable improvement in the strength occurs, compared with when the hole is first made, even though the defect is still visible on radiograph. This adaptation probably involves an addition of some callus around the hole and a smoothing of the sharp edges and small cracks created by the drill. This is a good illustration of how the process of fracture treatment has to be regarded as a dynamic process where the system adapts over time.

Bone screws are important and commonly used devices. As we have seen, they attach the device to the bone, and they are also used directly to fix bone fragments. The analysis of a bone screw alone is a difficult challenge, because the geometry of the interface is so complex. The basic contributors to the mechanical behavior are the nominal diameter of the screw, the design of the threads, the material properties of both the screw and the bone, and the length of engagement of the screw. A simple formula for the pullout strength of a single bone screw is

$$F = L \cdot C \cdot S \cdot G$$

where F = pullout force, L = length of engagement of the screw, C = the outer circumference of the screw, S = the shear strength of the bone, and G = a geometric factor, which is less than unit and which accounts for the thread profile and depth. This formula is based on the assumption that the bone will shear at the outer diameter of the screw, which is a good assumption for most circumstances.

Usually, a cortical bone screw is placed in a predrilled hole. The performance of the screw, at least initially, is also determined by the pilot hole diameter. For cancellous bone, with much lower density, the screw may be self-tapping. If a bone screw is used to fix two fragments, it is important to have the screw threads engage only the second fragment of cortex, in order to get good compression of the fragments.

When a bone plate is attached with screws, the loads on the screws are determined by the position on the plate, the local bone properties, and other factors, such as the amount of tightening and the design of the holes in the plate. As illustrated in Figure 8.11, if the screws have various amounts of tension, the combination of their loads and the contact forces must balance the bending moment transmitted across the plate. Obviously, this is a complex loading state, in which the actual forces (and moments) in each screw are difficult to predict.

FIGURE 8.11 A bone plate sustaining a bending moment across a fracture site in a long bone. If the entire moment across the comminuted fracture site is carried by the plate, as shown in (b), then static equilibrium requires that the screw forces, plus contact forces, generate a couple equal and opposite to the applied moment. The net sum of the forces must be zero, so the magnitude of the distributed contact forces (represented by a single resultant force F_c) must be equal to the sum of the three screw forces.

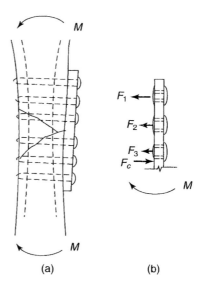

8.11 | Other Issues and Complications

The simple models introduced in the previous section describe the basic behavior of various fracture fixation schemes and identify the critical issues that must be considered in analysis and design of these bone-implant systems. However, they are rather simple models, and *in vivo* systems may differ from them in a number of ways.

Consider three examples. First, when fractures occur near joints, the bone involved is cancellous bone, so the fracture amounts to many local structural failures of trabeculae. Treatment in this case can vary from the use of screws to stabilize fragments to the introduction of bone grafts to replace major defects and cavities in the trabecular bone. Second, in spine fractures, several vertebral elements may be involved. Plates and rod systems are often used to stabilize these fractures. Plates and screws are also used frequently for complicated fractures of the skull and facial bones. The structural behavior of each of these systems is more complex than those analyzed in this chapter, but the basic principles still apply. In particular, all fixation systems must provide sufficient stability of the fracture to allow the normal callus tissues to survive and mature into bone resembling the original bone.

In some difficult fractures, a device alone cannot provide the necessary stability, and there is a need for material augmentation. In some cases, bone is obtained from other parts of the body and used to help reconstruct large bony defects. In addition, a number of artificial graft materials have been introduced. The use of either natural or artificial graft materials complicates the structural behavior of the bone–device–graft system. Further complications are introduced when artificial materials are used as scaffolding upon which new bone is built during the healing process. The analysis and design of these important constructs have been studied intensively, but involve issues that are beyond the scope of this text.

8.12 | Summary

The biomechanics of fracture treatment is a classic application in biomechanics. Some basic rules are well understood, and some of the most important mechanics issues can be understood in the context of relatively simple models. Even though more complex models than those presented here may be required for difficult fractures, the basic requirements are the same in complex and simple analyses. Therefore, a thorough understanding of the models presented provides a framework for developing analyses of more complex systems.

8.13   EXERCISES

8.1 Internal fracture fixation is used to provide bending and torsional rigidity to a bone while the fracture heals. Bone plates are often used to accomplish this. However, when the bone heals, the plate shares the load and may cause bone resorption beneath the plate. If too much resorption occurs, the bone may refracture when the plate is removed. Another possibility is that the plate will take more and more of the load, and the plate will fracture before it can be removed.

In this exercise, you are to model the bone-plate system as a metal plate attached to an intact (healed) femur. The nominal loading on the femur includes both bending and axial loads. The basic question to be addressed is, How are the stresses under the plate affected by the design of the plate and the material(s) from which the plate is made?

Specifically,

(a) Determine the stresses as a function of the bending and axial rigidity of the plate relative to the bone.

(b) Interpret your general results in terms of specific changes in material properties (e.g., using titanium alloy instead of stainless steel).

8.2 Consider a cylindrical model of a bone with outside radius r_O and inside radius r_m. A compressive load, P, is applied to the bone along its centroidal axis (the axis of symmetry). A bone plate with a rectangular cross section is added to the intact bone. The same axial load is applied along the centroidal axis of the bone.

(a) Describe in detail the steps you would go through to calculate the stress in the bone immediately beneath the plate if the normalized equation in the text were not available. Be sure to list the equations you would use for each step.

(b) Sketch the stress distributions in bone before the plate is attached, and in the bone and the plate after the plate is attached to the bone.

(c) Briefly explain why the stress in the bone changes as it does after the plate is attached.

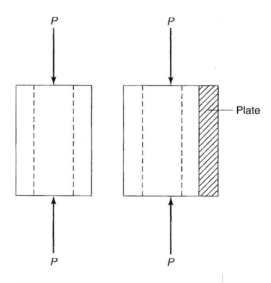

FIGURE P 8.2

8.3 The following equation is for the stress in the bone in the presence of a fracture fixation device, such as an IM rod or a bone plate:

$$\sigma_B = -\frac{P}{A_B}$$

$$\left[\frac{1}{1 + \rho_A} + \frac{\left(\alpha - \dfrac{\rho_A}{1 + \rho_A}\gamma \right)\dfrac{t_B}{r_o}}{\dfrac{1}{4}(1 + \beta^2)(1 + \rho_I) + \gamma^2\left(\dfrac{\rho_A}{1 + \rho_A} \right)} \right]$$

Here, αr_o locates the load P with respect to the neutral axis of the bone. (If $\alpha = 0$, the load is applied along the axis of the bone).

(a) What does this equation reduce to for pure bending of the bone with device?

(b) Write down the expressions for ρ_A and ρ_I, and define all the terms in these expressions.

8.4 Consider an intact bone with a fracture plate attached. On a plot, show how $\hat{y}/r_o$ varies as a function of $E_D A_D/E_B A_B$ for a reasonable value of $\bar{y}_D/r_o$. Assume that the bone is a hollow cylinder with inside radius, r_m, and outside radius, r_o. The location of the neutral axis, $\hat{y}$, and the location of the centroid of the plate, $\bar{y}_D$, are measured with respect to the axis of the bone.

8.5 On the graph for Exercise 8.4, show points representing plates made of stainless steel and Ti6Al4V. Choose reasonable values of b/r_o, h/r_o, and h/r_o to make your calculations.

8.6 A plate is added to a bone as shown in Figure P 8.6.

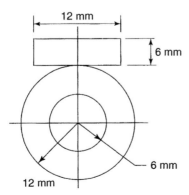

12 mm

6 mm

6 mm

12 mm

FIGURE P 8.6

(a) Compare the minimum bending stiffness of the plate with the bending stiffness of the bone. Use a modulus of $E_{\text{plate}} = 120,000$ MPa, and $E_{\text{bone}} = 15,000$ MPa

(b) Compare the bending strength of the plate about its weakest axis with the bending strength of the bone. Use strength values of $\sigma_{\max_{\text{plate}}} = 500$ MPa, and $\sigma_{\max_{\text{bone}}} = 80$ MPa.

(c) Calculate the bending stiffness of the combined plate and bone, when bending occurs in the plane of symmetry.

8.7 The axial rigidity of a homogeneous beam (e.g., a bone or a fracture fixation plate) is the product (area) × (modulus). The bending rigidity is the product (moment of inertia) × (modulus).

(a) For the bone and the plate of Exercise 8.6, how do the axial and bending rigidity of the (single) plate and bone compare?

(b) How might you design a plate that has a reduced axial rigidity, but maintains its bending rigidity about its least stiff axis?

8.8 A substantial increase in the stiffness of a plated fracture can be achieved by using two plates (Figure P 8.8). For the dimensions of bone (circular cross section) and plates given, determine the bending rigidity for bending in the plane of symmetry for bone plus one plate or two plates. Assume that the moduli for bone and plate are $E_B = 15,000$ MPa; $E_P = 130,000$ MPa.

8.9 A fracture fixation plate typically is not designed to sustain the entire bending load experienced by a bone on which the plate might be used. In its use, its placement can strongly influence the performance of the construct. Answer the following questions with words, sketches, and/or equations:

(a) Why is the plate typically not designed to be as strong or as stiff as the bone?

(b) How should the plate be applied to allow it to function adequately?

8.10 Fracture plates are essentially rectangular in cross section, for obvious reasons. Their bending rigidity about either principal axis is defined by EI_{xx} or EI_{yy}. The flatter the plate, the poorer is its torsional rigidity. The torsional rigidity can be approximated by

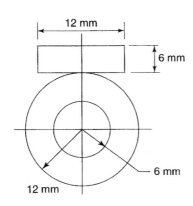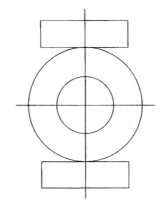

FIGURE P 8.8

the product GJ^*, where

$$J^* = ab^3\left[\frac{16}{3} - 3.36\frac{b}{a}\left(1 - \frac{b^4}{12a^4}\right)\right],$$

where $2a$ = width, $2b$ = height, $a \geq b$.

For a rectangular plate of width 12 mm and height 6 mm, compare the value for GJ^* to the torsional rigidity of a circular cross section of the same area.

Draw a sketch to show where the maximum shear stress would occur on the rectangular cross section due to an applied torque.

8.11   A bone is modeled as a hollow circular cylinder of outer radius $R = 13$ mm and inner radius $r = 8$ mm. To stabilize a fracture, an 8 mm intramedullary rod is placed in the bone. If the bone has a modulus $E = 15$ GPa, and a yield stress $S = 100$ MPa, would a rod of stainless steel ($E = 200$ GPa, $S = 400$ MPa) be as strong as the bone in bending? as stiff in bending?

8.12   A 10 mm stainless steel ($E = 200,000$ MPa) intramedullary rod is placed in a bone ($E = 15,000$ MPa) with a 10 mm inside diameter and a 16 mm outside diameter.

(**a**) Compare the bending rigidity of the bone and the rod.

(**b**) Compare the maximum stress for a given applied moment for the bone and the bone plus the rod.

8.13   One of the problems with internal fracture fixation plates is that they tend to shield the bone from its normal stresses as healing progresses. One idea that has been advanced to avoid this problem is to design plates with lower stiffness. See if you can come up with a realistic idea for a design of a plate with lower stiffness. Identify the problems and the design criteria that you would need before you started the design process.

9

Total Hip Replacements

The analysis and design of hip replacements, like all joint replacements, involves functional and structural issues. The hip is a ball and socket joint that provides flexion–extension, abduction–adduction, and internal–external rotations of the femur with respect to the pelvis, while transmitting substantial loads. In a total hip replacement, both sides of the joint are replaced by a new ball and socket. In some cases, this is done by replacing only the surfaces. In most cases, the surface of the acetabulum is replaced, and the head and neck of the proximal femur are removed and replaced by a prosthetic head and neck that are attached to an intramedullary fixation stem.

In this chapter, we address both functional and structural issues. Since the relative motion between the articulating surfaces of the highly conforming ball and socket is prescribed by geometry, our focus is primarily on how changing the centers of the articulating surfaces with respect to the pelvis and the femur affects the forces transmitted across the joint (Section 9.1). The knowledge of the muscle forces and the forces on the prosthetic components can then be used to address structural questions about fixation (beginning in Section 9.2) and bearing surface damage (Chapter 11). Although the discussion here is specifically about hip replacements, the general principles apply to other joint replacements as well. Upper extremity joint replacements, such as finger joints, elbow joints, and the humeral components for shoulder joints, frequently employ fixation stems. All of these bone-stem systems can be analyzed by the approaches presented in this chapter for analyzing and designing femoral components for hip replacements.

9.1 | Function: Kinematics and Loads

Kinematics

The range of motion is constrained by bony impingement between the femoral neck and the acetabulum and the soft tissue around the joint. When the natural joint is replaced by a prosthetic ball and socket, the kinematics of the proximal femur with respect to the pelvis may undergo substantial modification, depending upon the position of the head of the femoral component with respect to the femur and the position of the acetabular component with respect to the pelvis. For joint replacement patients with normal anatomy, the goal is to position the components to retain the normal kinematic and structural relationships. This allows each muscle to continue to operate at the same point on its length–tension curve and maintains normal muscle excursions.

If the normal anatomical geometry is reconstructed during joint replacement surgery, the rotational ranges of motion of the hip replacement will be similar to those of the natural joint. If the normal anatomical geometry is not reconstructed, the kinematics may be restricted. For example, the neck of the femoral component may impinge on the rim of the acetabular component and tend to lever the head out of the socket, increasing the risk of dislocation. The tendency to dislocate is a function of head size, acetabular cup geometry, and the geometry of the prosthetic femoral neck.

For some hip replacement patients, however, the joint anatomy is not normal because of disease, damage, or congenital deformities. In such cases, the surgeon may choose to change the positions of the femoral and acetabular components relative to their preoperative positions to increase the mechanical advantage of muscles about the joint or to provide more normal kinematics between the femur and the pelvis. There are, of course, constraints on how much the joint system can be modified. For example, the amount that the resting length of a muscle can be altered may be limited because of the changes these modifications may introduce in the length–tension behavior of the muscle. Furthermore, increasing leg length may also increase the length of associated nerves, which can be damaged if stretched too much.

Loads

Loads on the Proximal Femur and Pelvis   Like other natural joints, the force system at the hip joint is statically indeterminate; more forces act across the joint than can be determined from the equations of equilibrium. To obtain forces that can be used for analysis and design of joint replacements, the indeterminate system is usually reduced to a solvable set of forces that can be calculated by quasi-static equilibrium analyses (see Chapter 2). Figure 9.1 shows a two-dimensional model of the pelvis for single leg stance during normal gait. In two dimensions, there are only three equations of equilibrium. Consequently, there can be only three unknowns.

The abductor force M, the joint force J, and the weight of the body less the weight of the supporting leg, W_s, constitute a three-force system acting on the pelvis that must be concurrent for equilibrium. The point of concurrence is determined by the intersection of the lines of action of W_s and either M or J. The direction and magnitude of W_s are, of course, known completely. If the direction of either M or J is known, then the magnitudes of M and J can be determined analytically from the equations of equilibrium, or graphically by constructing a vector diagram.

We can obtain reasonable estimates of the directions of M and J from the characteristics of the joint. The direction of M can be estimated from joint anatomy, and the direction of J can be estimated from the bony morphology of the femoral head and neck. The force M shown in Figure 9.1 is the resultant of the abductor muscle forces and acts on the tip of the greater trochanter. One can estimate the direction of

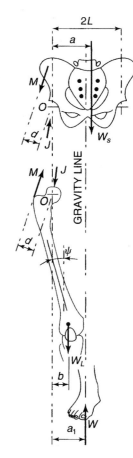

FIGURE 9.1 Two-dimensional model of the pelvis and lower leg in single stance gait. From McLeisch, R.D., and Charnley, J. (1970), "Abduction forces in the one legged stance." *J Biomechanics* 3:191–209.

the resultant in a frontal plane if the direction of the abductor tendon is known. Then the concurrency point can be found, and the magnitudes of M and J can be determined. The alternative approach is to determine the line of action of J first, and then determine the line of action of M and the magnitudes of M and J. The direction of J can be determined from a knowledge of the internal structure of the femoral head and neck and an understanding of how loads are transferred through regions with varying structural stiffness.

In a structure with parallel load paths, the stiffest path carries the greatest load. A radiograph of the femoral head shows a region of dense cancellous bone extending from the surface of the femoral head, through the head center, to the cortex at the calcar (Figure 9.2). To distinguish a difference in density of bony regions on a radiograph, the apparent density of the bone must differ by a factor of about two. If the elastic modulus is proportional to the square of the apparent density, then the modulus must differ by a factor of at least four between the two regions.

The impact of this observation can be seen by considering a two-material column that consists of a stiff inner core and an outer layer of the same cross-sectional area, but an elastic modulus one-fourth as stiff (Figure 9.3). If the column is loaded axially, the displacements of the core and the outer layer are equal, which leads to these relationships for displacement:

$$\Delta_c = \Delta_o = \frac{P_C L}{E_C A_C} = \frac{P_O L}{E_O A_O}$$

Since the lengths and areas of the core and outer layers are the same, it follows that

$$\frac{P_C}{P_O} = \frac{E_C}{E_O} = 4$$

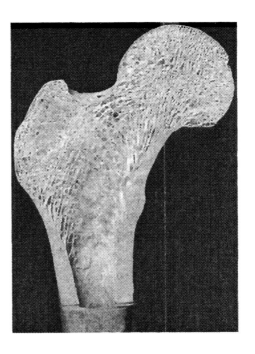

FIGURE 9.2 Cross-sectional view of the proximal femur. A dense region of cancellous bone transfers load from the surface of the head to the dense cortical bone at the calcar.

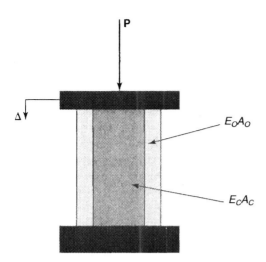

FIGURE 9.3 Cross section of a hollow cylinder with a stiff core.

Thus, we see that "load follows stiffness"; when the load paths are parallel, the stiff core carries 80 percent of the load.

Similarly, we conclude that the stiff core of cancellous bone in the femoral head is the primary load carrier between the joint surface and the calcar region of the femur. Consequently, the line of action of J must lie along this region of dense cancellous bone, which is consistent with the direction determined from an instrumented femoral component (Figure 9.4).

Figure 9.4 also shows that the point of application of the head force does not change substantially during the stance phase of gait. Similar observations have been

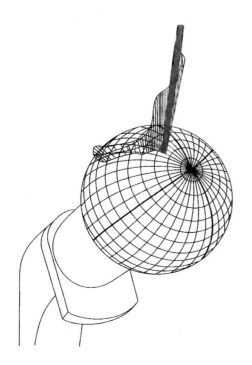

FIGURE 9.4 The load acting on the femoral head during a cycle of normal gait determined with an instrumented prosthesis. [Davy et al., *J Bone J Surg Am (January)* 1988, 70(1):45–50.] The magnitude and location of the resultant force on the head varies over the gait cycle. During the stance phase, the force is largest, but moves very little with respect to the femoral component.

FIGURE 9.5 The load (top) and load angle (bottom) of the femoral head on the acetabular cup. The angle varies about 12 degrees during the heavily loaded portion of the cycle, which is greater than the variation of the load of the cup on the head seen in Figure 9.4. From Pedersen, D.R., Brand, R.A., and Davy, D.T. (1997). "Pelvic muscle and acetabular contact forces during gait," *J Biomechanics*, 30:959–965.

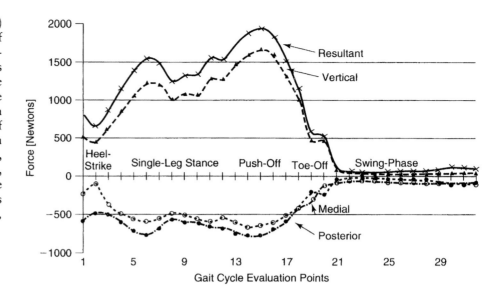

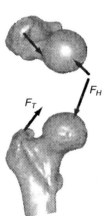

FIGURE 9.6 To make analysis easier, the complex loading on the proximal femur may be reduced to two forces: the compressive load on the femoral head F_H, and the tensile load on the greater trochanter F_T. Note in the top view that the forces act to produce a twisting moment about the axis of the femur.

made for other activities, such as stair climbing or walking on a ramp, where the tilt of the ramp is perpendicular to the direction of travel. Therefore, for most activities of daily living, only one load path is needed—the dense cancellous bone between the head center and the calcar. If the point of application of J on the head is approximately stationary, however, then the direction of J must vary considerably with respect to the acetabular cup (Figure 9.5).

Three-dimensional reduction models can also be used to determine the forces acting on the proximal femur (Figure 9.6). The three-dimensional analysis makes it possible to obtain estimates for six unknown forces rather than three. On the basis of models such as these, the magnitude of the joint force has been estimated to be about 2.5 times body weight (consistent with experimental results) and the abductor muscle force to be about 1.8 times body weight.

The tensile muscle force and the compressive joint force act as a couple on the proximal femur to produce a substantial bending moment in the femoral shaft. The resulting stresses are tensile on the lateral side and compressive on the medial side. The existence of the tensile strains on the lateral side for peak loading during normal gait has been confirmed by *in vivo* strain gage studies.

The muscle and joint forces are not coplanar (Figure 9.6). Three-dimensional analyses of hip forces with only a joint force and abductor force acting on the proximal femur show that these forces produce a twisting moment about the longitudinal axis of the femur. As a result, the internal forces and moments at a distal section of the femur include bending in two planes, twisting about the femoral axis, and compressive and shear forces.

The direction of the head load with respect to the femur has important implications for the design of total hip replacements. The joint force on the femoral component of a total hip replacement (Figure 9.6) has a posteriorly directed component, which tends to twist the prosthesis with respect to the femur. Consequently, the interface (or interfaces) between the implant and the bone must be able to transmit torsional loads as well as bending and axial loads.

Loads as a Function of Head and Cup Placement   The loads on the proximal femur with prosthesis will be the same as those on the normal femur if the normal geometry has been recreated when the prosthetic components are implanted. If, however, the geometry is changed, then the loads will also be changed. For example, if the distance, d, between the hip joint center and the line of action of the muscle force (Figure 9.1), M, is decreased, then the ratio a/d will increase and the muscle and joint forces will increase. This is a very important aspect of musculoskeletal joints. Joint forces and the kinematics of a joint are coupled—changing one will change the other. In the case of the hip joint, the relative motions of the articulating surfaces remain unchanged; a ball and socket joint is replaced by a prosthetic ball and socket. But, if either the position of the head with respect to the femur or the position of the acetabulum with respect to the pelvis is changed, then the lines of action and the magnitudes of the muscle and joint forces will be changed.

The position of the femoral head with respect to the femur can be defined in two ways. First, the head position can be determined by the use of radial coordinates—the angle of the head–neck axis with respect to the femoral axis and the distance from the intersection of the head–neck axis and the femoral axis to the head center. Second, the position can be described in terms of rectangular coordinates—head offset from the femoral axis, and head height above the intersection of the head–neck axis and the femoral axis. It is often convenient in analyses of joint force to write the appropriate equations in terms of changes in position of the centers of the head and the acetabulum with respect to the femur and pelvis, respectively, rather than in terms of positions measured with respect to other landmarks on the respective bones.

Prosthesis systems have been developed with the use of both radial and rectangular coordinates. Radial coordinates are the most common because, in most hip replacement systems, the femoral component has a fixed neck angle. For modular components (Figure 9.7), where different heads can be used with the same neck, the

FIGURE 9.7 Two modular femoral components for cementless fixation. Modular heads are attached to the tapered trunions. The proximal geometry is essentially the same; distal geometry is chosen by the surgeon. (Reproduced with permission of Exactech Corporation.)

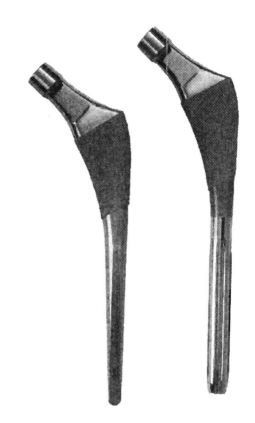

neck length is controlled by choosing the appropriate femoral head (with or without a skirt). The skirt can be thought of as a portion of the neck that is attached to the prosthetic head, which fits over the trunion of the femoral component. An added advantage of modular femoral components is that the head and stem can be made of different materials—CoCr heads can be used on titanium stems, and ceramic heads can be used on metal stems. For monoblock components, where the head and stem are made from one piece of material, a range of prostheses with different neck lengths must be available to the surgeon, and the inventory of fixation stems will be larger.

9.2 | Fixation: Femoral Stems

In principle, only the damaged surface of the femoral head needs to be replaced. The goal of surface replacements is to make use of the natural femoral neck to transfer the head load to the shaft of the femur. But surface replacements with metal heads and polyethylene acetabular surfaces have not been consistently successful. The large head size requires thin polyethylene components on the acetabular side (unless metal on metal bearings are used), and the stiff femoral component may shield the underlying cancellous bone from stress. Because of the lack of consistent clinical results for surface replacements, the entire head and neck are usually replaced in total hip arthroplasty. The prosthetic head is attached to the femur by a fixation stem. Stems of various lengths have been used. Some designers have advocated saving the femoral neck, but usually the neck is resected at its base. The femoral component, therefore, consists of a head, together with a neck that is attached to a distal stem which extends down into the medullary cavity some distance below the lesser trochanter (Figure 9.8).

The portion of the prosthesis in the medullary cavity generally tapers from proximal to distal. If cement is used for fixation, a cavity is machined in the bone that has the same shape as the stem, but is larger than the stem. The cavity is filled with bone cement, and the stem is inserted. A distal plug may be used to keep the cement from extruding farther down the canal than necessary, and centralizing spacers may be employed at the distal stem tip to provide a cement mantle that is as uniform as possible. When the cement has cured, the bone–cement–stem system forms a three-material composite beam.

If cementless fixation is used, then the stems are generally larger in cross section, and the cavity is machined so that the prosthesis fits precisely into the bone, at least in certain portions of the metaphyseal region. The shape of the prosthesis is determined so that intimate contact occurs between the prosthesis and the bone, where bone ingrowth or ongrowth is desired. Two types of designs are used, one symmetric and one anatomic. The anatomic designs are unsymmetrical, with wedge-shaped metaphyseal regions to facilitate load transfer and to provide stability of the implant while ingrowth or ongrowth occurs.

For both cemented and cementless designs, the loading of the proximal femur is radically altered when the femoral component is implanted. In the normal femur, the head and neck act as a compression strut that loads the cortex of the cortical bone directly; the internal cross section of the cortex is loaded. In the proximal femur with prosthesis, the load is transferred to the bone through the endosteal surface of the cortical shell. In cementless designs, this may be by direct contact between the prosthesis and the cortex; in cemented designs, load is transferred through the cement mantle to the endosteal surface.

After a prosthesis is implanted, the load carried by the bone is decreased, because it now shares the load with the stem (and the cement for cemented stems). According to composite beam theory (see Section 5.2), the amount of load carried by each component of the beam depends upon the relative structural rigidities of the components. For example, the bending moment carried by the ith component of the composite beam is given by

$$\frac{M_i}{M} = \frac{E_i I_i / E_B I_B}{1 + E_C I_C / E_B I_B + E_P I_P / E_B I_B}$$

Here, the bending rigidities of the cement and the prosthesis have been normalized with respect to the bone. The next example shows that the structural rigidity of the cement in the equation for M_i/M can usually be neglected.

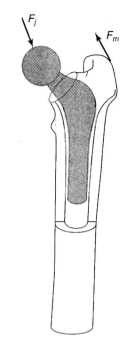

FIGURE 9.8 The loads on the proximal femur are not coplanar. The head load has a posteriorly directed component that causes twisting about the femoral axis, as well as bending in two planes.

EXAMPLE 9.1 Moments in a Three-Material Composite Beam

Question Consider a three-material composite beam consisting of cortical bone, a cement mantle, and the prosthesis. What are the moments carried by the bone, cement, and stem as a function of the size of the prosthesis with respect to the medullary cavity?

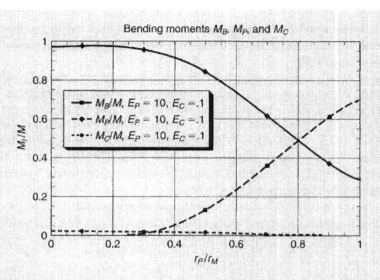

FIGURE 9.9 The portion of the total moment, M_i/M, in a bone-cement-stem system carried by the bone, cement, and prosthesis.

Solution For simplicity, we assume that the structure can be described by concentric circular cross sections. The graph shows the moments carried by the bone, the prosthesis, and the cement when $E_P/E_B = 10$, $E_C/E_B = .1$, and $r_O/r_M = 1.5$. The preceding equation for M_i/M can be specialized for the bone, cement, and prosthesis. For example, for bone the equation becomes

$$\frac{M_B}{M} = \frac{1}{1 + E_C I_C/E_B I_B + E_P I_P/E_B I_B}$$

The moments of area can be written in terms of the ratio of the radius of the prosthesis to the radius of the medullary cavity, and the moment ratios can be plotted as a function of r_P/r_M (Figure 9.9). As the size of the prosthesis increases, the moment carried by the bone decreases and the moment carried by the stem increases. The cement carries at most about 2 percent of the total moment. For most hip stems, the size range of the stem with respect to the bone can be approximated by $.5 < r_P/r_M < .7$ with concentric circular cross-sectional geometry. Within this range, the bone is carrying the majority of the load. However, when the stem fills the cavity, $r_P/r_M = 1.0$, and the stem carries about two thirds of the load and the bone only one third.

If the load carried by the cement is neglected, the portion of the moment carried by the bone is given by

$$\frac{M_B}{M} = \frac{1}{1 + E_P I_P/E_B I_B}$$

Figure 9.10 shows that when the structural stiffness of the stem is increased by increasing the elastic modulus of the stem with respect to the bone, the bone carries less of the load.

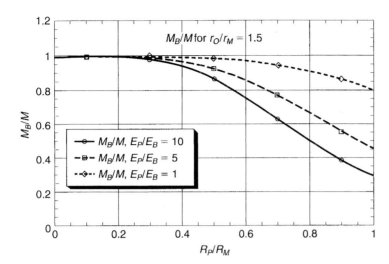

FIGURE 9.10 The load carried by the bone varies with the stiffness of the prosthesis. As the ratio of the stiffness increases, the amount of the load carried by the bone decreases.

The bone-stem system can be divided into proximal, central, and distal zones. The load sharing between components described by the equation for M_i/M is valid only in the central portion of the fixation stem, because beam theory does not apply near abrupt changes in loading or geometry. In the proximal zone, the loads proximal to the metaphyseal region, which are carried entirely by either the femoral neck or by the greater trochanter, are transferred gradually to the bone-stem composite. As a result, the load carried by the proximal medial cortex is generally less than that predicted by beam theory. In the distal zone, loads shared by the bone-stem composite are transferred to the bone alone, and stress concentrations can occur because of the abrupt changes in material properties and geometry of the composite beam near the tip of the fixation stem.

When the load on bone is changed, bone remodeling may occur. If the load is decreased, as it is near the calcar, both the size of the bone cross section and the bone modulus may decrease over time, leading to an increase in the relative structural rigidity of the prosthesis with respect to the bone. If this occurs, the load carried by the bone may be further decreased, potentially leading to a vicious cycle in which further bone is lost. At the stem tip, however, bone apposition may occur because of the stress concentration there, or because of the increased deformation due to the localized contact.

Failure Modes

Fundamentally, failures in a bone-implant system, as in any structure, occur because the stresses on a component or interface exceed the strength. For example, fixation stem failures have occurred in otherwise intact hip replacements due to cyclic loading that occurred during the normal activities of daily living or due to combinations of cyclic loads and large one-time loads that resulted in plastic deformation and tensile residual stresses.

But, failures can also occur because the strength of the bone or the strength of the bone–implant interface has degraded over time. This may be due to bone remodeling resulting from the altered loading on the femur or to biological reactions to debris. For

TABLE 9.1

Characteristic Failure Modes and Analysis Methods for Cemented Femoral Stems		
Zone	Characteristic Failures	Analysis Methods
Proximal zone	Cement fracture	BOEF
	Bone–cement interface failure	FEM
	Bone resorption	
Central zone	Stem fracture	CBT
		BOEF
		FEM
Distal zone	Cement fracture	BOEF
	Bone fracture	FEM

example, debris from damaged bearing surfaces may migrate to the bone–implant interface. When sufficient debris has accumulated, the body attacks it and, in the process, releases agents that attack bone at the bone–implant interface, where it is most vulnerable. The result is an increased risk of infection and interface failure, or loosening.

In the absence of gross interface failure secondary to debris, the proximal, central, and distal zones have characteristic failure modes, as shown in Table 9.1. The location of a failure within a particular zone depends, of course, upon the structural characteristics of the bone and the implant, and upon the loading on the system due to the structural configuration established during surgery. Composite beam theory (CBT) can be used to analyze stresses in the central zone, but does not apply to the transition zones, where either beam on elastic foundation theory (BOEF) or finite element analysis (FEM) must be used to determine load transfer and stresses.

9.3 | Stresses in the Central Zone

The stresses in the central zone due to bending and axial load can be determined with the use of composite beam theory. The derivations of the equations used in this section are presented in Section 5.2.

The central zone stresses in prosthesis and bone due to axial load are given by

$$\sigma_p = \frac{PE_P}{E_B A_B + E_C A_C + E_P A_P}$$

and

$$\sigma_B = \frac{PE_B}{E_B A_B + E_C A_C + E_P A_P}$$

The prosthesis stresses in the central zone due to bending are given by

$$\sigma_P = \frac{ME_P t_P}{E_B I_B + E_C I_C + E_P I_P}$$

Similarly, the bone stresses due to bending are given by

$$\sigma_B = \frac{M E_B t_B}{E_B I_B + E_C I_C + E_P I_P}$$

In these equations,

E_i is the elastic modulus of the ith component of the beam,

P is the total axial load acting on the composite beam at the section of interest,

M is the total bending moment acting on the composite beam at the section of interest,

A is the cross-sectional area of the ith component of the composite beam,

I_i is the second moment of the ith area, computed with respect to the neutral axis of the composite beam, and

t_i is the distance between the neutral axis of the composite beam and the point of interest in the ith material.

Note that I_i and t_i are computed with respect to the neutral axis of the composite structure, which is given by

$$\hat{y} = \frac{E_B A_B \bar{y}_B + E_C A_C \bar{y}_C + E_P A_P \bar{y}_P}{E_B A_B + E_C A_C + E_P A_P}$$

where

$\bar{y}_i$ is the location of the centroid of the ith component with respect to arbitrary reference axes,

$\hat{y}$ is the location of the neutral axis of the composite (modulus weighted centroid) with respect to the reference axes, and

A_i is the area of the ith component.

When the centroidal axes of the components of the beam coincide, $\hat{y}$ equals $\bar{y}$, and I_i is equal to $\bar{I}_i$. If the axes do not coincide, the parallel axis theorem must be used to compute the I's for the stress equations.

The tensile stresses in the bone, cement, and prosthesis are shown in Figure 9.11 for bending alone and for bending with an axial compressive load. As one would expect, the tensile stresses are reduced when the axial load is included, but only by about 10 percent. The stresses in the stem and the bone are dominated by the bending stresses (Figure 9.11).

If we normalize the stresses in the cement and the stem with respect to the fatigue strength of the materials, Figure 9.12 is obtained. Early stems were made from stainless steel, which has the lowest strength to stress ratio. Considerably better strength to stress ratios are obtained with the CoCr and Ti alloys currently used for implants. Note, however, that when a CoCr alloy stem is porous coated, the strength–stress ratio is reduced considerably.

We turn now to cementless stems. Two types have been used for femoral components in total hip replacements—press fit stems without porous layers for bone ingrowth, and stems with porous layers for bone ingrowth. The stem shown in Figure 9.13 is a press fit stem without a porous layer, but it does have fenestrations

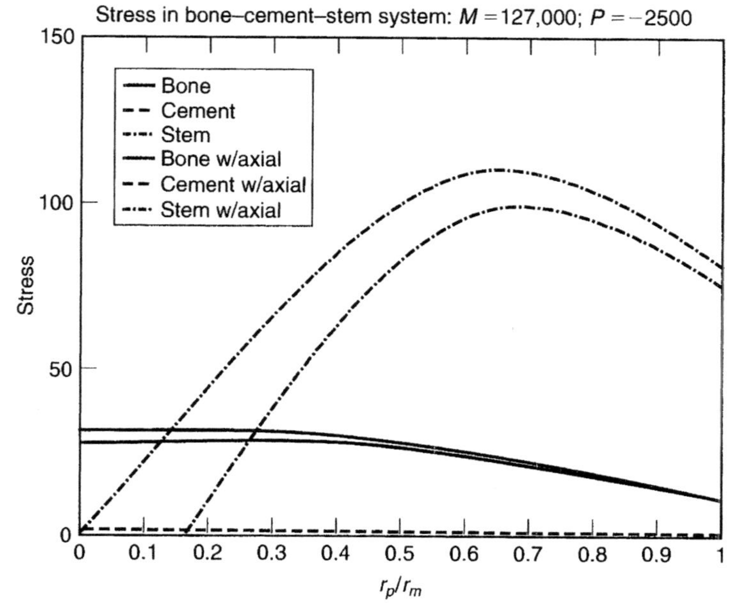

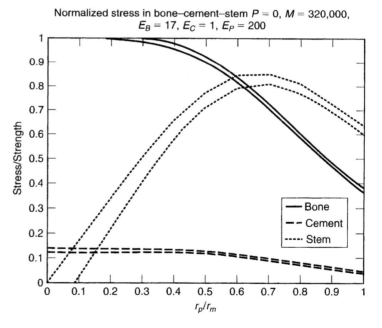

FIGURE 9.11 The stresses due to bending dominate in the central zone. The inclusion of the compressive stress due to axial load decreases the maximum stresses in the bone and the stem by about 10 percent.

FIGURE 9.12 Normalized stresses on the lateral side. The bone stress is normalized by the bone stress without prosthesis; the stem stress is normalized by the fatigue strength of CoCr alloy (325 MPa); the cement stress is normalized by the fatigue strength of PMMA (20 MPa).

(windows) into which bone may grow. This device was one of the earliest stemmed devices and similar stems are still used for hemiarthroplasty, where only the femoral head is replaced and the natural acetabulum is retained. Load transfer from the prosthesis to the bone can occur in three ways: wedging of the proximal portion of the stem into the canal, contact between the collar and the bone at the calcar, and bone ingrowth into the fenestrations in the stem. Clinical studies have shown that all three possibilities occur *in vivo*. Therefore, one cannot predict the

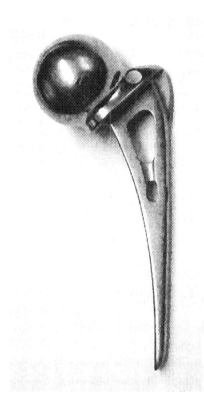

FIGURE 9.13 An early uncemented femoral component
used for hemiarthroplasty.
The large head contacts the
cartilage of the native socket.

load transfer mode that will occur in a particular patient; it depends upon bone
quality and the bone geometry created at the time of surgery. In the absence of bone
ingrowth into the fenestrations, it should be noted that wedging and collar load
transfer are mutually exclusive. Collar contact can occur only if there is no wedging.
If wedging occurs, there can be little, if any, contact between the collar and the bone.

The stem shown in Figure 9.14 is a successor to the stem of Figure 9.13. It is also
a symmetric design. Approximately two-thirds of current versions of the stem, including the proximal wedged portion, are coated with layers of beads for bone ingrowth.
You will notice that, like the stem in Figure 9.13, this prosthesis has a proximal
wedge, a collar, and the possibility for bone ingrowth. The same uncertainties about
load transfer also exist here. One way of making the fixation more predictable is to get
a tight fit between the distal stem and the bone. This is the surgical goal that the pro-
ponents of this device recommend. It can be shown that this may result in load bypass
of the proximal bone, which in some cases can lead to bone resorption in this region.

The stem shown in Figure 9.15 is an anatomic stem. It is an asymmetric,
bone-priority prosthesis. It is designed to transfer load to particular regions of the
proximal femur via three wedges: an A–P wedge, an L–M wedge, and a wedge in
the transverse cross section of the metaphyseal portion of the implant. There is no
collar, so all of the load on the prosthesis is transferred by the wedging action.
Furthermore, only the proximal portion of the prosthesis is coated—in this case
with a rough, plasma-sprayed surface. This surface is not porous, so bone interlock
is achieved by bone ongrowth, whereby the bone contacts the rough surface with
minimal sliding between the implant and the bone.

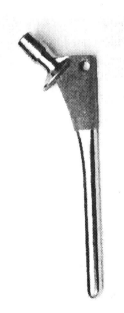

FIGURE 9.14 A descendent
of the stem in Figure 9.13. In
later versions two-thirds or
more of the stem has a porous
coating for bone ingrowth.

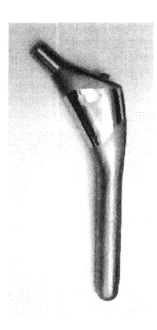

The trade-off between having a collar without wedging or porous ingrowth and having a proximal coating for porous ingrowth is demonstrated by the designs shown in Figure 9.16. The goal is to determine which design has the lowest bending stresses in the distal stem, the one with a proximal-medial collar (Figure 9.16, left) or the one with the proximal porous coating (Figure 9.16, right). To address this problem, we assume that there are only three forces acting on the prosthesis *in vivo*: (i) the joint contact force, which has known magnitude H and acts at a known angle θ, as shown; (ii) a distal contact force D that is horizontal and acts at Point d, but has an unknown magnitude; and (iii) a proximal supporting force P that acts through either Point a (if a collar is used) or Point b (if porous coating is used). The magnitude and direction of the proximal support forces for the two cases are not known. The solution of this problem is left as an exercise for the reader. It can be solved without writing any equations by modeling the implant as a three-force member, and by drawing the appropriate vector diagram.

FIGURE 9.15 An anatomical femoral stem that transfers load through a triple-action wedge. The shiny portion of the metaphyseal region is plasma coated for bone ongrowth to enhance fixation.

9.4 | BOEF and FEA Models for Bone-Stem Systems

Composite beam theory is applicable for cross sections away from abrupt changes in geometry, material properties, or loading. If, however, we want information about load transfer or stresses in the transition zones of a bone-implant system, the structure must be modeled in other ways. We have two choices: beam on elastic foundation theory (BOEF) or finite element analysis (FEA). In this section, we focus on the modeling of these systems without getting into detailed solutions.

Beam on elastic foundation analysis is a good next step in the process of understanding the mechanics of fixation stems like those used on femoral components for hip and elbow replacements. As discussed in Section 6.1, the stem and the bone are idealized as beams that are connected by an elastic layer, or "foundation." The foundation transmits loads from one beam to the other, so that bending moments and shear and axial forces vary along the length of each beam. In the axisymmetric BOEF model of a

FIGURE 9.16 Two proposed designs for a hip implant, one with a proximal–medial collar (left) and the other with proximal porous coating (right).

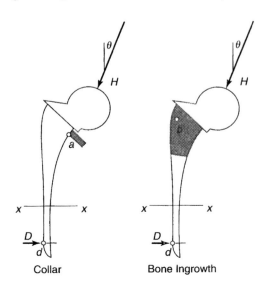

Collar   Bone Ingrowth

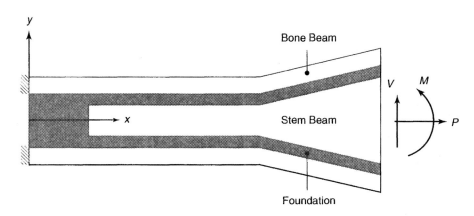

y

Bone Beam

x

Stem Beam

V   M

P

Foundation

FIGURE 9.17 An axisymmetric BOEF model of a bone with a fixation stem.

bone with prosthesis (as shown in Figure 9.17), the load is applied only to the prosthesis (stem beam) at the right-hand end. The bone is fixed at the left end.

Each beam deflects when the prosthesis is loaded and deforms the "foundation" layer between them, which transfers load through the layer from one beam to the other. The usual beam theory equations, for example,

$$\sigma = -\frac{Mt}{I}$$

are used to compute stresses once the bending moment, M, has been determined by solving the governing BOEF equations for displacement, $v(x)$, and then computing

$$M = EI\frac{d^2v}{dx^2}$$

As suggested by Figure 9.17, EI is not a constant along the length of the bone-implant system; EI for both the bone and the stem varies with length. In this case, the governing equations can be solved numerically.

EXAMPLE 9.2 BOEF Analysis of a Bone-Stem System

Question   A study was designed to examine the effects of changing the stiffness of the central portion of the distal stem for a hip prosthesis (Figure 9.18). Both computational (BOEF and FEA) and experimental (Figure 9.19) studies were done. Artificial femurs were used to eliminate the variations that occur from bone to bone when cadaver specimens are utilized. What is the process for determining the structural characteristics of this system if BOEF theory is to be used for the analysis?

Solution   Several things should be noted. First, the system was cementless. Contact between the implant and the bone occurred only in the proximal and distal portions of the device; there was no connection between the central portion of the distal stem and the bone. Second, loading was applied to both the head of the prosthesis and the greater trochanter.

To model this system, a more general BOEF model of the bone-stem composite was used that included bending and axial loading (upper portion of Figure 9.20). Models such as these can be solved with one-dimensional finite element techniques.

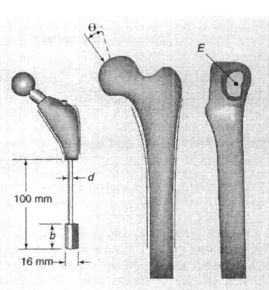

FIGURE 9.18 BOEF and FEA was used to model this bone-stem system used to examine experimentally the effects of reducing the cross section of the prosthesis in the central region of the distal stem. An artificial femur was used for this study. From Chang, P.B., Williams, B.J., Santner, T.J., and Bartel, D.L.(1999). "Robust Optimization of Total Joint Replacements Incorporating Environmental Variables," *J Biomech Eng* 121:304–310.

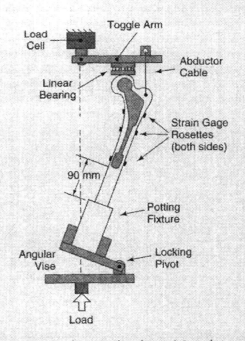

FIGURE 9.19 The experimental setup for determining the mechanics of the bone-implant system shown in Figure 9.18. From Chang, P.B., Williams, B.J., Bawa Bhalla, K.S., Belknap, T.W., Santner, T.J., Notz, W.I., and Bartel, D.L.(2001). "Robust Design and Analysis of Total Joint Replacements: Finite Element Model Experiments with Environmental Variables," *J Biomech Eng* 123 (3):239–246.

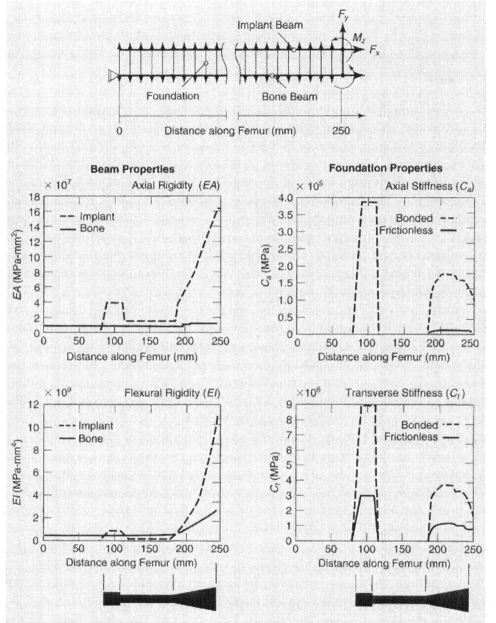

FIGURE 9.20   A BOEF model of a proximal femur with prosthesis. The abductor force on the greater trochanter and the head load on the prosthesis produce bending, axial, and transverse loads on the bone and prosthesis, respectively. Chang, P.B., Williams, B.J., Santner, T.J., and Bartel, D.L.(1999). "Robust Optimization of Total Joint Replacements Incorporating Environmental Variables," *J Biomech Eng* 121:304–310.

First, consider the proximal loading. Forces act on both the head and the greater trochanter. The line of action of the abductor force acts away from the centroid of the bone beam, which results in a bending moment and axial and

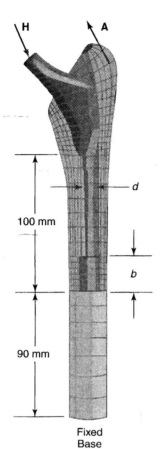

H   A

d

100 mm

b

90 mm

Fixed
Base

FIGURE 9.21 Three-dimensional model of the bone-implant composite studied in the experiment shown in Figure 9.19. From Chang, P.B., Williams, B.J., Bawa Bhalla, K.S., Belknap, T.W., Santner, T.J., Notz, W.I., and Bartel, D.L.(2001). "Robust Design and Analysis of Total Joint Replacements: Finite Element Model Experiments with Environmental Variables," *J Biomech Eng* 123 (3):239–246.

transverse loads acting on the bone, as shown in the upper portion of the figure. Similarly, the load on the prosthetic head has axial and transverse components and produces a moment with respect to the centroid of the stem beam, along with axial and transverse loads.

In general, the properties of the bone, implant, and the interface layer, *EI, EA, c_t*, and *c_a*, vary with distance along the femur. The structural rigidities of the stem can be determined from drawings or measurements of the stem; the rigidities of the bone can be determined from CT scans or from approximations to the geometry obtained from plane radiographs. The stiffnesses of the interface layer can be determined from the equation for *C_t* (presented in Section 6.1) for cemented stems, or assumptions about the interface, as was done in this example. The structural rigidities used in this study are shown in left-hand graphs in Figure 9.20; the transverse and axial stiffnesses of the elastic foundation are shown in the right-hand graphs in Figure 9.20.

The closed-form solutions of the moments and forces in the stem and bone presented in Section 6.1 can be solved only for simple cylindrical geometries. Therefore, models like this one, where the geometry varies along the length of the bone-implant system, were solved numerically with one-dimensional finite element techniques, as mentioned previously. The BOEF model was validated by the experimental analysis.

The advantage of BOEF as a solution is that it is computationally inexpensive. This particular model was used to test a statistically based optimal design algorithm for determining the influence of design and environmental variables, a process which required hundreds of analyses and would have been too expensive computationally to do with a finite element model of the system. Once the validity of the optimization algorithm had been determined, a finite element model (Figure 9.21) of the bone-implant system was incorporated, which provided further detail.

BOEF can also be used to model cementless stems. One way of doing this is to consider the bone to be made up of two regions: a thin region adjacent to the stem that is loaded transversely, and the remainder of the cross section, which resists bending loads. The thin layer adjacent to the stem contributes little to the bending stiffness and can therefore be subtracted from the overall cross section without loss.

EXAMPLE 9.3 Inner Layer of Bone as the Elastic Foundation

Question To examine the approach just described, assume that a thin layer of the bone is "removed" to play the role of the foundation in BOEF theory. What is the reduction of the bending rigidity of the bone if the layer of bone is removed?

Solution Consider an idealized cementless system with perfect ingrowth where the cross-sectional geometry is described by concentric circular cylinders. The ratio of bending rigidity of the bone with the layer removed to the bending rigidity of the bone with no layer removed is given by

$$\frac{EI_{\text{layer}}}{EI_{\text{nolayer}}} = \frac{r_o^4 - (r_m + \Delta)^4}{r_o^4 - r_m^4}$$

For outside and inside radii of bone given by

$$r_o = 26 \text{ mm}, r_m = 24 \text{ mm}$$

and layer thickness

$$\Delta = 1 \text{ mm}$$

this ratio is 0.96. Thus the bending stiffness is only reduced by 4 percent if the inside 1 mm of the cortex is considered to be the elastic foundation.

One could use a similar approach to see the effects of having a fibrous tissue interface between the stem and the bone by merely changing the material properties of the 1-mm-thick interface layer. The finite element model used in conjunction with the experimental study (see Figure 9.21) incorporated an artificial bone that had two regions with homogeneous properties—to represent cortical and cancellous bone, respectively.

In Figure 9.22, a real bone was CT scanned to determine the geometry and material properties of the proximal femur. The elastic modulus of the bone was determined from a modulus–density relationship and assigned on an element-by-element basis. The geometries of the two designs were based on actual implants, and a 2-mm-thick coating of cement was added to the implant. Interface elements were incorporated between the cement and the implant and between the cement and the bone to model bonded interfaces and no-tension interfaces with coulomb friction. In the model shown in Figure 9.22, the dark gray area of the proximal stem could be bonded or unbonded, depending upon whether or not the stem was precoated at the factory. The loading of this model consisted of a head load and a load on the greater

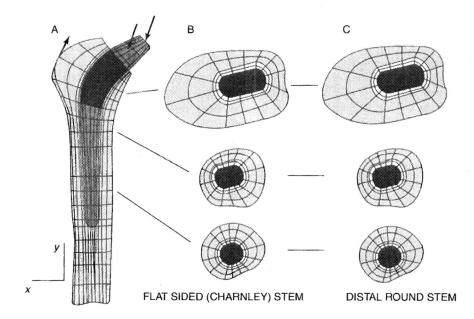

A   B   C

y

x

FLAT SIDED (CHARNLEY) STEM   DISTAL ROUND STEM

FIGURE   9.22 Proximal femur with a cemented prosthesis. The upper portion of the distal stem has flat sides for Design B, but is circular for Design C. From Chang, P.B., Mann, K.A., and Bartel, D.L. (1998). "Cemented Femoral Stem Performance Effects of Proximal Bonding, Geometry, and Neck Length," *Clinical Orthopaedics and Related Research* 355:57–69.

trochanter, which were not coplanar. Note that two head loads are shown to model the effects of two neck lengths. Thus, the design characteristics that could be investigated with this model included a flat-sided or distal round stem; a short or long neck length; and a bonded or unbonded proximal stem. By varying the load, environmental variables, such as patient weight and activity, can also be studied.

Models of the type shown in Figure 9.22 and their cementless counterparts are highly nonlinear contact problems because of the bone–cement and stem–cement interface characteristics. Additional nonlinearities are introduced if the elastic–plastic behavior of cancellous bone tissue is included in the model or if some model is introduced to represent damage due to cement failure. One needs a thorough understanding of nonlinear mechanics both to create these models and to interpret the results obtained from the finite element solutions.

9.5 | Summary

A total hip replacement is a ball and socket joint. The joint force and muscle forces depend upon the location of the center of the femoral head with respect to the femur and on the center of the acetabulum with respect to the pelvis. The joint force can be estimated by the quasi-static methods described in Chapter 2. The maximum resultant force across the joint is about 2.5 times body weight for normal gait. For activities of daily living, the location of the resultant joint force on the femoral head moves little, but moves considerably with respect to the socket.

Components may be fixed to the bone either with bone cement (Chapter 7) or by bone ingrowth or ongrowth to the prosthesis itself via porous or rough coatings on the prosthesis. Most femoral components are modular and consist of a combined stem and neck, to which various femoral heads may be attached at the time of surgery. The most common structural failures of the proximal femur with prosthesis are fracture of the fixation stem in the central zone, interface failures in the proximal and distal transition zones, and bone resorbtion due to stress shielding. The stresses associated with these failure modes can be computed by composite beam theory, beam on elastic foundation theory, or finite element methods.

9.6 EXERCISES

9.1 Fixation stems for femoral components may be made from either CoCr or titanium alloy. Produce a graph of M_i/M versus r_P/r_M, like that presented in Figure 9.9, that shows how the moments in the bone, cement, and prosthesis vary with material for $r_O/r_M = 1.5$.

9.2 The diameter and thickness of the cortex of the femur change with age. Produce a graph of M_i/M versus r_P/r_M, like that presented in Figure 9.9, that shows how the moment carried by the bone and the stem vary for $r_O/r_M = 1.5$, 1.4, and 1.3.

9.3 Reproduce the graph shown in Figure 9.12, but for titanium alloy rather than CoCr.

9.4 On a single graph of bending stress versus r_P/r_M, like that presented in Figure 9.11, show curves for bending stress alone when the stem is made from CoCr or from Ti alloy.

9.5 On a single graph of bending stress versus r_P/r_M, like that presented in Figure 9.11, show curves of bending stress alone for $r_O/r_M = 1.5$, 1.4, and 1.3 when the stem is made of CoCr alloy.

9.6 Solve Exercise 9.5 for the case where the stem is made of Ti alloy.

9.7 Fixation stems on femoral components for total hip replacements come in a variety of shapes. One possible design for a cemented stem is shown in Figure P 9.7. Use composite beam theory to decide on the material; the dimension d that locates the flat with respect to the center of the circular portion of the prosthesis; and r_p, the size of the prosthesis. Assume that the circular portion of the prosthesis is centered inside the bone. The dimensions used in the analysis should be normalized with respect to the radius of the medullary cavity of the bone.

What advantages and disadvantages do you see for this shape, compared with a rectangular shape that is tall in the lateral–medial direction and short in the anterior–posterior direction?

9.8 Calculate the maximum tensile stress in the Ti alloy prosthesis ($E_s = 100$ GPa) at section X–X for the model shown in Figure P 9.8. Perform your calculations for two cases:

(a) The stem is well fit so that there is ideal load sharing between the bone and prosthesis.

(b) The stem is fixed distally (below section X–X), but loose proximally, so that load sharing is negligible.

Assume a joint contact force J of 3285 N and an abductor force A of 2455 N. The coordinates (x, y) of

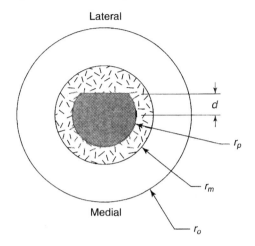

Lateral

Medial

d

r_p

r_m

r_o

FIGURE P 9.7

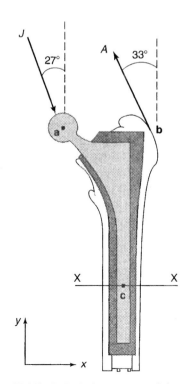

J

$27°$

A $33°$

a

b

X —— X

c

y

x

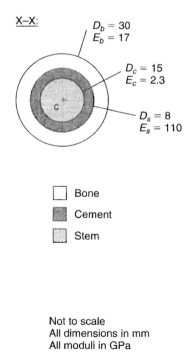

X–X:

$D_b = 30$
$E_b = 17$

$D_c = 15$
$E_c = 2.3$

c

$D_s = 8$
$E_s = 110$

☐ Bone

▨ Cement

☐ Stem

Not to scale
All dimensions in mm
All moduli in GPa

FIGURE P 9.8 Cemented hip prosthesis, showing cross section at mid-diaphysis with dimensions and material properties. (D = outside diameter; E = Young's modulus; subscripts b, c, and s refer to the bone, cement, and stem, respectively.)

points *a* (the femoral head center), *b* (the assumed single attachment point of the abductors), and *c* (the center of the cross section at X–X) are (26.5, 311), (95.9, 301), and (71.4, 200), respectively.

9.9   For the model shown in Figure P 9.8, and assuming composite beam behavior, plot a graph of the maximum bending tensile stress in the stem at section X–X as a function of the stem diameter for variations in the stem diameter from 6 to 15 mm. On the same graph, plot curves for periosteal bone diameters of 25, 30, and 35 mm, both for Ti alloy ($E_s = 110$ GPa) and CoCr ($E_s = 200$ GPa) stems.

9.10   You are a prosthesis designer working in an orthopaedic section of a hospital, and a surgeon has asked you to identify, for a specific patient (i.e., the bone dimensions and material properties are fixed), whether there are any stem sizes that should *not* be used (within the feasible range of stem sizes that do not require reaming of the diaphysis), either with Ti alloy or CoCr stems. Provide an answer based in part on the results from the following analysis:

Assuming composite beam behavior, derive an expression for the maximum value of the (maximum tensile bending) stress in a cemented stem as a function of the stem diameter. From this expression, identify the stem diameter that results in maximum stem stresses for Ti alloy and CoCr stems (for the bone size, bone material properties, and loading conditions, as shown in Figure P 9.8).

9.11   The risk of fatigue fracture of a prosthesis can be expressed as the ratio of the maximum tensile stress in the prosthesis to its fatigue strength. Assume that the maximum tensile stress can be calculated from composite beam theory, and (worst case scenario) that the loading in the mid-diaphysis is relatively strenuous ($M = 150$ N-m). For a well fit (i.e., stem diameter in the mid-diaphysis equals the bone endosteal diameter) sintered device with a fatigue strength of 300 MPa,

(a)   plot graphs of critical bone size (i.e., the periosteal bone diameter at which the risk of fatigue fracture is unity for a given stem size) versus stem diameter (independent variable, range 10–18 mm) for Ti alloy and cast CoCr stem materials (assume that the endurance limits of these sintered devices are the same);

(b)   from these graphs, identify the bone diameter for each of the preceding stem materials, for which there

should never be a risk of fatigue fracture of the stem under the given loading conditions.

(c)   How could this information be useful in a clinical setting?

9.12   Bone density in the mid-diaphysis decreases with implantation of a hip prosthesis, particularly for a cementless design. One could argue therefore that it might be beneficial to have a design with a biomechanical behavior which is relatively insensitive to reductions in bone density—at least in that situation, what you have in the short term is a good indication of what you will have later in the long term.

(a)   Assuming composite beam behavior for a well fit cementless hip prosthesis, derive an equation that can be used to quantify the sensitivity S of stem bending stresses σ_{stem} to changes in bone modulus E_{bone}, where

$$S = \frac{d\sigma_{stem}}{dE_{bone}}$$

(b)   According to your equation, would stem stresses change more with a unit reduction in bone modulus for

 (i)   a Ti alloy or CoCr prosthesis?
 (ii)   a large or small diameter prosthesis?
(iii)   a large or small diameter bone?
 (iv)   a cemented or cementless prosthesis?

(c)   What design parameter could be used to minimize this sensitivity?

9.13   The total hip replacement femoral component shown in Figure P 9.13 is fixed with bone cement. The cement mantle is 3 mm thick. Determine how much the bending and axial stresses are reduced *at midstem* by the implant.

Assume the following in your analysis:

The load is parallel to the stem, as shown.

All cross sections are circular. The original bone inner diameter was 18 mm.

The bone modulus of elasticity is 18,000 MPa, the implant modulus is 110,000 MPa, and the cement modulus is 3000 MPa.

9.14   There is considerable uncertainty about the *in vivo* loads that act across joint replacement implants. As a result, several different loads have been used to test implant designs. Assuming the geometry of the

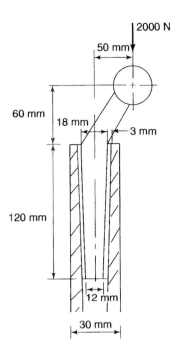

FIGURE P 9.13

implant and bone in the preceding problem, discuss the effects of the two loading conditions on stresses in the implant, cement, and bone. (AX, axial load, ML, medial to lateral load, AP, anterior to posterior load)

Case 1	Case 2
$AX = 1920$ N	$AX = 1920$ N
$ML = 420$ N	$ML = 0$
$AP = 400$ N	$AP = 400$ N

9.15   One of the problems with implants, including total joint replacements and internal fracture fixation devices, is that they "stress shield" the bone. Some of the load that is normally transferred through the bone is taken by the implant, reducing the stresses for the bone. One proposed solution is the "isoelastic prosthesis," which attempts to match the bone stiffness with the prosthesis stiffness. For the construct shown in Figure P 9.13, the bending stiffness of the implant matches the bone stiffness—that is, $E_P I_P = E_B I_B$—at the top of the stem.

(a)   How much is the maximum bending stress reduced at the top of the stem for this "isoelastic" design?

(b)   How do the bending stiffnesses of the implant and bone compare at the bottom of the stem?

(c)   How does the axial stiffness (stiffness due to pure axial loads) of the implant and bone compare at the top of the stem?

Assume that all cross sections are circular. Assume a modulus of 15,000 MPa for the bone.

CHAPTER 10

Total Knee Replacements

The knee joint is one of many joints in the body that is constrained primarily by the soft tissues surrounding the joint. Two obvious exceptions in the appendicular skeleton are the hip joint and the ulnar–humeral joint, where the bony anatomy provides the primary kinematic constraint. The hip joint is a ball and socket joint; the joint between the ulna and the humerus is a loose hinge. When we discussed the hip joint in Chapter 9, we could ignore the soft tissue structures around the joint, but in the knee, these structures must be taken into account. Therefore, we must first take a more detailed look at the anatomy of the joint before we can discuss joint function.

The knee is a tricompartmental joint consisting of the femur, tibia, and patella (Figure 1.11 and Figure 10.1). The femoral condyles contact the tibial plateaus through the medial and lateral menisci (MM and LM) that serve to make the joint more conforming. The patella, a sesamoid bone, articulates with the femur in the trochlear groove (patellar surface of femur in Figure 1.11). Its motion is guided partly by the geometry of the groove and partly by the action of the quadriceps muscle group.

The femoral–tibial joint is held together by the cruciate ligaments (ACL and PCL) and collateral ligaments (MCL and LCL) and by the joint capsule. The cruciate and collateral ligaments are the primary passive stabilizers of the joint. The cruciate ligaments provide anterior–posterior constraint; the collateral ligaments provide varus–valgus constraint in the frontal plane.

The articulating surfaces of the condyles, plateaus, patella, and trochlear groove are covered with articular cartilage, which may be idealized as a biphasic material consisting of a viscoelastic, porous solid, plus a fluid. This combination produces superb joint lubrication when the articular cartilage is healthy. The joint can become painful if trauma or disease damages the articular cartilage. Damage to cartilage may also be secondary to injuries to other joint structures, such as ligaments or menisci, that cause a change in the normal kinematics of the knee joint.

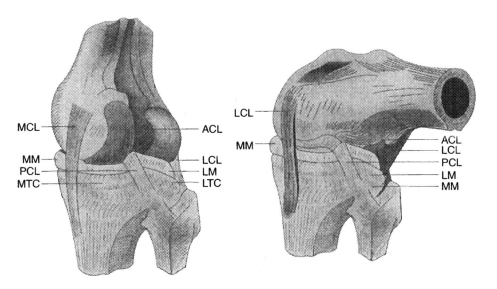

FIGURE 10.1 Knee anatomy showing the major soft tissue structures. (From Kapandji, *The Physiology of the Joints*, vol.2. Churchill Livingstone, New York, 1987.)

10.1 | Knee Function

Kinematics

The femoral–tibial joint has six degrees of freedom—three rotations and three translations. The primary motion, of course, is flexion and extension. Normal knee flexion ranges from zero degrees (full extension) to 160 degrees in a fully flexed knee. A small amount of hyperextension, on the order of 3–5 degrees, is also possible.

Rotation of the femur about the longitudinal tibial axis also occurs. This is greatest when the knee is flexed and least when the knee is in full extension. A small varus–valgus rotation of the femur with respect to the tibia can occur to provide unequal loading of the tibial plateaus without liftoff. The articular cartilage is compressed on one plateau and relaxed on the other. The largest varus–valgus rotations can result in liftoff of one condyle from the plateau when the loads on the lower extremity produce large varus–valgus moments. Varus–valgus motion can be constrained by the collateral ligaments, by co-contraction of the quadriceps and hamstrings muscle groups, or by some combination of the two.

The anterior–posterior translations are constrained by the cruciate ligaments and the geometry of the condyles, plateaus, and menisci. The lateral–medial translations are small. The posterior cruciate ligament constrains the femur to move posteriorly with respect to the tibia during flexion. This posterior motion maintains or increases the moment arm of the quadriceps mechanism with respect to the contact points on the tibia and allows for a greater range of motion by minimizing the possibility of bony impingement and soft tissue entrapment behind the knee. During normal activities such as gait, the AP motion of the lateral condyle is greater than the motion of the medial condyle for activities that include rotation of the femur about the tibial axis.

FIGURE 10.2 Reduced force set at the knee in the sagittal plane due to a functional load on the foot at heel strike. (From Burstein, A.H., and Wright, T.M., "Biomechanics," in *Surgery of the Knee*, ed. Insall, J.N., et al. Churchill Living-stone, New York, 1993.)

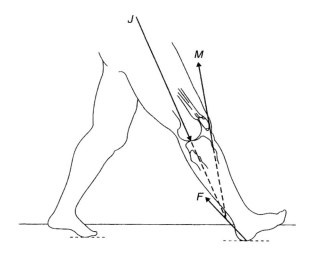

Injury or disease may result in the loss of ligament function. For example, if the anterior cruciate ligament is ruptured, anterior motion of the proximal tibia with respect to the femur will increase. Similarly, if posterior cruciate function is lost, the posterior motion of the proximal tibia with respect to the femur will be increased, which will reduce the quadriceps moment arm and decrease the range of motion of the knee in flexion. As will be discussed in more detail subsequently, the design goals for knee replacements depend upon the amount of constraint available from soft tissue structures of the knee, which can vary from patient to patient.

Loads and Moments

Motion analysis has been used to determine the resultant forces and moments acting across the knee joint (Figure 10.2). The quadriceps and hamstrings provide extension and flexion moments, respectively. The peak axial joint load, which approximates the contact force if soft tissue loading is negligible, has been determined to be three to four times bodyweight during normal gait. As a result, four times bodyweight is a commonly used value for the femoral–tibial contact force when designing total knee replacements.

EXAMPLE 10.1 Forces at the Knee Joint

Question What are the magnitudes of the joint force J and the patellar ligament force M for the situation shown in Figure 10.2? Assume that the force F of the floor on the foot is 1000 N.

Solution The simplest approach in this case is to simply create a vector diagram, as shown in Figure 10.3. The direction of the force of the foot on the floor is assumed to be measured by a force platform; the direction of the patellar ligament force can be estimated from the anatomy of the knee. Since the lower leg, the free-body diagram for this problem, is a three-force member if the weight of the leg is neglected, the direction of the joint force, J, is determined. A vector diagram can be drawn whose sides are parallel to the known force directions. The values of M and J can be scaled with respect to the value of F.

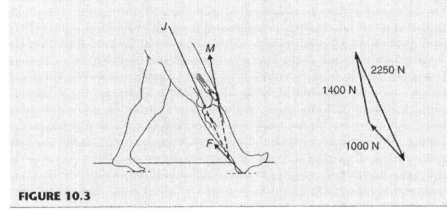

FIGURE 10.3

The muscle forces acting across the knee, the cruciate and collateral ligaments, and the menisci provide joint stability. As described in Chapter 2, the resultant forces and moments required for dynamic and quasi-static equilibrium can be determined from overall joint behavior—for example, flexion and extension of the knee joint. There are, however, other relative motions that can occur between the distal femur and the proximal tibia (A–P and L–M sliding and tilting of the femur with respect to the tibia). If the knee is not in stable equilibrium, small changes in the force environment may lead to relative large motions between the contacting surfaces. People with ruptured ligaments sense this as the "knee giving way" under certain loading conditions. The joint is stable when small changes in force result in only small changes in relative motion.

An interesting case in point, and one of importance to the designers of total knee prostheses, is the stable equilibrium of the knee joint under varus or valgus loading. During normal gait, a medially directed force acts on the foot (Figure 10.4). This force is not large, but has a large moment arm, which produces a substantial varus moment at the knee. Larger medially directed forces might occur in traumatic situations. The moment necessary for varus–valgus stability is provided by redistribution of the joint force between the medial and lateral compartments, the collateral and cruciate ligaments, and the co-contraction of the quadriceps and hamstrings muscles. Note that if the moment is too large to be developed by compression of one compartment and relaxation of the other, one of the collateral ligaments will be loaded, possibly in combination with co-contraction of the hamstrings and quadriceps groups.

The patellar–femoral loads are also large. It can be shown, through relatively simple two-dimensional analyses, that the sagittal plane component of the resultant of the patellar–femoral force and the tibial–femoral force, R, acts approximately along the femur (Figure 10.5).

FIGURE 10.4 A lateral to medial force acts on the foot during normal gait and produces a varus moment at the knee joint that leads to unequal forces in the lateral and medial tibial plateaus. (From Burstein, A.H., and Wright, T.M., "Biomechanics," in *Surgery of the Knee*, ed. Insall, J.N., et al. Churchill Living-stone, New York, 1993.)

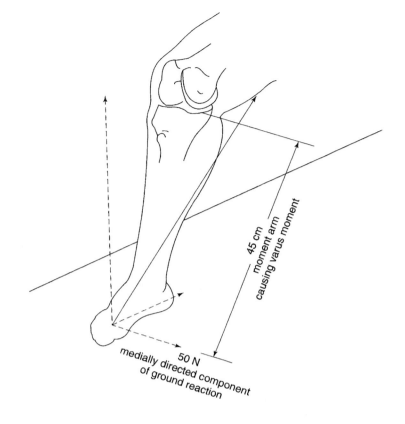

FIGURE 10.5 The resultant force of the patellar– femoral force and the tibial– femoral force acts along the femur. The case shown is for rising out of a chair. (From Dawson, J.E., "Effects of Loading and Fixation on Interface Stresses and Load Transfer in Total Joint Arthroplasties," PhD diss., Cornell University, 1991.)

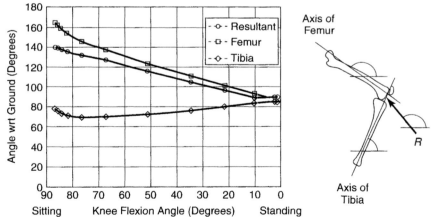

10.2 | Knee Structure

Bony Architecture

Like other long bones, the distal end of the femur and the proximal end of the tibia consist primarily of cancellous bone covered by a thin shell of bone that gets thicker toward the central shaft. The load transfer from the joint surfaces to the cortical

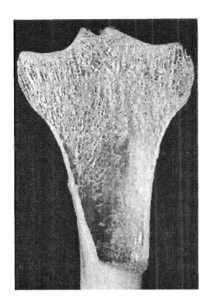

FIGURE 10.6 Cross-sectional view of the proximal tibia. Regions of dense cancellous bone transfer the condylar forces distally to the cortical shell. The cancellous bone between these two regions is much less dense and of little consequence structurally.

bone in the proximal tibia has been studied the most, because tibial loosening of prosthetic components has been a greater problem than femoral loosening.

Figure 10.6 shows a coronal slice of the proximal tibia. The cancellous bone texture is oriented in the proximal–distal direction. The densest (stiffest) cancellous bone is located at the joint surfaces; the density decreases from proximal to distal. Near the joint surface, the outer shell of the bone is very thin and has properties similar to cancellous bone tissue. The outer shell thickens toward the diaphysis, where it is fully dense cortical bone.

Load Transfer from the Articulating Surface to the Cortical Bone

The morphology of the proximal tibia provides insight as to how joint loads are transmitted to the tibial shaft. Most proximally, the load is carried entirely by the cancellous bone because the outer shell is thin, has properties similar to cancellous bone, and consequently, low structural stiffness. As mentioned previously, in parallel structures the stiffest component (in this case, the proximal cancellous bone) carries the greatest portion of the load. From proximal to distal, the cancellous bone becomes less dense (less stiff) and the outer shell becomes thicker (stiffer). Consequently, the amount of load carried by the cancellous bone decreases from proximal to distal; and the amount carried by the outer shell increases to the point where there is no more cancellous bone, and the shell (diaphysis) carries the entire load (Figure 10.6).

10.3 | Knee Replacements

The goal is to create a bone-implant system that provides normal function for the life of the patient. This involves design of the prosthetic components and the surgical procedures necessary to implant the devices. In knee joints, the problem of providing normal function is somewhat more complex than in hips, because soft tissues provide most of the kinematic constraint. The prosthetic components must provide adequate range of motion and transmit normal joint loads. Furthermore, the components must work in concert with existing soft tissue structures—ligaments, capsule, and muscles. In general, if normal function is to be maintained, the components must provide substitute function for the ligaments that are lost. In addition, the forces acting across the joint will be most nearly normal if the muscle resting length and excursions are the same as those for the normal anatomy.

Design for fixation, on the other hand, is somewhat simpler than for hip joints, because the typical components are surface replacements. As a result, the bone tissue in the proximal tibia and distal femur are loaded by the prosthetic components, similar to the way it is loaded in the normal joint. The most vulnerable bone is the cancellous bone in the proximal tibia. Another structural concern is the damage that can occur to the articulating surfaces of the polyethylene component. The contact surfaces are generally nonconforming. High stresses may cause failure on a micro or macro scale, and the debris generated may lead to increased risk of late loosening.

Types of Replacements

All knee designs are total joint replacements, in the sense that both contacting surfaces are replaced. There are several ways to categorize these designs. Most designs are tricompartmental. That is, the surfaces of the tibia, femur, and patella are all replaced. Here, we will refer to these designs as bicondylar, with the understanding that the inferior surface of the patella is almost always replaced as well. Unicondylar designs are sometimes used instead of bicondylar designs when only one compartment of the joint (lateral or medial) is affected. In this approach, only surfaces of the femoral condyle and the tibial plateau in the affected compartment are replaced. The function of the unicondylar joint depends upon having normal cruciate and collateral ligaments. Unicondylar replacements present special design challenges in order to provide both function and fixation. We will not address these issues specifically; the methods for studying fixation and contact stresses in bicondylar designs are directly applicable to the analysis and design of unicondylar devices, as well.

Bicondylar designs may be classified according to the amount of constraint the components provide. For example, if both the cruciate and collateral ligaments are missing or insufficient, the components must provide stability in both the sagittal and coronal planes. If only the cruciate ligaments are lost and the collateral ligaments are healthy, then the components need only to provide substitute cruciate ligament function.

Even if all the ligaments are healthy, it may be advantageous to sacrifice the cruciate ligaments and to provide their function through features of the device. This approach was originally introduced to increase the amount of exposure available to the surgeon to make it easier to properly prepare the fixation surfaces. The first designs of this type became known as total condylar designs. The femoral components had sagittal plane geometry that approximated the shape of the natural condyles; the tibial plateaus were dished to provide constraint in the anterior–posterior directions. The constraint provided by these designs was generally sufficient to provide substitute anterior cruciate ligament function, but was not adequate for posterior cruciate function. As a result, posterior cruciate ligament substituting designs were introduced, which have a spine or post on the tibial component and a cam in the femoral component, to provide substitute posterior cruciate function (Figure 10.7).

The alternative to a posterior cruciate ligament substituting design is a posterior cruciate ligament retaining design. This approach sacrifices the anterior cruciate ligament, but retains the posterior cruciate ligament. The basic idea behind this concept is to allow normal anatomical structures to provide the constraint whenever possible. The design of these devices must accommodate the posterior cruciate ligament both structurally and kinematically. The tibial component must have a posterior notch so that the ligament will not impinge on the component, and the articulating surfaces must be shaped and positioned to avoid overconstraint, while still providing normal relative motion.

The choice between posterior cruciate ligament retaining and substituting designs has been controversial. Through the 1990s, more posterior cruciate ligament retaining designs were used than substituting designs, but since then there has been a trend toward substituting designs because of the more consistent performance these designs produce.

The most constrained devices that have been used for knee replacement are single axis hinges. These were introduced as salvage devices for knees with completely compromised ligament function. Single axis devices were unsuccessful for two reasons. First, the axis of rotation of the knee moves with respect to the tibia during flexion and cannot be replaced by a fixed axis if the soft tissue structures are to function normally. Second, the fixed axis causes all joint loads to be transmitted through the prosthesis and eliminates load sharing between the prosthesis and soft tissues. As a result, the fixation interfaces are put at risk, and the incidence of loosening is greatly increased if these devices are used. Consequently, when hinges are used for salvage procedures, contemporary designs incorporate some joint laxity to lessen the risk of loosening.

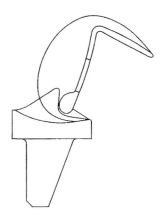

FIGURE 10.7 Total condylar with substitute posterior cruciate function. When the cam contacts the post the contact point between the femoral and tibial components moves posteriorly.

Function

As we have seen already, the relative motion and the joint loads are coupled for both normal and artificial skeletal joints. Changing one will inevitably change the other. The relative motion of the joint components is, therefore, controlled by the loads acting across the joint, by the geometry of the articulating surfaces, and by the soft tissues around the joint.

The geometry of knee joints varies widely from design to design. Some have symmetric femoral and tibial components, so they can be used for both left and right knees (Figure 10.8). Some are unsymmetrical to better approximate the normal geometry, with the underlying assumption that the kinematics will be more like normal motion if the artificial joint geometry mimics that of the natural knee

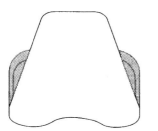
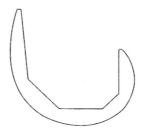

FIGURE 10.8 A double radius condylar knee. In this case, the two radii are equal, and the knee is symmetric. Contact occurs between toroidal surfaces.

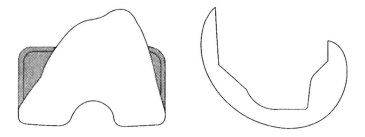

FIGURE 10.9 A single radius condylar knee. Both condylar surfaces are described by a single radius in the lateral–medial plane to increase conformity and allow for small misalignments.

(Figure 10.9). Unsymmetrical knees require larger operating room inventories, because both right and left knees must be available.

In posterior cruciate ligament substituting designs, the tibial surfaces are generally dished. In general, the tibial surfaces of posterior cruciate ligament retaining knees have been made flatter than those for posterior cruciate ligament substituting knees to avoid overconstraint. This results in less conforming contact, which, as we will see later, increases the risk of surface damage. Dished articulating surfaces are also used in some posterior cruciate ligament retaining designs. These provide more conforming contact to reduce contact stresses and will not overconstrain knee motion if the sulcus (low point) of the surface and the joint line are properly positioned.

We will consider two types of contacting surfaces that have been used successfully. For the first, the surfaces of the femoral and tibial components are both toroidal (Figure 10.8). For the second, the geometry is more complex. The lateral–medial geometry of the femoral and tibial articulating surfaces is highly conforming (Figure 10.9); both plateaus are described by a single lateral–medial radius.

The anterior–posterior geometry of both of these designs approximates the geometry of the normal condyles. Consequently, both designs can provide nearly normal knee flexion. Furthermore, either design concept can accommodate posterior cruciate ligament retaining or posterior cruciate ligament substituting features. Both require sacrifice of the ACL and provide ACL substitute function through upwardly curving posterior tibial contact surfaces.

These two design concepts deal with one of the most important design requirements in different ways. As has been described previously, even during normal gait there are varus–valgus moments at the knee that tend to cause small angular displacements in a frontal plane. Because the contacting components in an artificial knee joint are much stiffer than the articular cartilage in a normal knee, liftoff may occur for smaller varus or valgus moments. If the articulating surfaces are flat, extreme edge loading can occur, which generally increases the risk of bone failure beneath the prosthesis and surface damage to the polyethylene. If liftoff occurs in a toroidal bicondylar knee, edge loading is limited, because the load will be applied through the center of the contacting tibial plateau. The single radius knee allows some lateral–medial angulation before liftoff can occur, which increases the moment required for liftoff. With proper design, extreme edge loading can also be avoided, even if liftoff occurs.

Structure

Loads on the femoral and tibial components occur at points of contact—between the patella and femur, and between the tibia and femur. As seen in Figure 10.5, the resultant force acting on the femoral component lies approximately along the femoral axis. As a result, the resultant force moves little with respect to the femoral component. It is essentially a varying compressive force. On the other hand, the force on the tibia moves with respect to the tibial plateau during flexion–extension. Interestingly, the incidence of loosening has been much greater for tibial components than for femoral components. Consequently, we will concentrate on femoral–tibial contact, which involves contact between the condyles and plateaus, and for posterior cruciate ligament substituting devices, contact between a cam in the femoral component and a spine on the tibial component.

Condyle–plateau contact occurs between a convex metal component and a concave polyethylene component for both design concepts. Contact between the femoral components and the patellar component or upper constraint spine may involve contact where both the metal and polyethylene surfaces are convex. We will have more to say about contact and the stresses they produce in the polyethylene in later sections. The magnitudes of these forces can be approximated from quasi-static analysis of the lower extremity during functions such as normal gait, rising from a chair, or stair ascent or descent.

There are three structural considerations—component failure, fixation, and surface damage. Surface damage will be discussed in Chapter 11. Failures of femoral and tibial components are rare. Component failure can occur if proper attention is not paid to design. For example, the relatively thin metal trays for posterior cruciate ligament retaining tibial components failed due to combinations of tray design and material properties. Some porous coated trays for bone ingrowth fixation were particularly susceptible, because the process used to apply the porous coating resulted in reduced fatigue strength of the metal substrate (CoCr) or stress concentrations due to notch sensitivity (Ti alloy). In addition, high stresses could occur at the corner of the posterior cruciate ligament notch and near the junction of the tray and fixation pegs. The stresses were worst when these two regions coincided.

But on the tibial side, the most common source of failure of the joint replacement is by crushing the cancellous bone under the tray. When the proximal tibia is resected, the stiffest and strongest subchondral cancellous bone is removed. Note that the strains will be larger for the same stress and the risk of failure will be increased. The remaining cancellous bone must carry the compressive loads and transmit them to the cortical shell below the joint line. At this level of the tibia, the endosteal bony shell is thin and its properties are closer to those of cancellous than cortical bone. Therefore, as in the normal proximal tibia near the joint line, the cancellous bone carries the lion's share of the load. The endosteal shell carries very little, because, at this level, its structural rigidity is small with respect to that of the cancellous bone. One conclusion is that the amount of bone that is resected should be minimized so that the stiffest and strongest bone is retained.

The tibial component of an early knee design incorporated a semicircular disc imbedded in each condyle in contact with a short beam supported by cancellous bone. These did not work well, because the cancellous bone was not able to support the loads and because of the surgical challenges to get four individual components aligned properly. Furthermore, the patella was not replaced. From these early designs, tibial components have evolved to include a tray that covers the proximal tibia with either a central large fixation peg or smaller fixation pegs located beneath the lateral and medial plateaus. The components may be made entirely of polyethylene or may consist of a polyethylene insert supported by a metal tray with a metal fixation peg (or pegs). The tibial component is often attached to the bone with bone cement (PMMA). Cementless fixation can be accomplished with the use of porous coatings on the pegs and on the inferior surface of the metal tray. In some of these metal-backed designs, the initial stability of the trays has been enhanced with screws that fasten the tray to the bone.

Bone Loading by BOEF   We can consider the tibial component, in general, to be a plate supported by an elastic foundation of cancellous bone. Overall, the stiffness of the plate depends upon its geometry, the fixation peg configuration, and whether or not it is metal backed. Furthermore, the bending structural rigidity varies with position in the plate. For these reasons, and the fact that cancellous bone properties vary from point to point in the proximal tibia, finite element analysis must be used to understand the mechanics of this bone-implant system in detail. We can, however, get important insights into the interactions between the implant and the bone by using beam on elastic foundation analysis.

Figure 10.10 shows an idealization of the proximal tibia with prosthesis. The dashed lines show an anterior–posterior slice. A similar slice could be used in a lateral–medial direction. We can think of these slices as beams supported by an elastic foundation of cancellous bone, to examine the general behavior of the tibial component under load. If both plateaus are loaded, the BOEF model for the lateral–medial direction will have two loads, one for each condyle. If liftoff occurs, only one plateau is loaded and the BOEF configuration will be like that shown in Figure 10.11, which also applies for a BOEF model in the anterior–posterior direction. The load moves with respect to the beam in the anterior–posterior direction because the contact point between the femoral and tibial components moves during normal activities, such as gait and stair ascent or descent. Therefore, we will want to investigate a variety of loading positions to determine the effects of loading on the bone (the elastic foundation).

We will first consider the case of a beam with a central load (Figure 10.12). This is an idealization of an anterior–posterior slice of a tibial tray, when the contact point between the femur and the tibia is in the middle of the articular surface. In beam on elastic foundation theory, the amount of deformation is determined by the

FIGURE 10.10 The tibial plateau is a variable stiffness plate supported by an elastic foundation. Basic behavior can be understood by considering a slice of the plateau as a beam on an elastic foundation.

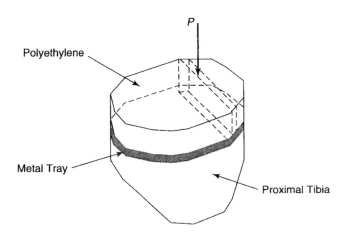

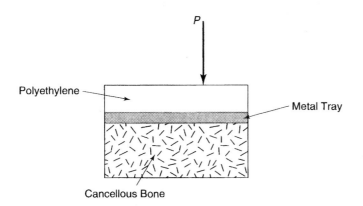

FIGURE 10.11 A BOEF idealization of a metal-backed tibial component.

load P, the bending rigidity EI of the beam, and the stiffness k of the foundation. The loading on the foundation is given by

$$q(x) = kv(x)$$

where $v(x)$ is the displacement of the beam at x and $q(x)$ is the load per unit length on the foundation at x. In other words, the force per unit length of the beam on the foundation is directly proportional to the displacement of the beam at that point. The deflection of the beam varies along its length, with greatest displacement being generally in the region of the load, as we would expect (Figure 10.12). For the case shown here, where the beam is loaded at its center, the maximum deflection occurs directly beneath the load. In Figure 10.13, the foundation modulus is constant, but the load is applied at three positions along the beam. The maximum deflection occurs near the load, but not necessarily immediately beneath the load. In these analyses, we have assumed that the beam is bonded to the foundation. The upward

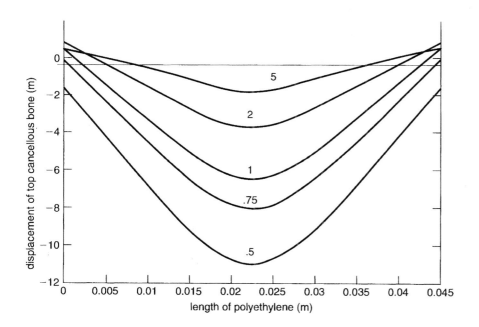

FIGURE 10.12 Deflection of a centrally loaded beam for different foundation stiffness, k. As k decreases, the maximum deflection increases.

FIGURE 10.13 Deflection of a beam loaded at .2L, .3L, and .5L. The greatest deformation is near where the load is applied; the greatest liftoff occurs away from the load. Displacement is in units of 10^{-5} m.

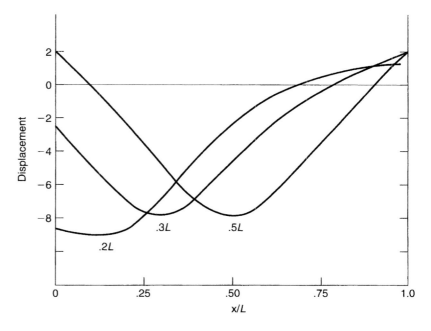

displacement indicates that there is tensile force applied to the foundation near the ends of the beam.

Figure 10.14 provides an interesting way of looking at the deformation of the beam. The ratio of end to center deflection is plotted against the stiffness parameter, λL, for the beam–foundation combination. As shown in Section 6.1,

$$\lambda = \sqrt[4]{k/4EI}$$

For small values of λL, the deformation ratio is one; the end deflection is the same as the center deflection, and the beam displaces into the foundation as if it were a rigid body. For values greater than $\lambda L \cong 3$, the deflection ratio is small—the end deflection is small with respect to the displacement at the center. When the ratio is positive, the force of the beam on the foundation is compressive along the entire length of the beam. When the ratio is negative, the beam is lifting off at the ends. In either case, for values of $\lambda L > 3$, the beam behaves like a flexible

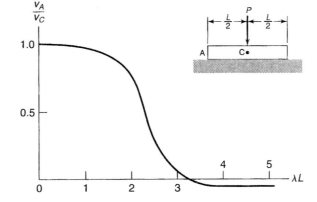

FIGURE 10.14 The ratio of end deflection to center deflection for a centrally loaded beam on an elastic foundation.

beam, and for values of $\lambda L < 1$, the beam behaves like a rigid beam. Note that the beam will behave more rigidly if EI is increased; if k, the foundation stiffness, is decreased; and if L, the length of the beam, is decreased. Thus, the stiffness of the structure is affected not only by the material properties of the beam and the bone, but by the cross-sectional geometry and the length of the beam as well.

For a rigid beam, the foundation displaces uniformly, and consequently, the loading on the foundation is distributed uniformly when the force on the beam is at the center. However, if the force is not centered, the beam will tilt, and the force on the foundation will be distributed nonuniformly, as shown in Figure 10.13. Notice that the farther the load is off center, the greater the compressive loading at the loaded end will be. However, the eccentric loading does not necessarily result in greater tensile loading away from the load (Figure 10.13).

These results provide several important insights into the fixation of tibial components. First, if a component is loaded toward the edge, the underlying cancellous bone beneath the load may be at risk. Second, edge loading increases the possibility of liftoff away from the load. If the implant–bone interface fails in tension, the compressive stresses on the bone will increase. Finally, the smallest maximum compressive stress occurs for rigid beam behavior with a centered load, because the stresses on the supporting cancellous bone are uniformly distributed. If, however, the rigid beam is subjected to off-center forces, the beam will tilt, and both compressive and tensile stresses at the beam–foundation interface will increase. These effects are moderated somewhat if the beam behaves more flexibly.

Bone Loading by Finite Element Analysis   To get more detail about the way contact loads are transferred through the tibial component to the underlying cancellous bone, finite element methods must be used. Figure 10.15 shows three designs of a posterior cruciate substituting tibial component; Figure 10.16 shows a relatively simple finite element model of the proximal tibia with prosthesis. In the finite element model, the cortical bone is represented by shell elements that increase in thickness from proximal to distal. The cement around the fixation peg and under the tray is also represented by shell elements. The cancellous bone and the implant are modeled with brick elements. The investigators knew from clinical experience that knee

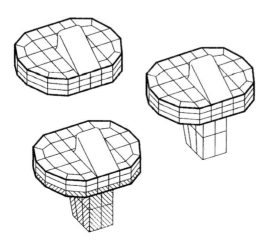

FIGURE 10.15 Three design configurations of standard tibial components: a polyethylene tibial component without a peg (upper model); a polyethylene tibial component with a polyethylene peg (middle model); a polyethylene tibial component with a metal tray and a metal peg (lower model). The total thickness of the plateau is the same for all three models, and the dimensions of the peg on the lower two models are the same. From Bartel, D.L., Burstein, A.H., Santavicca, E.A., and Insall, J.N. (1982). "Performance of the Tibial Component in Total Knee Replacement," *J Bone Jt Surg Am* 64:1026–1033.

FIGURE 10.16 Cross section of finite element model. The cortical shell and the cement layer are represented by shell elements. The cancellous bone modulus decreases from layer A to D (see Table 10.1).

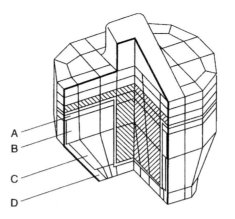

replacements of this type failed by crushing of the cancellous bone when the component was subjected to extreme edge loading. It is also known from stress analyses that the calculated interface stresses typically are within the strength of the materials, except for the cancellous bone (Figure 10.17).

Since the stresses in the cement and cortical bone were not of interest, these structures were not modeled in detail with brick elements. To do so would have required a considerably more complex finite element model. The decreasing stiffness of cancellous bone away from the joint line was included by choosing a different elastic modulus for each layer of cancellous bone, as shown in Figure 10.16 and Table 10.1. The spine shown in Figure 10.16 was not explicitly modeled. Instead, the resultant force and moment of the spine acting on the tray were applied to the upper surface of the constant thickness tray (Figure 10.18).

A wide range of loading conditions can occur during normal daily activities. In the best case, the femoral–tibial loading will be equally distributed between the two plateaus. Because of the built-in laxity of the joint, these loads can occur at different AP positions (Figure 10.18). But, as was discussed previously, normal

FIGURE 10.17 The loading range at tibia–tray interface is less than the strength range, except for cancellous bone in compression. Therefore, the cancellous bone is at the greatest risk for failure. (From Burstein, A.H., and Wright, T.M., *Fundamentals of Orthopaedic Biomechanics.* Williams & Wilkins, Baltimore, 1994.)

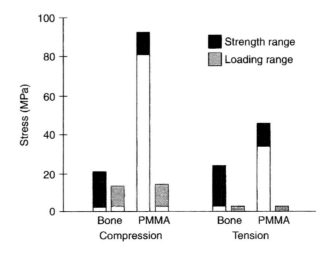

TABLE 10.1

Material Properties for the Model Shown in Figure 10.17

	Elastic Modulus (GPa)	Strength (MPa)
Metal (CoCr)	248	
Cortical Bone	17.2	
UHMWPE	1.72	
Cancellous Bone		
Layer A	.609	18.3
Layer B	.427	14.5
Layer C	.198	8.66
Layer D	.0609	3.95

Performance of the Tibial Component in Total Knee Replacement. *J Bone Jt Surg Am* 64:1026–1033.

Source: Bartel, D.L., Burstein, A.H., Santaricca, E.A., and Insall, J.N. (1982).

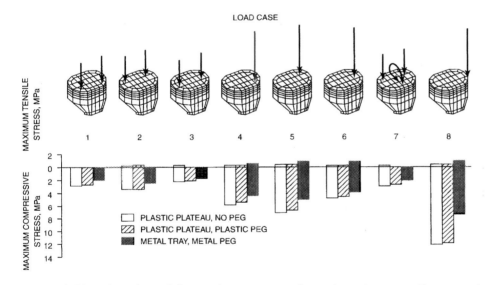

FIGURE 10.18 The values of the maximum compressive and maximum tensile stresses in the cancellous bone in the layer immediately beneath the plateau are shown in the bar graph. The maximum compressive stress always occurred in the cancellous bone near the location of the applied load. The maximum tensile stress always occurred in the cancellous bone at a location away from the applied load. The lengths of the vertical arrows indicate the magnitudes of the loads applied to the plateau. The total vertical load in each case was three times body weight (2280 newtons). In Case 7, the effect of loading the intercondylar spine is modeled by applying an equivalent shear and moment to the elements in the upper surface of the plastic component below the spine. (From Bartel, D.L., Burstein, A.H., Santavicca, E.A., and Insall, J.N. (1982). "Performance of the Tibial Component in Total Knee Replacement," *J Bone Jt Surg Am* 64:1026–1033.)

functional loads on the foot exist that cause the loads on the plateaus to be unevenly distributed. Therefore, the extreme case loading is for the entire load to be on one plateau. The worst case is loading on a single plateau applied in an extreme position (Figure 10.18).

EXAMPLE 10.2 Single and Double Plateau Loading

Question From the data provided in Figure 10.18, determine the increase in compressive cancellous bone stress when the load is applied to one plateau, instead of two. Is the difference a function of design? Briefly explain why the difference occurs.

Solution The maximum compressive stress when the load is applied to one plateau (Cases 4–6) is about twice the stress when the load is divided equally between both plateaus (Cases 1–3). This is true for all designs. The overall behavior of the tibial component under load can be approximated as a beam on an elastic foundation. The equation for the displacement of a finite beam on an elastic foundation given in Section 6.1 shows that the displacement is directly proportional to load. Since the stress of the beam on the foundation is proportional to the displacement, if the load is doubled, the stress will be doubled.

There are several interesting design questions that can be addressed with this model. First, what is the effect of having a metal backing and metal peg on the stresses in the cancellous bone? Second, what role does the peg play in an all-polyethylene component? Finally, does contact between the femoral component and constraint spine increase the risk of loosening by increasing the stresses on the cancellous bone?

The stresses shown in Figure 10.18 are the normal stresses acting on the cancellous bone in the longitudinal direction. The elastic modulus of the cancellous bone immediately beneath the tray is 609 MPa, which corresponds to a compressive strength of 18.3 MPa. For the load in the worst-case position (Case 8), the stresses exceed the strength of cancellous bone for all tray designs. The stresses are lowest, however, when the component is metal backed. This is generally true for all the loading cases shown, but the advantage of metal backing is greatest for the single plateau loading and extreme cases.

EXAMPLE 10.3 Effect of Peg in All-Polyethylene Components

Question Figure 10.18 shows that the central fixation peg does little, if anything, to reduce the stresses on the cancellous bone. Why is this the case? Would you expect the results to be different if the central peg were removed in favor of two smaller pegs, one under each plateau?

Solution To transfer load through the central peg, the peg would have to be stiffly coupled to the cortical shell. In this model, it is not stiffly coupled, and its role in relieving stresses on the cancellous bone beneath the tray is moderate. The reduction in stress that does occur is probably due to the resistance the peg provides to overall tilting of the component. The central peg also provides some resistance to torsion. Smaller pegs beneath the plateaus would also resist torsion and provide the ability to carry tensile loads across the implant–bone interface.

The use of the upper constraint spine to provide posterior cruciate ligament substitution is no disadvantage with respect to cancellous bone stresses. The stresses are about the same as they are for the other double plateau loading cases. The tilting moment introduced by the anteriorly directed force on the spine is counteracted by the tilting moment introduced by posteriorly applied contact forces. This result is also consistent with clinical studies that show no increase in radiolucencies beneath the plateau when the posterior cruciate ligament substituting design was used instead of the posterior cruciate ligament sacrificing design.

There is another very important design consideration. The model used in this analysis assumes bonding between the component and the cancellous bone. Therefore, these results apply only to knee replacements that satisfy these conditions. In most of the cases shown, tensile stresses are present. These occur away from the load, as we would expect from BOEF theory. From BOEF considerations, we also know that if the component is not fixed to the bone, the compressive stresses on the bone increase. Therefore, stresses on the cancellous bone are minimized if the bone–implant interface can transfer tensile loading. In successful cemented designs, this is achieved by providing undercuts or other features that create mechanical interlock between the cement and the device. This interlock between bone and prosthesis can also be achieved in cementless designs if adequate bone ingrowth occurs.

The ultimate goal is not the design of the components, per se, but the design of the bone-implant system. The final step in creating this system is the implantation of the devices by the surgeon. The results shown in Figure 10.18 emphasize three important points. First, it is important to balance the knee so that single plateau loading is avoided. Second, it is important to use techniques and devices that maximize interlock between the device and the bone. Finally, devices and techniques must be chosen that avoid edge loading.

Before we leave this section, something should be said about the validation of the model used. Strictly speaking, we cannot validate the model; we cannot show that the stresses predicted actually occur in the cancellous bone *in vivo* in a particular patient. But we can (and must) demonstrate that the results are consistent with clinical observations, if we are to draw clinically applicable conclusions. This was true for the model just discussed. Clinical failures in the cancellous bone occurred where the model predicted failure, and the upper constraint spine was not a problem clinically, again consistent with the results of this model. In any case, the greatest value of finite element models is to make A–B comparisons between design and clinical alternatives, not to predict absolute values of stresses in specific *in vivo* situations.

Long-Term Clinical Evaluation

The proof of the pudding lies ultimately in how well particular devices work in patients in the long term. The most commonly used approach for evaluating total joint replacement surgery is survival analysis. The end point measure of performance is revision. Based on analyses of known survivors at a particular point in time, the probability of survival can be determined, while taking into account joint replacements that have been lost to follow-up (censured data). These procedures are extremely helpful for determining survival for various designs and even the success rates for particular surgeons. But they provide little, if any, information about the reason for failure. For example, a poor functional design could survive because it was not being used and therefore didn't fail. Consequently, it is difficult at best to use these studies to determine the relationships between design and failure.

The most useful technique for relating design to failure is retrieval analysis. Devices removed from patients during revision procedures are retrieved and examined to determine failure modes. This, along with patient information, material evaluation, and structural analyses, can be used to determine reasons for failure and is an important part of the process of defining design goals to improve performance.

10.4 | Summary

The knee is a six-degree-of-freedom joint that is constrained by the collateral and cruciate ligaments, by the menisci, and by other soft tissue structures around the joint. In knee replacements, the problem of providing normal function is somewhat more complex than in hips, because soft tissues provide most of the kinematic constraint. The prosthetic components must work in concert with existing ligaments and, if normal function is to be maintained, the components must provide substitute function for ligaments that have been compromised. It is particularly important to maintain the function provided by the posterior cruciate ligament. This can be done either by retaining the ligament or by substituting for it by using a cam and post arrangement.

Knee replacement components are surface replacements. Therefore, the bone tissue in the proximal tibia and distal femur is loaded by the prosthetic components, similar to the way it is loaded in the normal joint. The most vulnerable bone tissue after knee replacement is the cancellous bone in the proximal tibia, where the stiffest and strongest bone is removed when the tibial plateaus are replaced.

10.5 EXERCISES

10.1 What are the relative advantages and disadvantages of using a condylar design for a total knee prosthesis instead of a hinged design? When might a hinged design be justified?

10.2 Based on the behavior of a composite beam bending on an elastic foundation, sketch a graph of the interface normal stresses (perpendicular to the plane of the interface) against the mediolateral position (x axis) for the tibial component shown in Figure P 10.2 when loaded with a central compressive force P. Contrast curves for an all-plastic component, a metal-backed component, and an all-metal component. Describe and

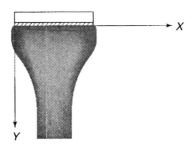

FIGURE P 10.2 Schematic of proximal tibia with a metal-backed tibial tray.

discuss the important characteristics of your graph in the context of design of total knee prostheses.

10.3 If the width (in the x direction) of the tibial component (in Figure P 10.2) is L, sketch typical interface stress distributions if P acts at $x = 0.75L$ ($x = 0$ on left-hand side, as shown). Contrast curves for an all-plastic component, a metal-backed component, and an all-metal component. Describe and discuss the important characteristics of your graph in the context of design of total knee prostheses.

10.4 A sectional view of a posterior cruciate substituting total knee replacement is shown in Figure P 10.4 along with the results from a finite element analysis. Successful designs must consider both functional and structural issues. Assume the tibial component has a metal tray and metal peg.

Contact between the upper constraint spine of the tibial component and the cam in the femoral component causes the tibial contact area on the articulating surface to move during knee flexion. What are the implications of this motion for the stresses associated with structural failure? Why?

10.4 In Figure P 10.4, the stresses on the cancellous bone are not changed much when the design is altered from an all-polyethylene component to one with a metal tray and peg. Use the concepts of beam on elastic foundation theory to explain why this is so.

10.5 The results shown in Figure P 10.4 can be used to argue that an all-polyethylene component may be used for clinical cases. On the basis of assumptions employed in the analysis, what conditions would have to be met for an all-polyethylene joint to function effectively?

10.6 On the basis of results of three-dimensional finite element stress analyses of the tibial component of a bicondylar knee prosthesis (Figure P 10.4),

(**a**) Discuss the advantages and disadvantages of metal backing from a stress perspective, considering a range of possible loading conditions.

(**b**) Explain what the main clinical advantage of using metal backing would be.

10.7 Using the data for the centrally loaded beam provided in Figure 10.13, plot the ratio of end to center displacement. Interpret your results in terms of Figure P 10.14. Is the beam on elastic foundation shown in Figure 10.13 behaving as a stiff or flexible structure? Why?

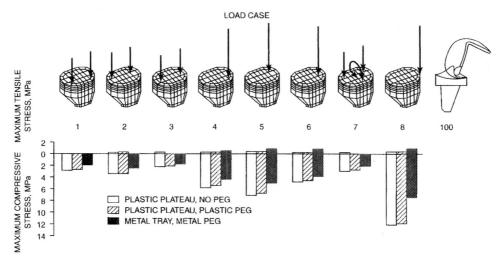

Eight cases representing different loading locations were investigated. The lengths of the vertical arrows indicate the magnitudes of the loads applied to the plateau. The total vertical load in each case was three times body weight (2280 newtons). The values of the maximum compressive and maximum tensile stresses in the cancellous bone in the layer immediately beneath the plateau are shown in the bar graph. The maximum compressive stress always occurred in the cancellous bone near the location of the applied load. The maximum tensile stress always occurred in the cancellous bone at a location away from the applied load. In Case 7, the effect of loads on the intercondylar spine is modeled by applying an equivalent shear and moment to the elements in the upper surface of the plastic component below the spine.

FIGURE P 10.4

10.8 A finite-length beam is supported by an elastic foundation. The 50-mm-long beam is made of polyethylene with modulus 1.0 GPa and has a cross section 10 mm high by 5 mm wide. It is supported by cancellous bone with modulus 800 MPa. Recall that $k \neq E$ for the foundation.

A 1000 N load is applied at the center of the beam. Using the equations in Section 6.1, determine the maximum stress in the beam and the loading on the foundation along the length of the beam.

10.9 Do Exercise 10.8 for cancellous bone of modulus 600 MPa.

10.10 Do Exercise 10.8 for the load applied at 12.5 mm from the left end of the beam.

10.11 Do Exercise 10.8 for cancellous bone of modulus 600 MPa and the load applied at 12.5 mm from the left end of the beam.

10.12 Do Exercise 10.8 for the case where the beam is a composite beam. The cross section comprises a 2-mm-thick layer of CoCr alloy next to the cancellous

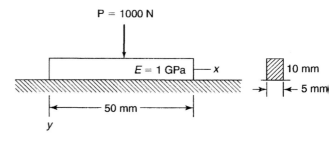

FIGURE P 10.8

bone with a polyethylene component bonded to the alloy. The cross section of the polyethylene is 5 mm × 8 mm. Determine the bending stress in the CoCr portion of the implant.

10.13 Do Exercise 10.9 for the case where the metal portion of cross section has a modulus $E = 3000$ MPa.

10.14 Do Exercise 10.9 for the case where the load is applied at 12.5 mm from the left end of the beam.

Articulating Surfaces

Total joint replacements have bearing surfaces that must transmit normal joint loads and motions. Low friction has been an important design objective for prosthetic joints for two reasons. First, if large shear forces due to friction are applied to the articulating surfaces, the risk of loosening may be increased. Second, the addition of frictional shear increases the stresses associated with surface damage due to contact, which can result in the release of wear debris to the surrounding tissue that also increases the risk of infection and loosening.

A number of material combinations have been tried since the earliest days of joint replacement surgery. Early on, metal on Teflon hip replacements were tried, but the Teflon cups degraded quickly and the arthroplasties failed, even though the combination provided a low-friction articulation. Metal on metal joints were also tried. The search for a low-friction articulation eventually led to bearing combinations of metal against polyethylene that were generally successful. Other material pairs are being developed and used—metal on polyurethane, ceramic on polyethylene, ceramic on ceramic, and metal on metal. All have potential advantages, but metal on polyethylene continues to be the most common bearing combination.

Most of the wear in metal–polyethylene joints occurs in the polyethylene component. Consequently, polyethylene wear has long been a concern at the articulating surfaces and, more recently, between polyethylene–metal interfaces in modular prostheses. In this chapter, we will focus on the articulating surfaces of polyethylene components. First, we will discuss briefly the role of debris in limiting the performance of joint replacements. Second, we will look at some general characteristics of the stresses resulting from contact between metal and polyethylene components. Finally, we will discuss the overall influence of design features on the contact stresses, because, in general, if the contact stresses are reduced, the specific stresses and stress combinations associated with surface damage will also be reduced.

11.1 | Damage Modes

Debris may be generated at both bearing surfaces during the normal functioning of a prosthetic joint, but the polyethylene component is the most abundant source of particles. Therefore, an important design goal is to minimize the amount of surface damage that occurs to the polyethylene articular surface during normal activities.

The biological reaction to debris is not just a question of biocompatibility. This phenomenon occurs for both metals and polymers that are biocompatible in bulk. A comprehensive discussion of biocompatibility is beyond the scope of this book. It is sufficient for our purposes to say simply that biocompatibility is a two-way street. First, the materials used must not harm the body, and second, the body must not harm the materials. Bulk polyethylene passes these criteria, but the biological response to very small debris particles of polyethylene is great and can ultimately lead to loosening of the implant.

In small amounts, particles can be eliminated through the perivascular lymph spaces. But when this transport system is insufficient to handle the volume, the biological response includes the release of agents that attack bone where it is most vulnerable—at the bone–implant interface. For example, in total hip replacements, osteolysis can occur around both the femoral and acetabular components. A joint replacement may function well for many years before sufficient debris has accumulated to initiate an osteolytic response.

The incidence of osteolysis is greatest in total hip replacements, but it also occurs in total knee replacements. The reasons why knees seem to be less susceptible are not completely known. The sensitivity of osteolysis to particle size or the rate at which particles are introduced to a particular site may be important. The efforts to eliminate this problem include designing joint replacements that minimize the stresses associated with surface damage and debris generation, developing more wear-resistant materials, and finding agents and processes that inhibit the biological response to debris.

The articulating surface is not the only place where damage can occur. Debris can also be generated at the polyethylene–metal interface in metal-backed components. The existence of gaps or other features necessary for interchangeable modular components can lead to relative motion between the polyethylene and the metal when the joint is loaded. Screws and screw holes may also cause problems. For example, if the polyethylene contacts a screw head, relative motion between the screw and the polyethylene may generate debris. Furthermore, in most designs employing screws for initial fixation, surgical flexibility is provided by having more holes than necessary. If the polyethylene rubs against the edge of a screw hole, debris may be generated. In addition, the unused screw holes provide channels for debris to migrate to the underlying bone.

The design of the polyethylene–metal interface in metal-backed components can also affect the contact stresses on the articulating surface. The stresses will be quite different if the polyethylene liner in an acetabular cup is in intimate contact with the backing than if it is not. Both the distribution and the magnitude of the contact stress will be affected. Initial conformity between the liner and the metal backing does not necessarily eliminate the possibility of wear at this interface. Wear can eventually occur in components that, to begin with, are perfectly conforming, because of *in vivo* changes in geometry and material properties that occur over time.

Frank fracture of the polyethylene component must also be avoided. This has occurred in cemented acetabular cups when grooves that provide interlock with the cement compromised the structural integrity of all-polyethylene acetabular cups and in uncemented cups when the polyethylene liner was supported only at the rim of the cup. The latter case is an example of how failure of the rim and subsequent dis-association of the polyethylene component from the metal backing can occur if the cup or the rim is too thin to support the load. Cracking and fracture have also been observed in tibial components for total knee replacements.

Wear at the liner–backing interface and frank fracture of polyethylene components are important design problems, but are beyond the scope of this chapter. Here, we restrict further discussion to the stresses associated with damage to the articulating surface of fixed bearing designs, where relative motion and large contact stresses are difficult to avoid if the joint is to provide normal anatomic function.

11.2 | Design: General Considerations

Stresses Caused by Contact

When contact occurs between metal and polyethylene components, both surfaces deform, but the deformation of the metal component is negligible and the metal component behaves like a rigid indenter. Thus, when an artificial joint is loaded, the polyethylene is squeezed between the rigid metal component and the supporting material (bone, cement, or metal backing), and in the region of contact, the articulating surface of the polyethylene is forced to conform to the shape of the metal surface. The resulting deformation causes compressive, tensile, and shear stresses in the polyethylene.

The magnitude of the stress depends on the magnitude of the joint load. As we have seen in previous chapters, these loads are large (3–5 times body weight). As a result, worst-case loads of 3000 N have been used to design polyethylene components. These large loads, in combination with the relative motion of the articulating surfaces, cause damage that increases with time of implantation (number of cycles of loading) and patient weight (magnitude). This provides strong circumstantial evidence that surface damage in total joint replacements is the result of fatigue processes.

The stresses associated with damage to the articulating surfaces occur both at the surface and within the polyethylene component. Two types of stresses can be applied to the surface—normal compressive stresses (contact stresses), and tangential shear stresses due to friction.

Metal and polyethylene were originally chosen for bearing surface materials to produce low-friction total joint replacements. When prostheses are properly manufactured (and undamaged), the friction between the metal and polyethylene components is quite small and may usually be ignored; the only stress acting on the surface in this case is the contact stress. However, if either one of the surfaces is damaged, the friction may be too large to ignore when stresses in the polyethylene are determined. Stresses due to friction, even though small, should also be included for undamaged polyethylene if the details of specific damage mechanisms are to be studied.

The stresses acting on the surface produce normal and shear stresses within the polyethylene. At the surface, the largest compressive stresses are the contact stresses that act perpendicular to the surface (Figure 11.1). They decrease nonlinearly with

FIGURE 11.1 Distributions of radial normal stresses due to contact. The maximum contact stresses will be over-estimated if a linear material model is used. (From Bicknall, VL, MS Thesis, Cornell University, 1984.)

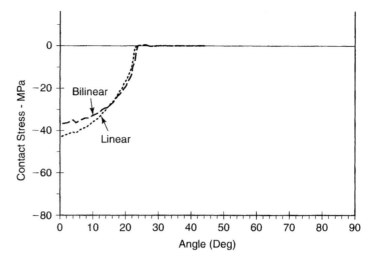

depth through the thickness of the polyethylene (Figure 11.2). Joint contact also produces compressive and tensile stresses within the polyethylene component that act tangent to the articulating surface. Tangential compressive stresses occur because the polyethylene under the center of the contact area expands radially as the component is compressed. This expansion is resisted by the surrounding material, and tangential compressive stresses are produced (Figure 11.3).

Joint contact also produces compressive and tensile stresses within the polyethylene component that act tangent to the articulating surface. Tangential compressive stresses occur because the polyethylene under the center of the contact area expands radially as the component is compressed. This expansion is resisted by the surrounding material, and tangential compressive stresses are produced (Figure 11.3).

Tangential tensile stresses near the articulating surface occur because the surface must stretch as the polyethylene conforms to the shape of the metal component when

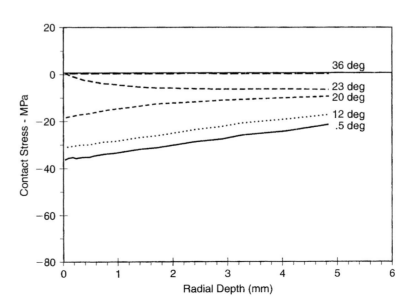

FIGURE 11.2 The radial stresses decrease with the depth. The angle is measured from the centerline for this axisymmetric model. (From Bicknall, VL, MS Thesis, Cornell University, 1984.)

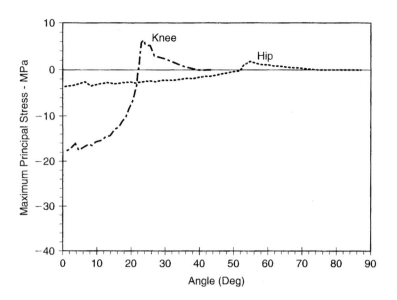

FIGURE 11.3 The maximum principal stresses act tangent to the surface for frictionless contact. The stresses for a knee are greater than the stresses for the hip, because knee contact is less conforming. (From Bicknall, VL, MS Thesis, Cornell University, 1984.)

the joint is loaded. The stretching occurs near the edge of the contact area (Figure 11.3). The resulting tensile stresses are largest at the surface of the component.

Surface damage is most likely due to combinations of stress components. The combined stresses associated with surface damage are the maximum principal stress (tangential stresses acting at the surface), minimum principal stress (the largest-magnitude compressive stress), and the maximum shear stress. The maximum shear stress occurs just below the surface (about 1 mm) for nonconforming joints such as knee joints and at the surface for conforming joints like hip joints (Figure 11.4).

The size distribution of the debris particles generated by these processes differs with the conformity of the joint. Although artificial joints produce a range of particle sizes, conforming joints such as hip replacements produce a number of smaller

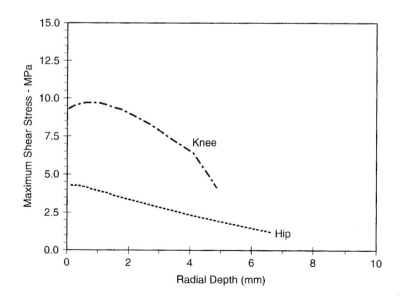

FIGURE 11.4 The maximum shear stress occurs about 1 mm below the surface for knee joints and at the surface for conforming joints. (From Bicknall, VL, MS Thesis, Cornell University, 1984.)

particles greater than the number of larger particles produced by nonconforming total knee replacements.

In knee joints, where pitting is one of the most frequently observed damage modes, the surfaces of the pits show the same characteristics observed on the fracture surfaces of crack propagation specimens tested in the laboratory. Pits may be formed when cracks propagate from the surface into the polyethylene or when subsurface cracks propagate toward the surface. In the first case, the important stresses are the maximum principal stresses; in the latter, the important stress is the maximum shear stress. In a knee joint, the contact area between the femoral and tibial components moves as the knee flexes and extends (Figure 11.5). Consequently, a point on the surface of the component will be subjected to varying stresses during the activities of daily living. The range (algebraic difference) of the stresses that act tangentially to the articulating surface (maximum principal stresses) varies between tension, when the point on the surface is at the edge of contact, and compression, when the point is at the center of contact. Although the damage to acetabular components is usually attributed to abrasive wear, fatigue processes similar to those that occur in knees may also be involved, but on a much smaller scale.

As mentioned previously, the maximum shear stress in nonconforming knee joints occurs about 1 mm beneath the articulating surface. This is about the same depth at which pitting and delamination occurs and provides circumstantial evidence that subsurface cracking is associated with these two failure mechanisms. Pits can occur when subsurface cracks turn and propagate toward the surface. Delamination occurs when the crack continues to propagate parallel to the surface, eventually resulting in the formation of a sheet of material.

If one examines the stresses at the edge of contact, it is clear why a crack propagating from the surface must turn. The tangential stresses at the edge of contact decrease rapidly with depth (Figure 11.6). They are tensile at the surface, but within less than a millimeter they become compressive. There are similar dramatic changes in the shear stresses at the edge of contact (Figure 11.7). For frictionless contact, the shear stress is zero at the surface, but reaches a maximum about 1 mm from the surface. We conclude that the maximum principal stress direction is also changing with

FIGURE 11.5 When the contact area moves on a tibial component, a point on the surface will be subjected to cyclic stresses in the tangential direction that range from compression, when the center of contact is at the point; to tension, when the edge of contact is at the point; to zero, when the contact area does not include the point.

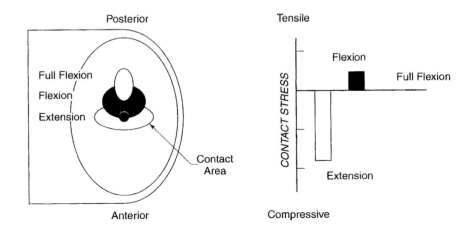

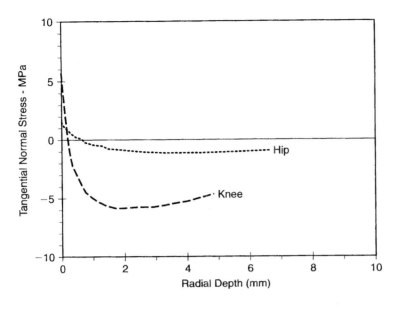

FIGURE 11.6 Tangential stresses at the edge of contact as a function of depth for geometries representing hip and knee components. (From Bicknall, VL, MS Thesis, Cornell University, 1984.)

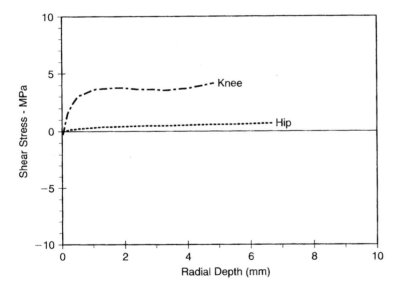

FIGURE 11.7 Shear stresses at the edge of contact as a function of depth for geometries representing hip and knee components. (From Bicknall, VL, MS Thesis, Cornell University, 1984.)

depth and that a crack propagating from the surface in such a changing stress field must turn.

Reducing Surface Damage

We can decrease the risk of surface damage by minimizing the stresses associated with the types of damage that can occur or by increasing the strength of the polyethylene. We know that abrasive wear which occurs in hip or knee joints can be minimized by a reduction in contact stress. Surface damage in knee joints has been associated with fatigue processes and crack propagation. Therefore, the stresses associated with fatigue processes involving crack propagation, the range of the maximum principal stress, and the magnitude of the maximum shear stress should also be minimized to decrease the risk of damage. Interestingly, both the range of the maximum principal stress and the maximum shear stress generally decrease when contact stress is decreased. Therefore, one can reduce the risk of abrasive wear and pitting and delamination by reducing the contact stress. The overall design goal, then, is to choose the geometry of the articulating surfaces and material properties of the polyethylene that minimize contact stress.

Minimizing Contact Stress

Contact stresses in acetabular components for total hip replacements and tibial components for total knee replacements are affected by changes in loading, conformity of the articulating surfaces, thickness of the polyethylene, and stiffness of the material. They may be determined with computational methods such as Hertz theory of elasticity, with finite element methods, or experimentally by the use of pressure-sensitive films. Computational methods have the advantage of providing stresses within the polyethylene, in addition to contact stress. But experimental methods provide contact stresses for actual geometries that may be difficult to approximate with idealized structural models.

Contact stresses increase with increasing load. If the same prosthesis (same conformity, thickness, and material) is used in patients with different weights, the stresses will be higher in the heavier patients. The stresses are not directly proportional to the load (Figure 11.8). As the load between the contacting surfaces increases, the contact area also gets larger. Because of this inherently nonlinear interaction between the load and the contact area, one must examine the effects of changes in conformity, thickness, and material for a particular joint load. The load should be representative of the largest loads expected for joint function. As mentioned earlier, a load of 3000 N has often been used for design purposes.

The contact stresses, of course, are not uniform over the contact area. The metal component of a total joint replacement is a rigid indenter. The contact stress will be greatest where the surface displacement of the polyethylene is greatest. Consequently, the displacement of the polyethylene surface in a direction normal to the surface will be determined by the shapes of the two contacting surfaces. For example, if the indenter and the polyethylene are both spherical, as they are in an ideal

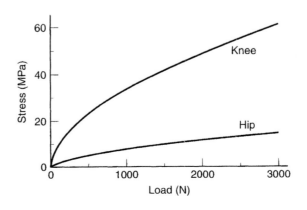

FIGURE 11.8 Contact stress as a function of load.

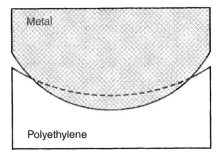

FIGURE 11.9 Contact between ideal spherical surfaces.

total hip replacement, then the maximum displacement of the polyethylene will occur at the center of contact (Figure 11.9). Therefore, the maximum contact stress will occur at the center of the contact area, and the minimum contact stress (zero) will occur at the edge of contact. Furthermore, the shape of the contact area in this ideal case will be circular.

If the surfaces are not spherical because of either design or manufacturing variations, then the maximum contact stress may not be at the center of the contact area. For example, in Figure 11.10 the indenter is spherical, but the acetabular surface has ripples in it. As a result, when the femoral head is pressed into the polyethylene, the largest displacement normal to the surface of the polyethylene component will be at locations like points A and C. Therefore, the greatest contact stresses will also occur at points A and C. The stress at point B in the contact area will be small, because the deformation (difference between the dashed and solid lines) will be small at this location. Surface waviness can be caused by normal variations in manufacturing processes. So it is not surprising that experimental measurements show variations from ideal contact shapes and ideal contact stress distributions.

Similar observations can be made for nonspherical contact geometries. For example, the articulating surfaces of the femoral and tibial components of some total condylar knee geometries are toroidal. For ideal geometry, the contact area for these designs will be approximately elliptical, but slight variations in surface geometry can produce substantial variations in the contact stresses and the shape of the contact area. Other knee designs have intentional variations in the articulating surface of the polyethylene component. These prostheses will have more pronounced variations in contact area geometry and contact stress than those with less complex surface shapes. Even though such variations in surface geometry can occur, the

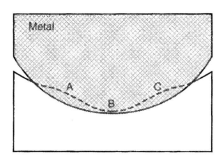

FIGURE 11.10 Contact between a spherical indenter and a polyethylene surface with ripples in it.

fundamental behavior of polyethylene components can be described in terms of the size of the contact area, on the basis of the ideal shapes of the articulating surfaces.

Changes in conformity, thickness, and material properties cause changes in the contact area. In general, changes that decrease the contact area will increase the stresses, because the same load must be distributed over a smaller region. The contact area decreases when the conformity between the articulating surfaces decreases, when the thickness of the material decreases, and when the stiffness of the material increases.

When the articulating surfaces are nonconforming, the contact area over which the stresses are distributed will be smaller, and the displacement of the surface at the center of contact will be greater, than when a more conforming geometry is used. Therefore, the maximum contact stress will be greater than for a more conforming geometry.

The effects of changes in thickness and elastic modulus on contact stresses may be understood as follows. Conceptually, the polyethylene may be considered to be supporting the metal indenter by a collection of parallel rods that are aligned along the direction of loading. (The rod analogy is, of course, limited, because shear stress cannot be transferred from one rod to another.) Each rod supports a portion, δP, of the total load P. The stiffness of a rod under axial load is given by

$$K_{rod} = \delta P / \Delta = \frac{EA}{L}$$

where Δ is the displacement of the rod, E is the elastic modulus of the rod material, Δ is the cross-sectional area of the rod, and L is the length of the rod, which corresponds to the thickness of the polyethylene component. It can be seen from this equation that the structural stiffness of the rod increases as the length of the rod decreases. In a similar way, the structural stiffness of polyethylene components increases with decreasing thickness. When the stiffness of the component increases, the indenter does not displace as much, the contact area decreases, and the contact stresses increase.

The rod analogy further shows that structural stiffness also increases when the elastic modulus of the rod material increases. Similarly, the structural stiffness of a polyethylene component increases when the elastic modulus of the polyethylene increases, leading to a decrease in contact area and an increase in contact stress.

Calculating Stresses in Polyethylene Components

Several methods are presented in Chapter 6 for computing stresses due to contact in polyethylene components. Hertz theory is the simplest, and the exercises at the end of the chapter provide opportunities to explore the concepts presented here quantitatively. In doing this, it must be realized that Hertz theory is quite limited (as discussed in Chapter 6), and the results obtained must be interpreted carefully.

Table 11.1 shows an example of how Hertz and FEA results differ for the same conceptual model, an axisymmetric representation of contact between a rigid metal indenter and a polyethylene component. The stress–strain relationship shown in Figure 11.11 was used for the FEA analysis.

For the conforming case, which approximates contact in a hip joint, the results are reasonably close for the 1000 N load. But Hertz theory overpredicts the maximum

TABLE 11.1

A Comparison of Maximum Contact Stresses Computed from Hertz Theory and Finite Element Analysis for the Same Axisymmetric Geometry[1]						
			1000 N		3000 N	
	R_i	R_p	Hertz	FEA	Hertz	FEA
Conforming	20	20.5	10	8	15	10
Nonconforming	20	40	120	45	170	50

[1]R_i is the radius of the metal indenter; R_p is the radius of the articulating surface of the polyethylene component.

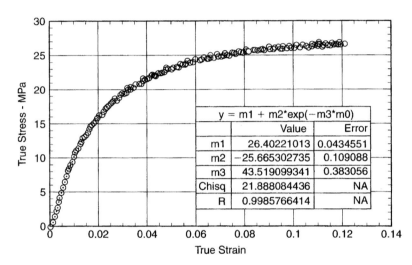

FIGURE 11.11   True stress–true strain behavior of UHMWPE.

contact stress substantially in the other cases shown in Table 11.1, in part because it is based upon linearly elastic material behavior, whereas the FEA results are for nonlinear behavior.

Stresses in Acetabular Components

The contact stresses for acetabular components are within the elastic limit of the polyethylene. Therefore, the intra-articular stresses can be computed from methods based on linear theory of elasticity. The diametral clearance is small—on the order of 0.1 to 0.2 mm. It can be shown that the contact stresses are independent of cup thickness and modulus for perfectly conforming spherical contact. This is consistent with observations of *in vivo* head penetration rates, which are constant with time after an initial wearing-in period. On the basis of contact stress alone, larger head sizes would be preferred. But it has been shown that wear at a point is proportional to pressure times sliding distance. Consequently, there is a trade-off between the relative sliding of the contacting surfaces and the contact stress, both of which are a function of diameter.

The maximum shear stress in polyethylene acetabular components occurs very close to the articulating surface. This is consistent with the observation that retrieved acetabular components have many fewer pits than tibial components for total knee prostheses, and delamination is rarely if ever seen in acetabular components. The fact that the maximum shear stress occurs at the surface in acetabular components has not yet been directly linked to the wear seen in these components. As noted previously, overall damage scores for acetabular components provide circumstantial evidence that the wear process is due to abrasion. It is possible that the large shear stresses at the surface may contribute to this process by fatigue failure on a microscale.

Stresses in Tibial Components

Even for the most conforming knee joints, the articulating surfaces are much less conforming than for total hip replacements. As a result, all of the stresses associated with surface damage are greater in tibial components than in acetabular components, because the contact areas are smaller for these less conforming devices. The stresses increase with decreasing thickness and increasing stiffness of the polyethylene. The stresses and strains are beyond the yield point for most knee designs in both flexion and extension. Therefore, analyses must account for the nonlinear behavior of polyethylene (Figure 11.11). For the more conforming total condylar type designs, the maximum strains will be in the 2–3 percent range. Figure 11.1 shows that for this type of design, the linear material model overestimates the maximum contact stress, but not by a lot. Such an approach is too conservative for less conforming designs, which must be based on nonlinear material behavior. An example of a finite element model that incorporated nonlinear material behavior is shown in Figure 11.12. Note that the maximum contact pressure (about 28 MPa) is the same order of magnitude as for the nonconforming case shown in Table 11.1 for the 3000 N load.

Most knee replacements use femoral condyles that approximate the anteroposterior geometry of the natural condyles of the knee. As a result, the anteroposterior geometry of the condyle is more or less fixed. This in turn defines the minimum anteroposterior radius of the tibial component—it can be no smaller than the largest radius of the femoral component. In practice, the anteroposterior radius of the tibia

FIGURE 11.12 A finite element model of a constrained condylar knee component, where a 3000 N load is applied to the medial plateau, along with a bending moment of 10 N-m in the medial direction.

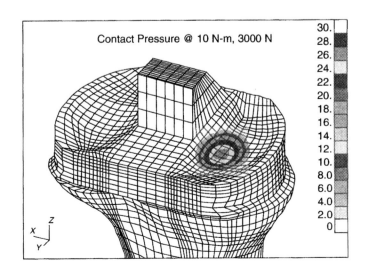

component is greater than the minimum allowable value, to provide some joint laxity in full extension. Good function of total knee replacements that spare the posterior cruciate ligament may require even larger anteroposterior radii on the tibial components, because when the surfaces are too conforming, the posterior ligament may not function properly. In some cruciate sparing designs, the posterior portion of the tibial plateau is flat or nearly flat. Consequently, anteroposterior conformity between the articulating surfaces may be further decreased.

These functional requirements limit what the designer can do to change the geometry in the anteroposterior direction. Consequently, changes in the lateral–medial geometry provide the greatest opportunities for increasing the conformity of the contacting surfaces (Figure 11.13). Conformity is maximized, and contact stresses are minimized, when the condyle and the plateau are flat in the lateral–medial direction, but this brings its own set of problems.

It is well known that there is a tendency for the lateral condyle to lift off because of medially directed loads on the foot during normal gait. When tilting occurs in a total knee replacement with articulating surfaces that are flat in the lateral–medial direction, two things happen. First, conformity between the femoral and tibial components is greatly decreased when the smaller radius on the outside of the prosthesis comes in contact with the polyethylene. As a result, the contact stresses and other stresses associated with surface damage may be dramatically increased. Second, with flat or nearly flat surfaces, tilting causes the contact area to move toward the edge of the polyethylene component. This can result in further increases in contact stress. In addition, the stresses associated with frank fracture of the component may also be increased. Edge loading is also a disadvantage because it is associated with increased stresses on the cancellous bone.

It is clear that articulating surfaces that are curved in the lateral–medial direction have distinct advantages because the contact area of the polyethylene does not shift to the edge when the femoral component tilts (Figure 11.14). When curved surfaces are used, maximum conformity will occur when the femoral and tibial radii in

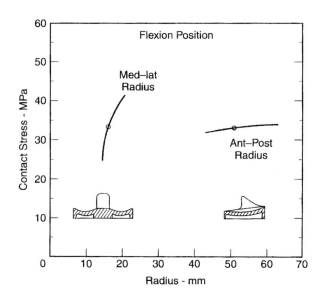

FIGURE 11.13 Stresses for a knee with toroidal contact. The dots indicate the nominal design. The effects of changing each radius were determined, while holding the other constant at the nominal design.

FIGURE 11.14 Knee with toroidal contact.

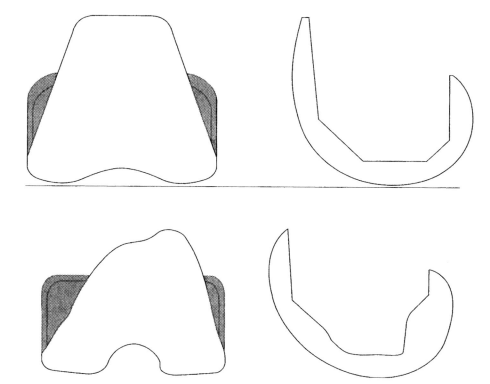

FIGURE 11.15 A total knee replacement. A single lateral–medial radius describes both the femoral and tibial surfaces. This design allows the some angular misalignment without liftoff.

the lateral–medial direction are the same. However, this decreases the rotational laxity of the knee joint about a tibial axis, which is necessary for the soft tissue structures around the joint to share load. If the soft tissue structures do not carry a portion of the load, then it will be transferred totally through the prosthetic components, and the risk of failure at the implant–bone interface will be increased. Therefore, the articulating surfaces in the lateral–medial direction must not be perfectly conforming. Radii must be chosen to minimize contact stress while providing an appropriate level of joint laxity.

An alternative approach is to use a single lateral–medial radius to describe the surfaces of both the femoral and tibial components (Figure 11.15). This provides the benefits of conformity while avoiding liftoff, by allowing small angular displacements to occur between the femur and the tibia to adjust the loading.

11.3 | Summary

In this chapter, we have focused on metal on polyethylene joints because they are the ones most frequently used. As mentioned earlier, other material combinations are used for bearing surfaces in joint replacements. In hip joints, these include metal on metal, ceramic on ceramic, and ceramic on polyethylene.

For metal on polyethylene contact, the deformation of the metal component is insignificant, compared with that of the polyethylene component—the metal component can be modeled as a rigid indenter. This is the basic assumption of the elasticity solution introduced in Chapter 6 and is often used in finite element analyses of polyethylene components. Both of these solutions must be solved computationally.

Hertz theory provides formulas for estimating stresses due to contact. Strictly speaking, the underlying assumptions of Hertz theory are not met in joint replacements. For example, the areas of contact are large with respect to the components, the material properties of the contacting materials may be very different, and the surface of contact is not planar. Even in metal on metal and ceramic on ceramic joints, where the material properties of the contacting components are the same, the assumptions about the size and flatness of the contact area are not satisfied (even approximately) for hip replacements. Nevertheless, the Hertz equations allow visualization of the roles of critical parameters and provide fundamental understanding of contact that helps interpret the results from the more computationally intensive methods, such as finite element analysis.

Surface damage in conforming joints like hip replacements is most likely due to abrasive wear. In knee replacements, the surface damage seen on retrievals can be associated with fatigue processes that create pits and delamination. These damage modes have been related circumstantially to the range of the principal stresses and the maximum shear stress. In general, these combined stress measures decrease when the contact stress is decreased. Therefore, at least to first order, decreasing the contact stresses in both hips and knees is a reasonable design goal. The problem is, of course, more complex than this, and the interested reader will want to consult with other references on the topic that go well beyond the introductory material in this book.

11.4   EXERCISES

11.1   Hertz contact theory can be used to determine the stresses due to contact between two spheres, which might be used approximate frictionless contact between the patellar and femoral components of a total knee replacement.

(a)   Show on a sketch how the stresses at the surface vary from the center of contact to the edge of contact.

(b)   Make a sketch of an infinitesimal element of material at the center of contact that shows the stress components. Identify the maximum principal stress, and write an expression for the maximum shear stress.

(c)   Sketch a graph that shows how the maximum contact pressure varies with load, and in a sentence explain why the curve has the shape it does.

11.2   Indicate whether the maximum contact stress in the artificial knee joint (Figure P 11.2) would increase or decrease if

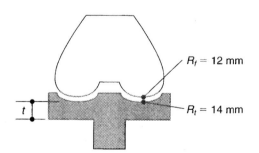

FIGURE P 11.2 R_f, R_t are the radii of the metal femoral (white) and plastic tibial (shaded) components, respectively; t is the average thickness of the plastic tibial component.

(a) R_f were increased (all else constant);
(b) R_t were increased (all else constant);
(c) t were increased (all else constant);
(d)   the modulus of the plastic were increased (all else constant).

11.3 Use Hertz theory to estimate the maximum contact pressure between a ball and a socket that are both made from CoCr alloy. The ball is 28 mm in diameter, and the diametral clearance varies from 0.0 to 0.5 mm. Make a plot that shows how the maximum contact pressure varies with clearance.

11.4 Use Hertz theory to estimate the maximum contact pressure between a ball and a socket that are both made from Al_2O_3 with modulus $E = 300$ GPa. The ball is 28 mm in diameter, and the diametral clearance varies from 0.0 to 0.5 mm. Make a plot that shows how the maximum contact pressure varies with clearance.

11.5 Use Hertz theory to estimate the maximum contact pressure between a CoCr ball and a polyethylene socket, where the diameter of the ball is 40 mm and the diameter of the cup is 80 mm, which approximates a knee joint in extension. Depending upon how the polyethylene is processed, its elastic modulus can vary between 750 MPa and 1500 MPa. Determine how the maximum contact stress varies as a function of modulus.

11.6 Use Hertz theory to estimate the maximum contact pressure between a CoCr ball and a polyethylene socket, where the diameter of the ball is 40 mm and the diameter of the cup is 40.4 mm, which approximates a hip replacement. Depending upon how the polyethylene is processed, its elastic modulus can vary between 750 MPa and 1500 MPa. Determine how the maximum contact stress varies as a function of modulus.

11.7 Use Hertz theory to estimate the maximum contact pressure between a CoCr ball and a polyethylene socket, where the diameter of the ball is 40 mm. Depending upon how the polyethylene is processed, its elastic modulus can vary between 750 MPa and 1500 MPa. Assume that the diametral clearance between the ball and the cup can vary from 0.0 to 0.5 mm. Determine how the maximum contact stress varies as a function of modulus for several values of clearance.

11.8 Use Hertz theory to estimate the maximum contact pressure between a polyethylene ball and a CoCr socket, where the diameter of the ball is 40 mm and the diameter of the cup is 80 mm, which approximates a knee joint in extension. Determine how the maximum contact stress varies with the radius of the cup over a range from 70 to 90 mm.

11.9 Example 6.3 in Chapter 6 shows that changing the elastic modulus of the ball from Ti to CoCr makes very little difference in the maximum compressive stress in the polyethylene.

(a) If the elasticity solution presented in Section 6.3 were used to estimate the maximum compressive stress in the polyethylene, would there be a difference in stress if the ball were changed from Ti to CoCr? Why or why not?

(b) What do the Hertz theory equations reduce to if the ball is rigid (i.e., $E_{Ball} \to \infty$)?

Suggestions for Further Reading

Chapter 1

Netter, F.H., *Atlas of Human Anatomy*. 1989, West Caldwell, NJ: CIBA-GEIGY Medical Foundation.

Simon, S.R. (Editor), *Orthopaedic Basic Science*. 1994, Rosemont, IL: AAOS.

Chapter 2

Winter, D.A., *Biomechanics and Motor Control of Human Movement*. 3d ed., 2004, New York: John Wiley & Sons.

Winters, J.M., and Crago, P.E. (Editors), *Biomechanics and Neural Control of Posture and Movement*. 2000, New York: Springer.

Nigg, B.N., and Herzog, W. (Editors), *Biomechanics of the Musculo-Skeletal System*. 2d ed., 1999, New York: John Wiley & Sons.

Rose, J., and Gamble, J.G., *Human Walking*. 2d ed., 1994, Baltimore: Williams and Wilkins.

Burstein, A.H., and Wright, T.M. *Fundamentals of Orthopaedic Biomechanics*, Chapter 3. 1994, Baltimore: Williams and Wilkins.

Chapter 3

Black, J., and Hastings, G., *Handbook of Biomaterial Properties*. 1998, London, UK: Chapman and Hall.

Carter, D.R., and Beaupré, G.S., *Skeletal Function and Form: Mechanobiology of Skeletal Development, Aging, and Regeneration*. 2001, Cambridge, UK: Cambridge University Press.

Cowin, S.C., *Bone Mechanics Handbook*. 2d ed., 2001, Boca Raton, FL: CRC Press.

Currey, J.D., *The Mechanical Adaptation of Bones*. 1984, Princeton, NJ: Princeton University Press.

Evans, F.G., *Mechanical Properties of Bone*. 1973, Springfield, IL: Charles C. Thomas.

Gibson, L.J., and Ashby, M.F., *Cellular Solids: Structures and Properties*. 2d ed., 1997, Cambridge, UK: Cambridge University Press.

Martin, R.B., Burr, D.B., and Sharkey, N.A., *Skeletal Tissue Mechanics*. 1998, New York: Springer.

Mow, V.C., and Hayes, W.C., *Basic Orthopaedic Biomechanics*. 2d ed., 1997, Philadelphia: Lippincott-Raven.

Martin, R.B., Burr, D.B., and Sharkey, N.A., *Skeletal Tissue Mechanics*. 1998, New York: Springer.

Currey, J.D., *Bones: Structure and Mechanics*. 2002, Princeton, NJ: Princeton University Press.

Chapter 4

Fung, Y.C., *Biomechanics: Mechanical Properties of Living Tissues*. 2d ed., 1993, New York Springer.

Black, J., and Hastings, G., *Handbook of Biomaterial Properties*. 1998, London, UK Chapman and Hall.

Humphrey, J.D., and Delange, S.L., *An Introduction to Biomechanics: Solids and Fluids Analysis and Design*. 2004, New York: Springer-Verlag.

McMahon, T.A., *Muscles, Reflexes, and Locomotion*. 1984, Princeton, NJ: Princeton University Press.

Mow, V.C., and Hayes, W.C., *Basic Orthopaedic Biomechanics*. 2d ed., 1997, Philadelphia Lippincott-Raven.

Mow, V.C., Ratcliffe, A., and Woo, S.L.Y., *Biomechanics of Diarthrodial Joint*s, Volumes 1 and 2; 1990, New York: Springer-Verlag.

White III, A.A., and Panjabi, M.M., *Clinical Biomechanics of the Spine*. 2d ed., 1990 Philadelphia: Lippincott-Raven.

Chapters 5, 6

Cook, R.D., and Young, W., *Advanced Mechanics of Materials*. 2d ed., 1998, Upper Saddle River, NJ: Prentice Hall.

Rivello, R.M., *Theory and Analysis of Flight Structures*. 1969, New York: McGraw-Hill.

Ugural, A.C., and Fenster, S.K., *Advanced Strength and Applied Elasticity*. 1995, Upper Saddle River, NJ: Prentice Hall.

Chapter 7

Ratner, B.D., Hoffman, A.S., Schoen, F.J., and Lemons, J.E. (Editors), *Biomaterials Science An Introduction to Materials in Medicine*. 1996, New York: Academic Press.

Mow, V.C., and Huiskes, R., *Basic Orthopaedic Biomechanics and Mechanobiology*. 3d ed., 2004, Baltimore: Lippincott Williams & Wilkins.

Burstein, A.H., and Wright, T.M., *Fundamentals of Orthopaedic Biomechanics*. 1994 Baltimore: Williams and Wilkins.

Morrey, B.F., *Joint Replacement Arthroplasty*. 3d ed., 2003, New York: Churchill Livingstone

Chapter 8

Tencer, A.F., and Johnson, K.D., *Biomechanics in Orthopedic Trauma: Bone Fracture and Fixation*. 1994, London, UK: M. Dunitz.

Muller, M.E., Allgower, M., Schneider, R., and Willenegger, H., *Manual of Internal Fixation* 3d ed., 2003, New York: Springer-Verlag.

Chapter 9

Charnley, J., *Low Friction Arthroplasty of the Hip: Theory and Practice*. 1979, Berlin Springer-Verlag.

Stillwell, W.T., *The Art of Total Hip Arthroplasty*. 1987, New York: Grune & Stratton, Inc

Chapter 10

Insall, J.N., and Scott, W.N., *Surgery of the Knee*. 3d ed., 2001, New York: Churchill Livingstone.

Chapter 11

Kurtz, S.M., *The UHMWPE Handbook: Ultra-High Molecular Weight Polyethylene in Total Joint Replacement*. 2004, New York: Academic Press, Inc.

Jacobs, J.J., and Craig, T.L. (Editors), *Alternative Bearing Surfaces in Total Joint Replacement*. 1998., West Conshohocken, PA: American Society for Testing and Materials.

Index